INTERNATIONAL SLEEP

Classification

	Page No.
1. DYSSOMNIAS	
A. Intrinsic Sleep Disorders	
1. Psychophysiologic Insomnia 307.42-0	28
2. Sleep State Misperception 307.49-1	32
3. Idiopathic Insomnia 780.52-7	35
4. Narcolepsy 347	38
5. Recurrent Hypersomnia 780.54-2	43
6. Idiopathic Hypersomnia 780.54-7	46
7. Post-traumatic Hypersomnia 780.54-8	49
8. Obstructive Sleep Apnea Syndrome 780.53-0	52
9. Central Sleep Apnea Syndrome 780.51-0	58
10. Central Alveolar Hypoventilation Syndrome. 780.51-1	61
11. Periodic Limb Movement Disorder 780.52-4	65
12. Restless Legs Syndrome. 780.52-5	68
13. Intrinsic Sleep Disorder NOS 780.52-9	
B. Extrinsic Sleep Disorders	
1. Inadequate Sleep Hygiene 307.41-1	73
2. Environmental Sleep Disorder 780.52-6	77
3. Altitude Insomnia 289.0	80
4. Adjustment Sleep Disorder. 307.41-0	83
5. Insufficient Sleep Syndrome. 307.49-4	87
6. Limit-setting Sleep Disorder. 307.42-4	90
7. Sleep-onset Association Disorder 307.42-5	94
8. Food Allergy Insomnia. 780.52-2	98
9. Nocturnal Eating (Drinking) Syndrome 780.52-8	100
10. Hypnotic-Dependent Sleep Disorder 780.52-0	104
11. Stimulant-Dependent Sleep Disorder 780.52-1	107
12. Alcohol-Dependent Sleep Disorder 780.52-3	111
13. Toxin-Induced Sleep Disorder 780.54-6	114
14. Extrinsic Sleep Disorder NOS 780.52-9	
C. Circadian-Rhythm Sleep Disorders	
1. Time Zone Change (Jet Lag) Syndrome 307.45-0	118
2. Shift Work Sleep Disorder 307.45-1	121
3. Irregular Sleep-Wake Pattern 307.45-3	125
4. Delayed Sleep-Phase Syndrome 780.55-0	128
5. Advanced Sleep-Phase Syndrome. 780.55-1	133
6. Non-24-Hour Sleep-Wake Disorder 780.55-2	137
7. Circadian Rhythm Sleep Disorder NOS 780.55-9	
2. PARASOMNIAS	
A. Arousal Disorders	
1. Confusional Arousals 307.46-2	142
2. Sleepwalking 307.46-0	145
3. Sleep Terrors 307.46-1	147
B. Sleep-Wake Transition Disorders	
1. Rhythmic movement Disorder 307.3	151
2. Sleep Starts 307.47-2	155
3. Sleep Talking 307.47-3	157
4. Nocturnal Leg Cramps 729.82	159

				Page No.

C. Parasomnias Usually Associated with REM Sleep
   1. Nightmares 307.47-0   162
   2. Sleep Paralysis 780.56-2   166
   3. Impaired Sleep-Related Penile Erections 780.56-3   169
   4. Sleep-Related Painful Erections 780.56-4   173
   5. REM Sleep-Related Sinus Arrest 780.56-8   175
   6. REM Sleep Behavior Disorder 780.59-0   177

D. Other Parasomnias
   1. Sleep Bruxism 306.8   182
   2. Sleep Enuresis 788.36-0   185
   3. Sleep-Related Abnormal Swallowing Syndrome 780.56-6   188
   4. Nocturnal Paroxysmal Dystonia 780.59-1   190
   5. Sudden Unexplained Nocturnal Death Syndrome 780.59-3   193
   6. Primary Snoring 786.09-1   195
   7. Infant Sleep Apnea 770.80   198
   8. Congenital Central Hypoventilation Syndrome 770.81   205
   9. Sudden Infant Death Syndrome 798.0   209
   10. Benign Neonatal Sleep Myoclonus 780.59-5   212
   11. Other Parasomnia NOS 780.59-9

3. SLEEP DISORDERS ASSOCIATED WITH MENTAL, NEUROLOGIC, OR OTHER MEDICAL DISORDERS

   A. Associated with Mental Disorders 290-319
      1. Psychoses 290-299   216
      2. Mood Disorders 296-301, 311   219
      3. Anxiety Disorders 300, 308, 309   224
      4. Panic Disorders 300   227
      5. Alcoholism 303, 305   230

   B. Associated with Neurologic Disorders 320-389
      1. Cerebral Degenerative Disorders 330-337   234
      2. Dementia 331   237
      3. Parkinsonism 332   240
      4. Fatal Familial Insomnia 337.9   245
      5. Sleep-Related Epilepsy 345   247
      6. Electrical Status Epilepticus of Sleep 345.8   252
      7. Sleep-Related Headaches 346   255

   C. Associated with Other Medical Disorders
      1. Sleeping Sickness 086   260
      2. Nocturnal Cardiac Ischemia 411-414   263
      3. Chronic Obstructive Pulmonary Disease 490-496   265
      4. Sleep-Related Asthma 493   269
      5. Sleep-Related Gastroesophageal Reflux 530.81   272
      6. Peptic Ulcer Disease 531-534   274
      7. Fibromyalgia 729.1   278

4. PROPOSED SLEEP DISORDERS
   1. Short Sleeper 307.49-0   282
   2. Long Sleeper 307.49-2   285
   3. Subwakefulness Syndrome 307.47-1   288
   4. Fragmentary Myoclonus 780.59-7   291
   5. Sleep Hyperhidrosis 780.8   293
   6. Menstrual-Associated Sleep Disorder 780.54-3   295
   7. Pregnancy-Associated Sleep Disorder 780.59-6   297
   8. Terrifying Hypnagogic Hallucinations 307.47-4   300
   9. Sleep-Related Neurogenic Tachypnea 780.53-2   302
   10. Sleep-Related Laryngospasm 780.59-4   304
   11. Sleep Choking Syndrome 307.42-1   307

THE INTERNATIONAL CLASSIFICATION OF SLEEP DISORDERS, REVISED
Diagnostic and Coding Manual

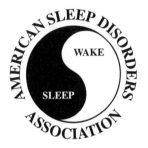

Produced by the
AMERICAN SLEEP DISORDERS ASSOCIATION

in association with the
EUROPEAN SLEEP RESEARCH SOCIETY
JAPANESE SOCIETY OF SLEEP RESEARCH
LATIN AMERICAN SLEEP SOCIETY

Copyright © 1990, 1997, American Sleep Disorders Association, 1610 14th Street NW, Suite 300, Rochester, MN 55901, U.S.A.

Copies of the manual are available from the American Sleep Disorders Assocation in the U.S.A.

All rights reserved. Unless authorized in writing by the ASDA, no portion of this book may be reproduced or used in a manner inconsistent with the copyright. This applies to unauthorized reproductions in any form, including computer programs.

Correspondence regarding copyright permissions should be directed to the Executive Director, American Sleep Disorders Association, 1610 14th Street NW, Suite 300, Rochester, MN 55901, U.S.A. Translations to other languages must be authorized by the American Sleep Disorders Association, U.S.A.

Recommended Citations
(Numerical)
American Sleep Disorders Association. International classification of sleep disorders, revised: Diagnostic and coding manual. Rochester, Minnesota: American Sleep Disorders Association, 1997.

(Alphabetical)
American Sleep Disorders Association.
ICSD - International classification of sleep disorders, revised: Diagnostic and coding manual. American Sleep Disorders Association, 1997.

Library of Congress Catalog No. 97-71405
International classification of sleep disorders, revised: Diagnostic and coding manual. American Sleep Disorders Association. Includes bibliographies and index.

1. Sleep Disorders–Classification. 2. Sleep Disorders–Diagnosis

Printed by: Davies Printing Company, Rochester, Minnesota
ISBN: 0-9657220-0-7

CONTENTS

Foreword	v
Preface	vii
Diagnostic Classification Steering Committee	ix
Alphabetical Listing of Participants	xiv
Introduction	1
The Axial System	13
International Classification of Sleep Disorders	15
Classification Outline	15
Criteria	21
Diagnostic Criteria	21
Minimal Criteria	22
Severity Criteria	22
Sleepiness	23
Insomnia	23
Duration Criteria	24
Dyssomnias	25
Intrinsic Sleep Disorders	27
Extrinsic Sleep Disorders	72
Circadian-Rhythm Sleep Disorders	117
Parasomnias	141
Arousal Disorders	142
Sleep-Wake Transition Disorders	151
Parasomnias Usually Associated with REM Sleep	162
Other Parasomnias	181
Sleep Disorders Associated with Other Disorders	215
Associated with Mental Disorders	216
Associated with Neurologic Disorders	234
Associated with Other Medical Disorders	259
Proposed Sleep Disorders	281
Classification of Procedures	311
ICSD Coding System	314
Axis A Modifiers	316
Diagnostic Criteria	316
Remission	316
Acute Onset	316
Severity	317
Duration	317
Symptom	317

Axis B	320
Procedures	320
Procedure Features	320
Axis C	322
Summary	323
Procedure Feature Codes	325
Data Base	329
Differential Diagnosis	331
Glossary	337
List of Abbreviations	
General Bibliography	352
Appendix A	355
ICSD Listing by Medical System	355
ICD-9-CM Listings	358
ICSD Alphabetical Listing	358
ICSD Numerical Listing	360
ICD-9-CM Sleep Listings	
Current Procedural Terminology (CPT) Codes	365
Clinical Field Trials	366
Appendix B	367
Introduction to the DCSAD First Edition	367
DCSAD–Classification Outline	378
Alphabetical Listing of DCSAD and Comparison with ICSD	381
Comparative Listing of DCSAD and ICSD	384
Index	389

FOREWORD TO THE REVISED EDITION

Since its introduction in 1990, the *International Classification of Sleep Disorders (ICSD)* has gained wide acceptance as a tool for clinical practice and research in sleep disorders medicine. The years between 1990 and 1997 have witnessed wide-ranging changes in sleep disorders medicine from many perspectives: the growth of managed health care; public health care reform; efforts to better integrate sleep disorders medicine into the community of medical specialties; major efforts at improving public awareness of the serious toll of sleep disorders; and–perhaps most importantly–a rapid growth in our understanding of the pathophysiology and effective treatment of sleep disorders.

Such changes present a fundamental challenge for any classification of diseases and disorders, including the *ICSD:* How often and how extensively should the classification be updated to reflect developments in the field? On the one hand, research and clinical developments have clearly changed the way we view many sleep disorders, most notably sleep-related breathing disorders. Some disorders in the *ICSD* may not be the distinct conditions conceptualized earlier (e.g., nocturnal paroxysmal dystonia), and other conditions *not* recognized in the *ICSD* (e.g., upper airway resistance syndrome, sleep-related eating disorders) may deserve their own listings. Such developments call for an in-depth revision of the classification system. On the other hand, frequent, major changes in a classification of disorders can be disruptive for both clinical and research practice. Maintaining a stable definition of a syndrome over a period of time is necessary to further define the reliability and validity of that disorder. Moreover, clinical and research progress has varied widely across disorders in the *ICSD*. Although we have greatly improved our knowledge about some sleep disorders, the essential features of other disorders (not to mention their epidemiology, pathophysiology, and treatment) remain in the realm of expert opinion. Ideally, substantive revisions are guided by a comprehensive analysis of applied, clinical, and basic research on the disorders themselves, as well as a clear understanding of which features of the classification work (and which don't work) in clinical and research practice. Expert opinion is always required, but should be secondary to empirical data.

At this point, the sleep disorders field has not conducted the type of rigorous re-examination needed to support a substantive revision of its diagnostic classification. As a result, this revision to the *ICSD* falls on the side of minor rather than major changes. Our intent in compiling this revision was to make the *ICSD* easier to use and more accurate, without altering the basic structure (or indeed, the vast majority of the text) of the classification. The revisions are summarized as follows:

1. The listing of disorders has been made accessible by printing it on the inside cover of the book. Diagnostic codes and page numbers are also included with this listing.
2. Text for individual disorders has been revised to clarify textual errors, standardize format across disorders, and correct minor factual errors.
3. Minor changes have been made to the text for a few of the disorders (e.g., obstructive sleep apnea syndrome, apnea of infancy, narcolepsy, fibrositis

syndrome) to reflect crucial developments since the first edition. Changes were made only if the fundamental accuracy of the original text was in question.
4. Code numbers for *ICSD* diagnoses, *ICD-9-CM* diagnoses, and *ICD-9-CM* procedures have been edited for accuracy.
5. The glossary has been revised editorially.
6. The index has been updated, expanded, and corrected for accuracy.
7. The authorship of the *ICSD* has been changed from "Diagnostic Classification Steering Committee, Thorpy MJ, Chairman" to "American Sleep Disorders Association." This change will make the *ICSD* more consistent with other diagnostic classifications such as the *Diagnostic and Statistical Manual, Fourth Edition* (American Psychiatric Association) and the *International Classification of Diseases* (World Health Organization).
8. The title of the classification has been modified to *The International Classification of Sleep Disorders, Revised* (*ICSD*-R). This should avoid any confusion stemming from the minor textual changes and change in authorship from the original volume.

Although these changes are relatively minor, they required the efforts of many individuals over a two year period. In particular, members of the ASDA Nosology Committee (Jack D. Edinger, Ph.D.; John L. Carroll, M.D.; Stuart Menn, M.D.; and Terry Young, Ph.D.), Publications Committee (Cynthia Dorsey, Ph.D.; Russell Rosenberg, Ph.D.; and Barry Krakow, M.D.) and Research Committee (Emmanuel Mignot, M.D., Ph.D.) reviewed and revised the text. Members of the ASDA Board of Directors provided guidance during the course of this project. And most particularly, Michelle Saxton-Felten and Judith Morton of the ASDA office and Catherine Friederich Murray provided the many long hours of expert editing which made this revision possible.

Daniel J. Buysse, M.D.
Chair, ASDA Nosology Committee
February, 1997

PREFACE

This classification, diagnostic, and coding manual represents a major four-year effort of many individuals. Sleep specialists and interested parties from around the world have actively participated in its development. National and international meetings have been held to openly discuss the ongoing developments. This manual will lead to more-accurate diagnoses of the sleep disorders, improved treatment, and stimulation of epidemiologic and clinical research for many years.

This manual would not have been possible without the tireless participation of the members of the Diagnostic Classification Steering Committee of the American Sleep Disorders Association. These committee members generously and selflessly gave of their time to accumulate the material for this volume. I would especially like to thank Howard P. Roffwarg, M.D., Chairman of the Sleep Disorders Classification Committee that produced the *Diagnostic Classification of Sleep and Arousal Disorders*, whose classification experience and contributions were invaluable.

The advisory committees consisted of many individuals who contributed to the manual by producing text, reviewing sections of text, or providing useful commentary. Many other contributors, most of whom are included in the list of contributors, provided helpful advice and comments. Some contributors, however, are unknown and, therefore, cannot be listed, but their contribution is gratefully acknowledged.

Carol Westbrook, Executive Director, and the staff of the American Sleep Disorders Association provided support and helpful advice throughout the long process of developing the text.

Karel M. Weigel, R.R.A., of the Council on Clinical Classifications; Robert H. Seeman, of the Commission on Professional and Hospital Activities; Patricia E. Brooks, R.R.A., of the Health Care Financing Administration; and Robert A. Israel, Deputy Director, Mary Sue Meads, R.R.A., and Delray Green, R.R.A., of the National Center for Health Statistics, were all helpful in providing advice regarding the use of terminology and coding. Robert Spitzer, M.D., editor of the *DSM-III-R* manual of the American Psychiatric Association, also provided helpful classification advice during the early stages of development of this manual.

I would like to thank Michel Billiard, M.D., representative of the European Sleep Research Society; Yutaka Honda, M.D., representative of the Japanese Society of Sleep Research; and Rubens Reimao, M.D., representative of the Latin American Sleep Society, for developing their respective societies' awareness of and participation in the production of this manual.

I would like to thank my wife Marie-Louise, not only for her support and encouragement throughout the long process of developing the manual, but also for her typing and editorial assistance. Careful and accurate secretarial assistance was also provided by Sonia Colon and Elaine Ullman.

The Diagnostic Classification Steering Committee actively solicits opinions, criticisms, corrections, and recommendations for improvement of this manual from all interested parties. Please forward comments, reprints, or other material to the Chairman, Diagnostic Classification Committee, American Sleep Disorders Association, 1610 14th Street, N.W., Rochester, Minnesota, 55901.

> Michael J. Thorpy, M.D.
> Chair
> Diagnostic Classification Steering Committee
> American Sleep Disorders Association

The diagnostic coding system reported in the *International Classification of Sleep Disorders* is presented solely for the purposes of communication between physicians and other healthcare workers and for database purposes. The coding system is not presented for third-party-payer reimbursement purposes or to be regarded as meeting the requirements for state or federal healthcare agencies, such as those of the Health Care Financing Administration. For such purposes, it is recommended that local and federal guidelines should be consulted and used whenever appropriate.

Diagnostic Classification Steering Committee of the American Sleep Disorders Association

CHAIR:

Michael J. Thorpy, M.D., *Director, Sleep-Wake Disorders Center, Montefiore Medical Center, Bronx, New York; Associate Professor of Neurology, Albert Einstein College of Medicine, New York*

COMMITTEE MEMBERS:

Roger J. Broughton, M.D., Ph.D., F.R.C.P.(C), *Professor of Medicine (Neurology), Pharmacology and Psychology, University of Ottawa, Ottawa, Canada; Director, Sleep Disorders Center, and Medical Director, Department of Clinical Neurophysiology and Neuropsychology, Ottawa General Hospital, Ottawa, Canada*

Martin A. Cohn, M.D., *Director, Sleep Disorders Center of Southwest Florida, Naples, Florida; Clinical Associate Professor of Medicine, University of Miami, Miami, Florida*

Charles A. Czeisler, Ph.D., M.D., *Director, Neuroendocrinology Laboratory, Division of Endocrinology, Brigham and Women's Hospital; Associate Professor of Medicine, Department of Medicine, Harvard Medical School, Boston, Massachusetts*

William C. Dement, M.D., Ph.D., *Professor, Department of Psychiatry and Behavioral Science, and Director, Sleep Disorders Clinic and Research Center, Stanford University School of Medicine, Stanford, California*

Richard Ferber, M.D., *Director, Center for Pediatric Sleep Disorders, The Childrens Hospital; Instructor in Neurology, Harvard Medical School, Boston, Massachusetts*

Christian Guilleminault, M.D., *Professor of Psychiatry and Behavioral Sciences, Stanford University School of Medicine; Staff Neurologist, Sleep Disorders Center, Stanford Medical Center, Stanford, California*

Peter J. Hauri, Ph.D., *Professor of Psychology, Mayo Medical School; Director, Insomnia Program, Sleep Disorders Center, Mayo Clinic, Rochester, Minnesota*

Max Hirshkowitz, Ph.D., *Scientific Director, Sleep Disorders and Research Center, Baylor College of Medicine; Co-Director, Sleep Research Laboratory, Veterans Administration Medical Center, Houston, Texas*

Ismet Karacan, M.D., *D.Sc., Director, Sleep Disorders Center, Veterans Administration Medical Center; Professor of Psychiatry and Director, Sleep Disorders and Research Center, Baylor College of Medicine, Houston, Texas*

Paul A. Nausieda, M.D., *Director, Wisconsin Institute for Neurological and Sleep Disorders, St. Mary's Hospital, Milwaukee, Wisconsin*

Ralph A. Pascualy, M.D., *Director, Sleep Disorders Center, Providence Medical Center, Seattle, Washington*

Charles F. Reynolds III, M.D., *Professor of Psychiatry and Neurology and Director, Sleep Evaluation Center, Western Psychiatric Institute and Clinic, University of Pittsburgh School of Medicine, Pittsburgh, Pennsylvania*

Howard P. Roffwarg, M.D., *Professor of Psychiatry, Director of the Sleep Study Unit, and Director of Research, Department of Psychiatry, University of Texas Southwestern Medical Center; Consulting Director, Sleep/Wake Disorders Center, Presbyterian Hospital of Dallas, Dallas, Texas*

Thomas Roth, Ph.D., *Director, Sleep Disorders Center, Henry Ford Hospital, Detroit, Michigan*

Daniel Wagner, M.D., *Assistant Professor of Neurology in Psychiatry, Cornell University Medical Center; Director, Sleep-Wake Disorders Center, New York Hospital (Westchester Division), White Plains, New York*

Vincent Zarcone, M.D., *Professor of Psychiatry (Clinical), Department of Psychiatry and Behavioral Sciences, Stanford University School of Medicine, Stanford; Staff Psychiatrist, Stanford Sleep Disorders Clinic, Stanford, Palo Alto, California*

Frank Zorick, M.D., *Medical Director, Sleep Disorders and Research Center, Henry Ford Hospital, Detroit, Michigan*

ADVISORY COMMITTEES:

Advisory committees were established in order to develop the text of the individual disorders. Headed by two members of the classification committee, the subcommittees consisted of individuals with clinical expertise in diagnosing one or more of the particular disorders in each group. The groups were organized along traditional systematic lines for ease of developing the texts. The groupings were not intended to convey the impression that the classification committee believes that any particular disorder solely pertains to one system. The groups could easily have been organized differently, but the groupings shown here were regarded as being preferable for the purposes of developing this manual. Most of the subcommittee members had the opportunity to view and comment on each disorder draft in their section.

Behavioral or Environmental Sleep Disorders

Vincent Zarcone, M.D., Chair
Frank Zorick, M.D., Co-Chair
Peter J. Hauri, Ph.D.
Richard Ferber, M.D.
Edward Stepanski, Ph.D.

Arthur J. Spielman, Ph.D.
Jack D. Edinger, Ph.D.
Andre Kahn, M.D. Ph.D.
Richard M. Coleman, Ph.D.

- Inadequate Sleep Hygiene
- Limit-setting Sleep Disorder
- Environmental Sleep Disorder
- Toxin-induced Sleep Disorder
- Insufficient Sleep Syndrome
- Sleep-onset Association Disorder
- Nocturnal Eating (Drinking) Syndrome
- Food-Allergy Insomnia

Psychiatric Sleep Disorders

Howard P. Roffwarg, M.D., Chair
Charles F. Reynolds III, M.D., Co-Chair
Wallace B. Mendelson, M.D.
Rosalind Cartwright, Ph.D.
Paul A. Nausieda, M.D.
Richard Allen, Ph.D.

James E. Shipley, M.D.
Peter J. Hauri, Ph.D.
Vincent Zarcone, M.D.
Stephen A. Burton, Ph.D., A.B.M.P.
Thomas Roth, Ph.D.
Hagop S. Akiskal, M.D.

- Sleep-state Misperception
- Psychophysiologic Insomnia
- Stimulant-dependent Sleep Disorder
- Psychoses
- Alcohol-dependent Sleep Disorder
- Panic Disorder
- Adjustment Sleep Disorder
- Anxiety Disorders
- Mood Disorders
- Alcoholism
- Hypnotic-dependent Sleep Disorder
- Idiopathic Insomnia

Respiratory-related Sleep Disorders

Martin A. Cohn, M.D., Chair
Christian Guilleminault, M.D., Co-Chair
Michael J. Thorpy, M.D
A. Jay Block, M.D.
Wolfgang Schmidt-Nowara, M.D.
Thomas G. Keens, M.D.

Stuart Quan, M.D.
Meir Kryger, M.D.
Colin Sullivan, M.B., Ph.D.
Eugene Fletcher, M.D.
Stuart J. Menn, M.D.
Toke Hoppenbrouwers, Ph.D.
Elio Lugaresi, M.D.

Primary Snoring

- Central Alveolar Hypoventilation Syndrome
- Sleep-related Abnormal Swallowing Syndrome
- Chronic Obstructive Pulmonary Disease
- Obstructive Sleep Apnea Syndrome
- Central Sleep Apnea Syndrome
- Sleep-related Asthma
- Sleep Choking Syndrome
- Sleep-related Laryngospasm
- Congenital Central Hypoventilation Syndrome
- Sudden Infant Death Syndrome
- Infant Sleep Apnea
- Altitude Insomnia

Neurologic Disorders

Christian Guilleminault, M.D., Chair
Paul A. Nausieda, M.D., Co-Chair
Jacques Montplaisir, M.D., Ph.D.
Mark Mahowald, M.D.
Yutaka Honda, M.D.
Elio Lugaresi, M.D.
Carlo A. Tassinari, M.D.
Michael Aldrich, M.D.
John M. Andrews, M.D.
Dudley Dinner, M.D.
Masaya Segawa, M.D.
K. Kayed, M.D.
Paul Saskin, Ph.D.
Donald Bliwise, Ph.D.

- Narcolepsy
- Posttraumatic Hypersomnia
- REM-Sleep Behavior Disorder
- Recurrent Hypersomnia
- Fatal Familial Insomnia
- Parkinsonism
- Sleep-related Headaches
- Sleeping Sickness
- Idiopathic Hypersomnia
- Sleep-related Epilepsy
- Nocturnal Paroxysmal Dystonia
- Dementia
- Cerebral Degenerative Disorders
- Electrical Status Epilepticus in Sleep

Circadian-Rhythm Sleep Disorders

Charles A. Czeisler, Ph.D., M.D., Chair
Daniel Wagner, M.D., Co-Chair
Peretz Lavie, Ph.D.
Timothy Monk, Ph.D.
Charles Pollak, M.D.
Gary S. Richardson, M.D.
Richard Ferber, M.D.

- Short Sleeper
- Shift-Work Sleep Disorder
- Advanced Sleep-Phase Syndrome
- Irregular Sleep-Wake Pattern
- Long Sleeper
- Delayed Sleep-Phase Syndrome
- Non-24-Hour Sleep-Wake Syndrome
- Time-Zone Change (Jet-Lag) Syndrome

Developmental or Neuropsychiatric Sleep Disorders

Richard Ferber, M.D., Chair
Roger J. Broughton, M.D., Ph.D., Co-Chair
German Nino-Murcia, M.D.*
Ernest Hartmann, M.D.
Vernon Pegram, Ph.D.
Piero Salzarulo, M.D.
Lawrence W. Brown, M.D.
Martin B. Scharf, Ph.D.
Masaya Segawa, M.D.

- Sleep Enuresis
- Sleep Terrors
- Rhythmic-Movement Disorder
- Benign Neonatal Sleep Myoclonus
- Sleep Paralysis
- Confusional Arousals
- Subwakefulness Syndrome
- Sleepwalking
- Nightmares
- Sleep Bruxism
- Sleep Starts
- Fragmentary Myoclonus
- Terrifying Hypnagogic Hallucinations
- Sleep Talking

Other Sleep-related Medical Disorders

Ismet Karacan, M.D., D.Sc., Chair
Ralph A. Pascualy, M.D., Co-Chair
Mark Pressman, Ph.D.
Anne M. Gillis, M.D., FRCP(C)
Max Hirshkowitz, Ph.D.
William Orr, Ph.D.
J. Catesby Ware, Ph.D.
Zenji Shiozawa, M.D.

Andre Kahn, M.D., Ph.D.
Christian Guilleminault, M.D.
Helmut S. Schmidt, M.D.
Harvey Moldofsky, M.D.
Rubens Reimao, M.D.
Richard Allen, Ph.D.
John Stirling Meyer, M.D.

- Restless Legs Syndrome
- Sleep-related Gastroesophageal Reflux
- REM-Sleep-related Sinus Arrest
- Sleep-related Painful Erections
- Pregnancy-associated Sleep Disorder
- Sudden Unexplained Nocturnal Death Syndrome
- Fibrositis Syndrome

- Nocturnal Leg Cramps
- Periodic Limb Movement Disorder
- Peptic Ulcer Disease
- Impaired Sleep-related Penile Erections
- Menstrual-associated Sleep Disorder
- Nocturnal Cardiac Ischemia
- Sleep Hyperhidrosis

INTERNATIONAL ADVISERS:

Draft material for this manual was periodically forwarded to the following international advisers for their comments or contributions. Many of the international advisers contributed drafts of individual disorders, communicated with their regional societies about the classification, or held a forum for discussion of the classification text material.

Michel Billiard, M.D., France
Jacques De Roeck, M.D., Ph.D., Belgium
Yutaka Honda, M.D., Japan
Andre Kahn, M.D., Ph.D., Belgium
Elio Lugaresi, M.D., Italy
Markku Partinen, M.D., Ph.D., Finland
David J. Parkes, M.D., F.R.C.P., England

Rubens Reimao, M.D., Brazil
Bedrich Roth, M.D.,* Czechoslovakia
Eckart Rüther, M.D., West Germany
Colin Sullivan, M.B., Ph.D., F.R.A.C.P. Australia
Gordon Wilderschiodtz, M.D., Denmark
Enrique M. Soltanik, M.D., Argentina

*Deceased

Alphabetic Listing of Participants in the Development of the *International Classification of Sleep Disorders*

The following alphabetic list contains the names of the contributors to the development of the classification. The classification committee apologizes for not listing those many other individuals whose names are not known to the committee and who may have contributed in direct or indirect ways.

Michael Aldrich, M.D.
Richard Allen, Ph.D.
John M. Andrews, M.D.
Gabriele Barthlen, M.D.
Michel Billiard, M.D.
A. Jay Block, M.D.
Roger J. Broughton, M.D., Ph.D.
Lawrence W. Brown, M.D.
Bernard Burack, M.D.
Stephen A. Burton, Ph.D.,
Rosalind Cartwright, Ph.D.
Martin A. Cohn, M.D.
Richard M. Coleman, Ph.D.
Charles A. Czeisler, Ph.D., M.D.
William C. Dement, M.D., Ph.D.
Jacques De Roeck, M.D., Ph.D.
Dudley Dinner, M.D.
Jack D. Edinger, Ph.D.
Richard Ferber, M.D.
Eugene Fletcher, M.D.
Anne M. Gillis, M.D., FRCP(C)
Ron Grunstein, M.D
Christian Guilleminault, M.D.
Ernest Hartmann, M.D.
Peter J. Hauri, Ph.D.
Max Hirshkowitz, Ph.D.
Yutaka Honda, M.D.
Toke Hoppenbrouwers, Ph.D.
Andre Kahn, M.D., Ph.D.
Ismet Karacan, M.D., D.Sc.
K. Kayed, M.D.
Thomas G. Keens, M.D.
Robert Kowatch, M.D.
Meir Kryger, M.D.
Peretz Lavie, Ph.D.
Elio Lugaresi, M.D.
Mark Mahowald, M.D.
Wallace B. Mendelson, M.D.
Stuart J. Menn, M.D.
John Stirling Meyer, M.D.

Harvey Moldofsky, M.D.
Timothy Monk, Ph.D.
Jacques Montplaisir, M.D., Ph.D.
Paul A. Nausieda, M.D.
German Nino-Murcia, M.D.*
William Orr, Ph.D.
David J. Parkes, M.D., F.R.C.P.
Markku Partinen, M.D., Ph.D.
Vernon Pegram, Ph.D.
Charles Pollak, M.D.
Mark Pressman, Ph.D.
Rubens Reimao, M.D.
Charles F. Reynolds III, M.D.
Gary S. Richardson, M.D.
Howard P. Roffwarg, M.D.
Bedrich Roth, M.D.*
Thomas Roth, Ph.D.
Eckart Rüther, M.D.
Piero Salzarulo, M.D.
Paul Saskin, Ph.D.
Martin B. Scharf, Ph.D.
Helmut S. Schmidt, M.D.
Wolfgang Schmidt-Nowara, M.D.
Kose Segawa, M.D.
Masaya Segawa, M.D.
Zenji Shiozawa, M.D.
James E. Shipley, M.D.
Enrique M. Soltanik, M.D.
Arthur J. Spielman, Ph.D.
Edward Stepanski, Ph.D.
Colin Sullivan, M.B., Ph.D., F.R.A.C.P.
Carlo A. Tassinari, M.D.
Michael J. Thorpy, M.D.
Daniel Wagner, M.D.
J. Catesby Ware, Ph.D.
Gordon Wilderschiodtz, M.D.
Vincent Zarcone, M.D.
Frank Zorick, M.D.

*Deceased

INTRODUCTION

The *International Classification of Sleep Disorders (ICSD)* was produced by the American Sleep Disorders Association (ASDA) in association with the European Sleep Research Society, the Japanese Society of Sleep Research, and the Latin American Sleep Society. The classification was developed as a revision and update of the *Diagnostic Classification of Sleep and Arousal Disorders (DCSAD)* that was produced by both the Association of Sleep Disorders Centers (ASDC) and the Association for the Psychophysiological Study of Sleep and was published in the journal Sleep in 1979. This revision was made necessary by the description of many new disorders and the development of additional information on many of the originally described disorders.

This introduction describes the rationale behind the major changes that have been instituted in the diagnostic classification manual and briefly describes in a sequential manner the material contained in this volume. Because there are many changes from the 1979 classification, the steering committee strongly recommends that users of this manual read the introduction in its entirety.

A. The Revision Process

1. The Questionnaire Survey

In 1985, the ASDC initiated the process of revising the classification by establishing an 18-member Diagnostic Classification Steering Committee. The first meeting of this group was convened in July 1985 at the Annual Meeting of the ASDC in Seattle. The group decided to survey sleep specialists to determine the usefulness of the first edition of the classification and to assess the potential usefulness of a number of proposed changes. A detailed questionnaire was developed and distributed to members of the Clinical Sleep Society (CSS) in the United States and to sleep specialists around the world. In addition to specific questions, general comments and recommendations were solicited.

The response was excellent: 160 fully completed questionnaires were received and analyzed by computer. Every entry in the *DCSAD* was assessed for content and relevance in the practice of sleep disorders medicine. The basic structure of the classification system was reviewed, and areas requiring improvement were identified. New suggestions regarding structure were assessed. Most respondents regarded the original classification as very useful in the practice of sleep medicine, and most individual diagnostic entities were considered appropriate and relevant to clinical practice. Opinions differed, however, on both the overall classification structure and some of the individual diagnostic entries.

The four sections of the original classification provided a useful structure for developing a differential diagnosis. The first two categories, i.e., the disorders of initiating and maintaining sleep (DIMS) and the disorders of excessive somnolence (DOES), were very helpful in considering the differential diagnosis of patients presenting with one or both of those major sleep symptoms. However, disorders listed within the third section, the disorders of the sleep-wake schedule (DSWS), could also produce complaints of insomnia or excessive sleepiness, as could some of the disorders listed in the fourth section, the parasomnias. In addition, some diagnostic entries were listed in more than one section and consequently had two text entries and two code numbers.

Of the four main diagnostic categories, section C, the DSWS, was the most favored grouping, probably because of its pathophysiologic consistency due to the underlying chronophysiologic basis. Classifying the disorders by pathophysiologic mechanism was preferred, and to have divided the schedule disorders by primary complaint would have been less acceptable. Concern did arise that the parasomnia listing was long and did not have subcategory organization.

Most individual diagnostic entries were considered highly relevant and useful. When divergent opinions on usefulness were reported, the committee recommended that the information contained in the text of the individual disorder be substantially improved. The few unsatisfactory entries resulted from the text being out of date. Obsolete diagnostic entries are not included in the ICSD, and the texts of the related disorders were updated.

The survey also demonstrated that clinicians required more diagnostic information about respiratory and neurologic disorders, so these sections were expanded. In addition, integration of childhood sleep disorders into the overall classification system was recommended. A separate childhood sleep disorders classification was considered, but this separation may have produced an artificial distinction between the same disorder in different age groups. A number of new childhood sleep disorders are included, and many of the original texts are updated to include the relevant childhood information.

The questionnaire survey assessed the potential utility of an axial system for stating diagnoses, similar to that of the American Psychiatric Association's *Diagnostic and Statistical Manual of Mental Disorders (DSM-III)-R*. An axial system would be helpful for treatment planning and the prediction of outcome. A two- or three-axes system was preferred.

2. Development of the ICSD

Based upon the information obtained from the questionnaire survey, several different classification systems were reviewed, and additional proposals were solicited. A classification for statistical and epidemiologic purposes required that each disorder be listed only once. Organization on the basis of symptomatology was unsatisfactory because many disorders could produce more than one sleep-related symptom.

Seven major classification systems, with numerous minor revisions, were reviewed by the committee before agreement was reached on the final system. A structure organized pathologically and less symptomatically was sought. Because the pathology is unknown for most sleep disorders, however, the classification was organized in part on physiologic features, i.e., a pathophysiologic organization.

A more-traditional, system-oriented approach to classification would compartmentalize the sleep disorders in a manner that would inhibit a multidisciplinary approach to diagnosis. Training in sleep disorders medicine is multidisciplinary, and such an approach applied to classification would allow a synthesis of physiology, pathophysiology, and symptomatology.

The new classification system groups the primary sleep disorders under two subgroups: (1) dyssomnias, which include those disorders that produce a complaint of insomnia or excessive sleepiness, and (2) the parasomnias, which include those disorders that intrude into or occur during sleep but do not produce a primary complaint of insomnia or excessive sleepiness. The dyssomnias are further subdivided, in part along pathophysiologic lines, into the intrinsic, extrinsic, and circadian-rhythm sleep disorders. The distinction into intrinsic and extrinsic sleep disorders divides the major causes of insomnia and excessive sleepiness into those that are induced primarily by factors within the body (intrinsic) and those produced primarily by factors outside of the body (extrinsic). Nathaniel Kleitman initially proposed this grouping of the sleep disorders in his extensive monologue on sleep disorders that was published in 1939. This organization of the classification also preserves the integrity of circadian-rhythm sleep disorders, as was mandated by the questionnaire survey.

The primary sleep disorders (dyssomnias and parasomnias) are separated from the medical or psychiatric sleep disorder section. The use of the terms medical and psychiatric is not ideal but is preferred to the *ICD-9* use of terms organic and nonorganic. With advances in understanding the pathophysiologic bases of the sleep disorders, the primary sleep disorders may be organized along pathologically oriented lines in the future.

Subcommittees of the classification committee were established to develop the textual material for the individual sleep disorders. The sleep disorders were arbitrarily grouped into seven sections for ease in accumulating the text. Each subcommittee was headed by two members, who organized a group of up to 10 sleep specialists to develop the text of the disorders in each section. The members of the seven committees, listed at the beginning of this book, were selected for their expertise in the diagnosis and management of the particular disorders under review.

A group of international advisers was chosen to give diversified opinions and recommendations on the revision process. This group included members representing the European Sleep Research Society, the Japanese Society of Sleep Research, and the Latin American Sleep Society. In addition to the subcommittees and international advisers, many other sleep specialists offered suggestions on the organization of the classification and assisted in reviewing and developing text material.

B. ICD-9-CM

The classification committee developed the diagnoses and diagnostic codes in a manner compatible with the North American version of the *International Classification of Diseases (ICD-9-CM)*. The *ICD-9-CM* contains an expanded listing of the disorders included under the major sleep-disorder headings in the

World Health Organization's ninth revision of the *ICD-9*. The sleep-disorder diagnoses in *ICD-9-CM* are organized under two major headings, "The specific disorders of sleep of non-organic origin" (ICD #307.4) and "The sleep disturbances" (ICD #780.5). Subdivisions of these two *ICD-9-CM* categories are partly based upon the headings and disorders of the *1979 ASDC DCSAD*. The *ICSD* classification committee assigned a single *ICD-9-CM* code number to each disorder listed in the *ICSD*. Because the *ICD-9-CM* headings were listed within the unsatisfactory divisions of organic and nonorganic sections, the sleep disorders listed in the *ICSD* had to be coded under these headings (see *ICD-9-CM* main sleep listing in Appendix A). Sleep disorders coded in sections other than #307.4 and #780.5 retained their original *ICD-9-CM* code number in the new classification.

C. DSM-III-R

The revision of the American Psychiatric Association's *Diagnostic and Statistical Manual III* was under way when the *ICSD* was in development. *DSM-III-R* contains an abbreviated list of sleep disorders that serves the purposes of the overall *DSM-III-R* classification but is not compatible with the *ICSD*.

D. Organization of the ICSD

The *ICSD* consists of disorders primarily associated with disturbances of sleep and wakefulness, as well as disorders that intrude into or occur during sleep. The classification provides a unique code number for each sleep disorder so that disorders can be efficiently tabulated for diagnostic, statistical, and research purposes. The primary aim of the text is to provide useful diagnostic information. Diagnostic, severity, and duration criteria are presented, as is an axial system whereby clinicians can standardize the presentation of relevant information regarding a patient's disorder.

The axial system assists in reporting appropriate diagnostic information, either in the clinical summaries or for database purposes. The first axis, axis A, contains the primary diagnoses of the *ICSD,* such as narcolepsy. These diagnoses are stated according to the recommendations in the text material of this volume. The second axis, axis B, contains the names of the procedures performed, such as polysomnography, or the names of particular abnormalities present on diagnostic testing, such as the number of sleep-onset rapid eye movement (REM) periods seen on multiple sleep latency testing. The third axis, axis C, contains *ICD-9-CM* medical diagnoses that are not sleep disorders, such as hypertension. axis C contains other diagnoses that are relevant to the patient's medical assessment and are included for planning treatment or predicting patient outcome.

The axial system was organized so that a specific *ICD-9-CM* code number could be given on each axis. A specialized code number, the *ICSD* research sleep code, can be given for coding information to modify the sleep diagnosis, such as the main symptom, and the severity or duration of the disorder. *ICD-9-CM* code numbers can also be given for documenting sleep tests and procedures. Additional

ICSD sleep code numbers are available for documenting abnormalities detected during polysomnographic or other types of objective testing, such as the sleep-onset REM periods detected on multiple sleep latency testing.

1. Axis A

Axis A contains the primary sleep diagnoses of the *ICSD*. The classification is divided into four sections:

The first section, the dyssomnias, comprises disorders that cause a complaint of either insomnia or excessive sleepiness.

The second section, the parasomnias, comprises disorders that intrude into or occur during sleep and that are not primarily disorders of the states of sleep and wakefulness per se.

The third section, the medical or psychiatric sleep disorders, comprises the medical and psychiatric disorders that are commonly associated with sleep disturbance. Because most medical and psychiatric disorders can be associated with disturbed sleep or impaired alertness, only those with major features of disturbed sleep or wakefulness, or those commonly considered in the differential diagnosis of the primary sleep disorders, are included in this section.

The fourth section comprises the proposed sleep disorders. This section was developed in recognition of the new and rapid advances in sleep disorders medicine. New disorders have been discovered, and some questionable sleep disorders have been more clearly described. The presentation of these disorders will encourage further research to determine whether these are specific disorders in their own right or whether they are variants of other already classified disorders.

2. Axis B

Axis B lists tests and procedures that are performed in the practice of sleep disorders medicine. The main tests include all-night polysomnography and the multiple sleep latency test (MSLT). Other medical tests that commonly may be recommended for patients who have sleep disorders also are listed in axis B. Statement of the test name and code number is encouraged. Because knowledge of the objective features of many sleep disorders is still in its infancy, the axis B system provides a means whereby abnormalities detected during polysomnographic and other forms of testing can be stated and coded for statistical and database purposes. A standardized means of documenting this information will assist in allowing future research to determine which sleep abnormalities have particular diagnostic significance. Many sleep disorders clinicians will not want to code abnormal procedure features; therefore, this coding system is devised primarily for research purposes.

3. Axis C

Axis C comprises the medical and psychiatric disorders that are not primarily sleep disorders in themselves. It is recommended that the appropriate *ICD-9-CM* code number be used for coding these disorders. Any medical or psychiatric disorder that is relevant to a patient's clinical care should be stated and coded by the clinician.

E. Text Content

The text of each disorder has been developed in a standardized manner to ensure the comprehensiveness of descriptions and consistency among sections. The major heading of the disorder is followed by the *ICSD* code number in parentheses. The following subheadings are used in each text:

1. Synonyms and Key Words

This section includes terms and phrases that have been used or are currently used to describe the disorder. In the medical and psychiatric section, diagnoses are given, with their respective *ICD-9-CM* number given in parentheses; the names of disorders pertaining to the text that are included under a different *ICD-9-CM* code number are also included here. Other disorders included in *ICD-9-CM* under the overall diagnostic group heading or code number may be excluded from the text description and, therefore, may have a separate text; such disorders are indicated as being excluded from the text. When appropriate, an explanation is given for the choice of the preferred name of the disorder.

2. Essential Features

This section includes one or two paragraphs that describe the predominant symptoms and main features of the disorder.

3. Associated Features

This section contains those features that are often but not invariably present. It also includes complications that may be a direct consequence of the disorder.

4. Course

This section describes the usual clinical course and outcome of the untreated disorder.

5. Predisposing Factors

This section describes internal as well as external factors that increase the patient's risk of developing the disorder.

6. Prevalence

This section presents the prevalence of the specific sleep disorder, if the prevalence is known. The prevalence is the proportion of individuals who at some time have a disorder. For some disorders, the exact prevalence is unknown, and only the prevalence of the underlying medical disorder can be stated.

7. Age of Onset

This section includes the age range within which the clinical features first becomes apparent.

8. Sex Ratio

This section includes the relative frequency with which the disorder is diagnosed in each sex.

9. Familial Pattern

This section states whether the disorder is more common among biologically related family members than in the general population. The presence of a disorder in several family members, however, does not necessarily mean that the disorder has a genetic basis.

10. Pathology

This section describes, if known, the gross or microscopic pathologic features of the disorder. When the exact pathologic basis of the sleep disorder is not known, the pathology of the underlying medical disorder is presented.

11. Complications

This section includes other disorders or events that may develop during the course of the disorder. Separating complications from the associated features may be difficult for many disorders; therefore, the reader sometimes is referred to the section on associated features.

12. Polysomnographic Features

This section presents the characteristic polysomnographic features of the disorder, including the best diagnostic polysomnographic measures. Information may be presented on the number of nights of polysomnographic recording required for diagnosis and whether certain special conditions are necessary for appropriate interpretation of the polysomnographic results. Where appropriate, information is given on diagnostic features seen on the MSLT.

13. Other Laboratory Features

This section describes features of laboratory tests, other than polysomnographic procedures, that aid in either establishing the diagnosis or eliminating other disorders that may have a similar presentation. Such tests may include blood tests, electroencephalographic studies, brain imaging, and temperature recordings.

14. Differential Diagnosis

This section includes disorders that have similar symptoms or features and that should be distinguished from the disorder under discussion.

15. Diagnostic Criteria

The presence of diagnostic criteria in the *ICSD* is a major change from the *1979 DCSAD*, which did not contain specific diagnostic criteria for each individual disorder. Diagnostic criteria were considered by the classification committee to be helpful not only for clinical but also for research purposes. Criteria are presented that allow for the unequivocal diagnosis of a particular disorder. From these criteria, the minimal criteria necessary to make a particular diagnosis are presented. The final assignment of a particular diagnosis depends upon clinical judgment, and the criteria do not exclude those disorders in which there may be variability of the clinical features. However, the inclusion of guidelines for diagnostic purposes is useful for most clinicians, not only to aid in establishing a diagnosis, but also to provide a checklist of additional information required to substantiate an otherwise unclear diagnosis. These criteria should provoke discussion and appropriate clinical testing in field trials to refine and enhance their diagnostic reliability. Future editions of this manual will include revisions and adjustments of the criteria.

16. Minimal Criteria

The minimal criteria aid in the early diagnosis of a sleep disorder, usually before diagnostic testing. The main diagnostic criteria assist in making a final diagnosis; however, all the information required may not be available, and appropriate diagnostic testing, such as polysomnography, may not be widely accessible. Therefore, the minimal criteria are mainly for general clinical practice or for making a provisional diagnosis. For sleep specialists, most minimal criteria are unreliable for an unequivocal diagnosis and, therefore, are unacceptable for research purposes. The minimal criteria usually are dependent upon the available patient history and clinical features. Objective testing is included in the minimal criteria when it is essential to define a disorder.

17. Severity Criteria

Criteria have been developed to specify the severity of a disorder. A relatively simple three-part classification into "mild," "moderate," and "severe" is available for clinical- and research-coding purposes. For most disorders, an exact numerical value for differentiating severity levels was avoided. The severity criteria usually depend upon clinical judgment. As with the diagnostic criteria, ongoing research will refine the severity criteria.

18. Duration Criteria

Duration criteria allow the clinician to categorize how long a particular disorder has been present. Durations are grouped as "acute," "subacute," and "chronic," according to specific information given in the text of each disorder. Duration has relevance to clinical investigation and patient management. For example, the patient with a disorder of acute duration may be examined and treated differently from a patient presenting with the same but chronic disorder. As with the diagnostic and severity criteria, future research will refine the duration criteria.

19. Bibliography

Approximately five references selected from the world literature present the cardinal clinical and diagnostic features of the disorder. Classic articles from a variety of authors and sources have been selected, and the number of abstracts and review articles is limited.

F. Axis B: Procedure Codes

This section contains a listing of medical procedures with the corresponding *ICD-9-CM* code numbers. In order to allow greater specificity for tests used in the practice of sleep disorders medicine, an expanded code number is used.

G. ICSD Coding System

This section describes the *ICSD* coding system that has been developed specifically to code symptoms, the severity and duration criteria, and the features seen during polysomnographic testing.

1. Axis B: Procedure Feature Codes

Listed here are the normal and abnormal procedure features seen during polysomnography or during other tests that can be coded in the *ICSD* coding system.

2. Database

To facilitate record keeping of the sleep disorders encountered, a database system has been devised. The purpose of this database is to establish a format for epidemiologic tracking of sleep disorders at sleep disorders centers.

H. Differential-Diagnosis Listing

The *1979 DCSAD* demonstrated that a differential-diagnostic listing was useful for clinical and teaching purposes. A differential-diagnostic listing of the three main presenting sleep complaints is insomnia, excessive sleepiness, and symptomatic or asymptomatic abnormal events during sleep. These symptoms are used as subheadings, and the disorders are organized in a uniform manner in each section. The subgroups are partly descriptive and suggest a diagnosis from information available at initial presentation.

I. Glossary

An expanded and revised version of the glossary contained in the *1979 DCSAD* defines the terms used in the manual. Many new terms have been added, and some original terms have been redefined. The committee recommends that these terms and definitions be widely used and standardized. Approval for the reproduction of this glossary should be sought from the ASDA.

J. General Bibliography

A short bibliography is provided to assist in obtaining additional information on the disorders presented in the *ICSD*. The bibliography is not exhaustive and includes only books of classic importance or that provide current, additional clinical information. The *ICSD* is not intended to be comprehensive in its description of individual sleep disorders or to provide therapeutic guidelines. The primary aim of this manual is to provide diagnostic information; therefore, new research results and an in-depth discussion of pathophysiology are not presented here. The bibliography provides sources for obtaining that additional information.

K. Appendix A

1. Listing by Medical System

Grouping specific sleep disorders under associated medical specialties may be useful for categorization; however, many sleep disorders cannot be attributed to a single medical specialty, and, therefore, this listing cannot be unequivocal. Appendix A contains such a list according to the *ICD-9* headings. The first section, the mental disorders, is divided in an unconventional manner into five subsections: developmental sleep disorders, behavioral sleep disorders, circadian rhythm sleep disorders, environmental sleep disorders, and psychopathologic disorders. This subgrouping was chosen to organize the large number of disorders listed in the mental disorders section. The other sections conform to usual medical specialty practice.

2. ICSD Alphabetic Listing

An alphabetic listing of all disorders contained in the *ICSD* is presented with *ICD-9-CM* code numbers. This list assists the clinician in finding the appropriate code number for a specific sleep disorder.

3. ICSD Listing by ICD-9-CM Code Number

The disorders of the *ICSD* are presented in numerical sequence by *ICD-9-CM* code number, allowing the name of a sleep disorder to be determined from a known *ICD-9-CM* code number.

4. *ICD-9-CM* Main Sleep Listings

All relevant disorders listed in the *ICSD* are presented under the two main *ICD-9-CM* subheading code numbers, #307.4 and #708.5. The *ICSD* coding system is derived from this numerical list, which is a revision of that published in the official *ICD-9-CM* classification volume.

5. Common Procedural Terminology

The American Medical Association has published a list of the names and appropriate procedure-code numbers of services and procedures performed by physicians. The code numbers recommended by the American Medical Association for sleep disorders diagnostic testing are presented in this section. This list of code numbers is particularly useful for reimbursement coding purposes.

6. Field Trials

A brief review of the importance of field trials in maximizing the sensitivity and specificity of diagnostic criteria is presented.

L. Appendix B

Appendix B contains the following information directly pertaining to the first edition of the *DCSAD*, published in the journal *Sleep* in 1979:

1. Introduction

The original introduction of the *DCSAD* of 1979 is reprinted as background information on both the development of the classification of sleep disorders and the rationale behind the format of the initial classification.

2. ASDC Classification

This section contains the complete 1979 *DCSAD*, along with the ASDC codes and original *ICD-9-CM* code numbers.

3. Comparative Listing

A comparative listing of the *DCSAD* and the current *ICSD* is presented, as are the prior ASDC code numbers and the new *ICD-9-CM* code numbers used in the *ICSD*. This list aids the clinician familiar with the 1979 classification in finding the new terminology and code numbers.

4. Alphabetic Comparative Listing

In this section, the *DCSAD* is listed alphabetically together with the new ICSD terminology and recommended *ICD-9-CM* code numbers. The reader unfamiliar with the organization of the *DCSAD* classification can locate the new ICSD term and code number according to previous terminology.

M. Index

The index contains the *ICSD* diagnoses and diagnostic terms. In addition, this index contains terms that were previously used in the 1979 *DCSAD* and other terms that may have been replaced by new terminology.

Bibliography

Association of Sleep Disorders Centers. Diagnostic classification of sleep and arousal disorders, 1st edition, Prepared by the Sleep Disorders Classification Committee, H. P. Roffwarg, Chairman. Sleep 1979; 2: 1-137.

DSM-III-R: Diagnostic and statistical manual of mental disorders, 3rd edition. Washington, D.C.: American Psychiatric Association, 1987.

DSM-IV Sourcebook, Washington: American Psychiatric Association, 1994.

ICD-9-CM: Manual of the international classification of diseases, 9th revision, clinical modification. Washington, D.C.: U.S. Government Printing Office, 1980.

ICD-9-CM 1994, International classification of diseases, clinical modification, 4th edition, 9th revision. Salt Lake City: Medicode Inc., 1994.

ICD-9: Manual of the international classification of diseases, injuries, and causes of death. Geneva, Switzerland: World Health Organization, 1977.

THE AXIAL SYSTEM

The *International Classification of Sleep Disorders (ICSD)* uses a multiaxial system for stating and coding diagnoses both in clinical reports or for data base purposes. The axial system uses *International Classification of Diseases (ICD-9-CM)* coding wherever possible. Additional codes are included for procedures and physical signs of particular interest to sleep disorders clinicians and researchers. Modifying information, such as severity, duration, and symptoms, also can be specified and coded by a special ICSD sleep code, which is presented on page 314. Diagnoses and procedures are listed and coded on three main "axes."

The axial system is arranged as follows:

Axis A *ICSD Classification of Sleep Disorders*
Axis B *ICD-9-CM Classification of Procedures*
Axis C *ICD-9-CM Classification of Diseases* (nonsleep diagnoses)

Short Version

Most clinicians will not wish to either code or state modifiers but only will want to state the main diagnoses, procedures performed, and associated *ICD-9-CM* code numbers. A recommended short version of the axial system is presented here.

Axis A

Axis A comprises the main diagnoses of the *ICSD*. These disorders are described in the body of the text of this manual.

The main diagnostic code consists of the *ICD-9* three- or four-digit numeric code, e.g.,

    Narcolepsy   347
    Specific Sleep Disorders of Nonorganic Origin   307.4

The North American Clinical Modification version of *ICD-9* (i.e., *ICD-9-CM*) has expanded the four-digit code of the sleep disorders to the fifth digit to allow greater specificity, e.g.,

    Sleepwalking   307.46

The first edition of the *Diagnostic Classification of Sleep and Arousal Disorders (DCSAD)* expanded the five-digit rubric to the sixth-digit level for even greater specificity, e.g.,

    Sleep Terrors   307.46-1

The code numbers of the first edition of the *DCSAD* are retained in this classification where appropriate. Most of the *ICSD* code numbers are fully compatible with those of the first edition of the *DCSAD*.

More than one diagnosis can be stated on axis A; however, the diagnosis that is the focus of attention and treatment is listed first, with any additional diagnoses listed in order of clinical importance, e.g.,

Axis A	Narcolepsy	347
	Periodic limb movement disorder	780.52-4

For diagnoses that produce sleep disturbance but are not included in the dyssomnias, parasomnias, or proposed sleep disorders sections of the classification, the appropriate *ICD-9-CM* code number is used on axis A, e.g.,

Axis A	Fatal Familial Insomnia	337.9
	Sleep-related Asthma	493

Axis B

Axis B comprises the *ICD-9-CM's* classification of procedures. This listing is used to specify laboratory or operative procedures, e.g.,

Axis B	Polysomnogram	89.17
	Multiple Sleep Latency Test	89.18

Axis C

Axis C diagnoses are the "nonsleep" diagnoses (diagnoses other than the ICSD diagnoses) listed in the *ICD-9* or *ICD-9-CM* diagnostic classification of diseases. In North America, the use of the *ICD-9-CM* code number is preferred because it gives greater specificity; however, the *ICD-9* code number is adequate for use where access to the *ICD-9-CM* is limited. The *ICD-9-CM* code numbers are compatible with the *ICD-9* code numbers. The diagnoses and code numbers are listed in order of clinical importance to the patient, e.g.,

Axis C	Recurrent Depression	296.3
Hypertension		401

Summary (Short Version)

The clinician states the diagnoses in the clinical report in a manner similar to the following example:

Axis A	Narcolepsy	347
	Periodic limb movement disorder	780.52-4
Axis B	Polysomnogram	89.17
	Multiple Sleep Latency Test	89.18
Axis C	Recurrent Depression	296.3
	Hypertension	401

INTERNATIONAL CLASSIFICATION OF SLEEP DISORDERS

Classification Outline

1. Dyssomnias
   A. Intrinsic Sleep Disorders
   B. Extrinsic Sleep Disorders
   C. Circadian Rhythm Sleep Disorders
2. Parasomnias
   A. Arousal Disorders
   B. Sleep-Wake Transition Disorders
   C. Parasomnias Usually Associated with REM Sleep
   D. Other Parasomnias
3. Sleep Disorders Associated with Mental, Neurologic, or Other Medical Disorders
   A. Associated with Mental Disorders
   B. Associated with Neurologic Disorders
   C. Associated with Other Medical Disorders
4. Proposed Sleep Disorders

1. DYSSOMNIAS
   A. Intrinsic Sleep Disorders
      1. Psychophysiologic Insomnia 307.42-0
      2. Sleep State Misperception 307.49-1
      3. Idiopathic Insomnia 780.52-7
      4. Narcolepsy 347
      5. Recurrent Hypersomnia 780.54-2
      6. Idiopathic Hypersomnia 780.54-7
      7. Post-traumatic Hypersomnia 780.54-8
      8. Obstructive Sleep Apnea Syndrome 780.53-0
      9. Central Sleep Apnea Syndrome 780.51-0
      10. Central Alveolar Hypoventilation Syndrome 780.51-1
      11. Periodic Limb Movement Disorder 780.52-4
      12. Restless Legs Syndrome 780.52-5
      13. Intrinsic Sleep Disorder NOS 780.52-9

B. Extrinsic Sleep Disorders
  1. Inadequate Sleep Hygiene 307.41-1
  2. Environmental Sleep Disorder 780.52-6
  3. Altitude Insomnia 289.0
  4. Adjustment Sleep Disorder 307.41-0
  5. Insufficient Sleep Syndrome 307.49-4
  6. Limit-setting Sleep Disorder 307.42-4
  7. Sleep-onset Association Disorder 307.42-5
  8. Food Allergy Insomnia 780.52-2
  9. Nocturnal Eating (Drinking) Syndrome 780.52-8
  10. Hypnotic-Dependent Sleep Disorder 780.52-0
  11. Stimulant-Dependent Sleep Disorder 780.52-1
  12. Alcohol-Dependent Sleep Disorder 780.52-3
  13. Toxin-Induced Sleep Disorder 780.54-6
  14. Extrinsic Sleep Disorder NOS 780.52-9

C. Circadian-Rhythm Sleep Disorders
  1. Time Zone Change (Jet Lag) Syndrome 307.45-0
  2. Shift Work Sleep Disorder 307.45-1
  3. Irregular Sleep-Wake Pattern 307.45-3
  4. Delayed Sleep-Phase Syndrome 780.55-0
  5. Advanced Sleep-phase Syndrome 780.55-1
  6. Non-24-Hour Sleep-Wake Disorder 780.55-2
  7. Circadian Rhythm Sleep Disorder NOS 780.55-9

2. PARASOMNIAS

A. Arousal Disorders
  1. Confusional Arousals 307.46-2
  2. Sleepwalking 307.46-0
  3. Sleep Terrors 307.46-1

B. Sleep-Wake Transition Disorders
  1. Rhythmic movement Disorder 307.3
  2. Sleep Starts 307.47-2
  3. Sleep Talking 307.47-3
  4. Nocturnal Leg Cramps 729.82

C. Parasomnias Usually Associated with REM Sleep
  1. Nightmares 307.47-0
  2. Sleep Paralysis 780.56-2
  3. Impaired Sleep-Related Penile Erections 780.56-3
  4. Sleep-Related Painful Erections 780.56-4
  5. REM Sleep-Related Sinus Arrest 780.56-8
  6. REM Sleep Behavior Disorder 780.59-0

D. Other Parasomnias
  1. Sleep Bruxism 306.8
  2. Sleep Enuresis 788.36-0

3. Sleep-Related Abnormal Swallowing Syndrome 780.56-6
4. Nocturnal Paroxysmal Dystonia..................... 780.59-1
5. Sudden Unexplained Nocturnal Death Syndrome........ 780.59-3
6. Primary Snoring 786.09-1
7. Infant Sleep Apnea 770.80
8. Congenital Central Hypoventilation Syndrome 770.81
9. Sudden Infant Death Syndrome 798.0
10. Benign Neonatal Sleep Myoclonus 780.59-5
11. Other Parasomnia NOS 780.59-9

3. SLEEP DISORDERS ASSOCIATED WITH MENTAL, NEUROLOGIC, OR OTHER MEDICAL DISORDERS
  A. Associated with Mental Disorders..................... 290-319
    1. Psychoses...................................... 290-299
    2. Mood Disorders 296-301, 311
    3. Anxiety Disorders 300, 308, 309
    4. Panic Disorders 300
    5. Alcoholism 303, 305
  B. Associated with Neurologic Disorders 320-389
    1. Cerebral Degenerative Disorders.................. 330-337
    2. Dementia... 331
    3. Parkinsonism..................................... 332
    4. Fatal Familial Insomnia 337.9
    5. Sleep-Related Epilepsy 345
    6. Electrical Status Epilepticus of Sleep 345.8
    7. Sleep-Related Headaches........................... 346
  C. Associated with Other Medical Disorders
    1. Sleeping Sickness 086
    2. Nocturnal Cardiac Ischemia 411-414
    3. Chronic Obstructive Pulmonary Disease........... 490-496
    4. Sleep-Related Asthma 493
    5. Sleep-Related Gastroesophageal Reflux 530.81
    6. Peptic Ulcer Disease........................... 531-534
    7. Fibromyalgia 729.1

4. PROPOSED SLEEP DISORDERS
  1. Short Sleeper..................................... 307.49-0
  2. Long Sleeper...................................... 307.49-2
  3. Subwakefulness Syndrome 307.47-1
  4. Fragmentary Myoclonus 780.59-7
  5. Sleep Hyperhidrosis 780.8
  6. Menstrual-Associated Sleep Disorder 780.54-3
  7. Pregnancy-Associated Sleep Disorder 780.59-6
  8. Terrifying Hypnagogic Hallucinations 307.47-4
  9. Sleep-Related Neurogenic Tachypnea 780.53-2
  10. Sleep-Related Laryngospasm....................... 780.59-4
  11. Sleep Choking Syndrome 307.42-1

Classification

The *International Classification of Sleep Disorders (ICSD)* was produced primarily for diagnostic and epidemiologic purposes so that disorders could be indexed and morbidity and mortality information could be recorded and retrieved. This classification is not intended to provide a differential diagnostic listing of sleep and arousal disorders. A differential diagnostic listing is presented on page 331 and is included to assist the clinician in diagnosing disease related to one of three major sleep symptoms: insomnia, excessive sleepiness, or an abnormal event during sleep.

The *ICSD* is consistent in style with *International Classification of Diseases (ICD-9-CM)* classifications for disorders affecting systems such as the cardiovascular or respiratory.

The ICSD consists of four categories. The first category comprises the dyssomnias (i.e., the disorders of initiating and maintaining sleep and the disorders of excessive sleepiness). The second category, the parasomnias, comprises the disorders of arousal, partial arousal, or sleep stage transition, which do not cause a primary complaint of insomnia or excessive sleepiness. The third category, sleep disorders associated with mental, neurologic, or other medical disorders, comprises disorders with a prominent sleep complaint that is felt to be secondary to another condition. The fourth category, proposed sleep disorders, includes those disorders for which there is insufficient information available to confirm their acceptance as definitive sleep disorders.

Textual content is included for all the *ICSD* disorders that are listed in Axis A.

1. Dyssomnias

The dyssomnias are the disorders that produce either difficulty initiating or maintaining sleep or excessive sleepiness. This section is divided into three groups of disorders: intrinsic sleep disorders, extrinsic sleep disorders, and circadian rhythm sleep disorders.

1. A. Intrinsic Sleep Disorders

Intrinsic sleep disorders either originate or develop within the body or arise from causes within the body. Psychologic and medical disorders producing a primary sleep disorder are listed here. Disorders arising within the body that are not primary sleep disorders are listed under Section 3, sleep disorders associated with mental, neurologic, or other medical disorders.

1. B. Extrinsic Sleep Disorders

Extrinsic sleep disorders either originate or develop from causes outside of the body. External factors are integral in producing these disorders. Removal of the external factor usually is associated with resolution of the sleep disturbance unless another sleep disorder develops during the course of the sleep disturbance (e.g., psychophysiologic insomnia may follow removal of an external factor responsible for the development of an adjustment sleep disorder).

1. C. Circadian Rhythm Sleep Disorders

Circadian rhythm sleep disorders are disorders that are related to the timing of sleep within the 24-hour day. Some of these disorders are influenced by the timing of the sleep period that is under the individual's control (e.g., shift work or time-zone change), whereas others are disorders of neurologic mechanisms (e.g., irregular sleep-wake pattern and advanced sleep-phase syndrome). Some of these disorders can be present in both an intrinsic and extrinsic form; however, their common linkage through chronobiologic, pathophysiologic mechanisms dictates their recognition as a homogeneous group of disorders.

2. Parasomnias

The parasomnias (i.e., the disorders of arousal, partial arousal, and sleep-stage transition) are disorders that intrude into the sleep process and are not primarily disorders of sleep and wake states per se. These disorders are manifestations of central nervous system activation, usually transmitted through skeletal muscle or autonomic nervous system channels. They are divided into four groups: arousal disorders, sleep-wake transition disorders, parasomnias usually associated with rapid eye movement (REM) sleep, and other parasomnias.

2. A. Arousal Disorders

Arousal disorders are manifestations of partial arousal that occur during sleep. These disorders are the "classic" arousal disorders that appear to be primarily disorders of normal arousal mechanisms.

2. B. Sleep-Wake Transition Disorders

Sleep-wake transition disorders are those that occur mainly during the transition from wakefulness to sleep or from one sleep stage to another. Although under some circumstances these disorders can occur within specific sleep stages, this is usually the exception rather than the rule.

2. C. Parasomnias Usually Associated with REM Sleep

The parasomnias usually associated with REM sleep have their onset during the REM sleep stage; some of these REM sleep parasomnias do occur during other sleep stages, but this occurrence is rare.

2. D. Other Parasomnias

Other parasomnias are those parasomnias that do not fall into the categories of arousal disorders, sleep-wake transition disorders, or parasomnias associated with REM sleep.

3. Sleep Disorders Associated with Mental, Neurologic, or Other Medical Disorders

This section lists those disorders that are not primarily sleep disorders but are mental, neurologic, or other medical disorders that have either sleep disturbance or excessive sleepiness as a major feature of the disorder. This listing of mental, neurologic, or other medical disorders is not intended to include all mental and medical disorders that affect sleep or wakefulness. It does include, however, those disorders most commonly associated with sleep symptoms.

4. Proposed Sleep Disorders

This section lists those disorders for which there is insufficient information available to confirm the unequivocal existence of the disorder (e.g., subwakefulness syndrome). Most newly described sleep disorders fall under this category until replicated data are available in the literature (e.g., sleep choking syndrome). Some sleep disorders that are controversial as to whether they are the extremes of the normal range or represent a definitive disorder of sleep also are included here (e.g., short and long sleepers).

Symptom

The sleep symptom associated with the diagnosis can be stated on Axis A if desired (e.g., obstructive sleep apnea syndrome associated with excessive sleepiness). Statement of the symptom is essential for disorders listed in the medical or psychiatric section that are not preceded by the term *sleep-related*, such as depression, which should be stated with the major sleep symptom (e.g., depression associated with insomnia).

The symptom can be coded for research purposes by the ICSD code as described on page 317.

Criteria

Diagnostic Criteria

The diagnostic criteria have been developed to aid in the diagnosis of a particular disorder. They are dependent upon the information contained within the text of the disorder and should not be viewed as being entirely independent. For example, the criterion for cataplexy is dependent upon compatibility with the description of cataplexy given in the text.

The text for each disorder contains a list of criteria that have been organized according to the following format:

> The first item contains the ***principal complaint*** or form of presentation. Some disorders may be asymptomatic and have features observed by others, such as in periodic limb movement disorder, whereas many disorders are entirely dependent upon a principal complaint, such as a complaint of insomnia in idiopathic insomnia.
>
> The second item usually refers to the ***pathophysiologic abnormality*** underlying the disorder, as contrasted with the subjective complaint (e.g., frequent episodes of shallow breathing in the criteria for central alveolar hypoventilation syndrome and a delay in the timing of the major sleep episode in delayed sleep-phase syndrome).
>
> The third, and sometimes fourth and fifth items, are the ***associated features*** that aid in the diagnosis (e.g., removal of the allergen associated with improved sleep in food allergy insomnia, and the presence of sleep paralysis and hypnagogic hallucinations in narcolepsy).
>
> The next item is the ***objective documentation*** of the disorder or documentation that some other disorder does not produce the primary complaint (e.g., polysomnographic evidence of central sleep apneic episodes confirms a diagnosis of central sleep apnea syndrome).
>
> The following item indicates the ***medical and mental disorders*** that may or may not be present for the particular diagnosis to be made (e.g., a diagnosis of psychophysiologic insomnia cannot be made in the presence of a diagnosis of depression).
>
> The final criterion indicates the ***sleep disorders*** that may or may not be present in order for a diagnosis to be made (e.g., a diagnosis of sleep terrors can be made if nightmares coexist; however, a diagnosis of non-24-hour sleep-wake disorder cannot be made in the presence of a diagnosis of delayed sleep-phase syndrome).

The diagnostic criteria have been developed to aid in establishing the unequivocal presence of a particular disorder; they are not the minimal criteria necessary for diagnosis. The diagnostic criteria should be viewed as an aid to the clinician in deciding what factors must be present if there is some doubt about the existence of a disorder. The clinician's judgment is the final arbiter of whether a particular disorder is present, but the diagnostic criteria will help the clinician decide what additional information or testing is required to confirm a diagnosis. Research should be conducted only with patients who meet the full criteria for a disorder to ensure homogeneity of the sample population. The minimal criteria necessary for a diagnosis are given and described next.

Minimal Criteria

The minimal criteria are derived from the diagnostic criteria and represent those parameters required to make a particular diagnosis. The minimal criteria and the diagnostic criteria depend on the information contained within the text of the disorder. These criteria should not be viewed as being entirely independent. For example, the criterion of cataplexy is dependent upon compatibility with the description given in the text.

These criteria do not establish the unequivocal presence of the disorder but do enable the clinician to make a diagnosis when some information may not be available. For example, a diagnosis of narcolepsy can be made if the patient gives a history of typical sleepiness and cataplexy. The disorder is not unequivocally present, however, unless there has been objective documentation. In many situations, polysomnographic confirmation of narcolepsy is not available or feasible. The clinician does have the right, however, to make a diagnosis solely based upon the history of sleepiness and cataplexy.

Severity Criteria

The severity criteria have been established to aid in the determination of the severity of a particular sleep disorder. In most disorders, these criteria reflect the severity of the major presenting sleep symptom, such as the intensity of insomnia or excessive sleepiness. A guide for determining the severity of these two symptoms is presented here.

In a few disorders, additional information is supplied to aid in determining severity, such as the number of movements per hour of sleep (PLM index) in periodic limb movement disorder. These criteria should be considered in addition to the criteria for the primary symptom of either insomnia or excessive sleepiness. For most disorders, however, the classification committee specifically avoided providing numerical indexes to differentiate severity (e.g., in the sleep-related breathing disorders). This was done because a single numerical cut point (such as the apnea index) is often not an appropriate division between levels of severity, and clinical judgment of several indexes of severity is considered superior. Additional clinical information contained in the severity criteria indicates to the clinician which parameters should be considered in deciding the severity of the disorder.

It is emphasized that these criteria are a guide, are not absolute, and are to be applied in conjunction with consideration of the patient's clinical status. The criteria for sleepiness and insomnia are described next.

Sleepiness

Mild Sleepiness: This term describes sleep episodes that are present only during times of rest or when little attention is required. Situations in which mild sleepiness may become evident include but are not limited to watching television, reading while lying down in a quiet room, or being a passenger in a moving vehicle. Mild sleepiness may not be present every day. The symptoms of mild sleepiness produce a minor impairment of social or occupational function.

This degree of sleepiness is usually associated with a multiple sleep latency test (MSLT) mean sleep latency of 10 to 15 minutes.

Moderate Sleepiness: This term describes sleep episodes that are present daily and that occur during very mild physical activities requiring, at most, a moderate degree of attention. Examples of situations in which moderate sleepiness occur include during concerts, movies, theater performances, group meetings and driving. The symptoms of moderate sleepiness produce a moderate impairment of social or occupational function.

This degree of sleepiness is usually associated with an MSLT mean sleep latency of 5 to 10 minutes.

Severe Sleepiness: This term describes sleep episodes that are present daily and at times of physical activities that require mild to moderate attention. Situations in which severe sleepiness may occur include during eating, direct personal conversation, driving, walking, and physical activities. The symptoms of severe sleepiness produce a marked impairment of social or occupational function.

This degree of sleepiness is usually associated with an MSLT mean sleep latency of less than 5 minutes.

Insomnia

Mild Insomnia: This term describes an almost nightly complaint of an insufficient amount of sleep or not feeling rested after the habitual sleep episode. It is accompanied by little or no evidence of impairment of social or occupational functioning. Mild insomnia often is associated with feelings of restlessness, irritability, mild anxiety, daytime fatigue, and tiredness.

Moderate Insomnia: This term describes a nightly complaint of an insufficient amount of sleep or not feeling rested after the habitual sleep episode. It is accompanied by mild or moderate impairment of social or occupational functioning. Moderate insomnia always is associated with feelings of restlessness, irritability, anxiety, daytime fatigue, and tiredness.

Severe Insomnia: This term describes a nightly complaint of an insufficient amount of sleep or not feeling rested after the habitual sleep episode. It is accompanied by severe impairment of social or occupational functioning. Severe insomnia is associated with feelings of restlessness, irritability, anxiety, daytime fatigue, and tiredness.

The severity criteria can be coded for research purposes by the ICSD sleep code on Axis A. The code is specified according to the instructions given in the ICSD coding system section of this manual on page 317.

Duration Criteria

The duration criteria were established to allow the clinician to provide information about the course of the disorder in terms of the length of time that a particular disorder has been present. These criteria do not provide information on the rapidity of onset of a disorder. Such information can be conveyed by the use of the term *acute onset* placed in brackets after a diagnosis (see discussion under the ICSD coding system).

The duration criteria are presented under the subheadings of acute, subacute, or chronic. The duration that applies to each disorder is specified in the text for that particular disorder (e.g., acute duration for narcolepsy is the onset within 6 months of presentation, subacute presentation occurs within 6 to 12 months of the onset, and a chronic disorder has been present for at least 12 months).

The duration criteria can be coded for research purposes by the *ICSD* sleep code on axis A. The code is specified according to the instructions given in the *ICSD* coding system section of this manual on page 317.

DYSSOMNIAS

The dyssomnias are disorders that produce either excessive sleepiness or difficulty in initiating or maintaining sleep. They are primarily the disorders contained within the first two sections of the 1979 *Diagnostic Classification of Sleep and Arousal Disorders (DCSAD)*, i.e., the DIMS disorders, the disorders of initiating and maintaining sleep (insomnias), and the DOES disorders, the disorders of excessive somnolence. The dyssomnias are the major, or primary, sleep disorders that are associated with disturbed sleep at night or impaired wakefulness. The second section of the *International Classification of Sleep Disorders (ICSD)* comprises the parasomnias, which are sleep disorders that usually do not cause a complaint of either insomnia or excessive sleepiness.

One major difference between the disorders in the first two sections of the 1979 *DCSAD* and the dyssomnias of the *ICSD* is that mental, neurologic, and other medical disorders that secondarily produce sleep disturbance are listed separately as the third section of the *ICSD*. The medical and mental disorders were listed in the first two sections of the *DCSAD*. Because many mental, neurologic, and other medical disorders can produce either insomnia or excessive sleepiness, an exhaustive listing of all disorders is not provided. Only those disorders that are commonly seen in the practice of sleep disorders medicine are included within the section of sleep disorders associated with mental, neurologic, and other medical disorders. This division allows the dyssomnia section to comprise only the primary sleep disorders with characteristic sleep features. Without the sleep features, the dyssomnias would not exist. This distinction differentiates the dyssomnias from the mental, neurologic, and other medical disorders that can exist without the sleep disturbance being a fundamental part of the disorder.

The term *dyssomnia* is used in the *ICSD* in a slightly different sense than previously used. Formerly, the term dyssomnia was applied to any disorder of sleep or wakefulness and included parasomnias as well as medical and mental disorders that produce sleep disturbance. The more commonly used term *sleep disorder* is now used in this general way to refer to all types of sleep disorders. The American Psychiatric Association's *Diagnostic and Statistical Manual,* third revision *(DSM-III-R),* applies the term *dyssomnia* to those sleep disorders that can produce either insomnia or excessive sleepiness, and excludes the parasomnias but includes mental, neurologic, and other medical causes of sleep disturbance.

The dyssomnias include a heterogeneous group of disorders that originate in different systems of the body. For example, in narcolepsy, a primary disorder of the central nervous system is believed to be the cause, whereas in obstructive sleep apnea syndrome, a physical obstruction in the upper airway may be the sole cause. Some disorders that had been included in the first two sections of the *DCSAD* are now included in the proposed sleep disorder section (e.g., short sleeper and long sleeper).

The dyssomnias are divided into three major groups: intrinsic sleep disorders, extrinsic sleep disorders, and circadian rhythm sleep disorders. These separate divisions are provided to allow some organization of the disorders that can produce insomnia and excessive sleepiness. The divisions are based, in part, upon pathophysiologic mechanisms. Because the circadian rhythm sleep disorders share a common chronophysiologic basis, they were kept as a single group. Both intrinsic and extrinsic factors may be involved in some of the circadian rhythm sleep disorders; therefore, the relevant disorders are subdivided into the two types: intrinsic and extrinsic.

DYSSOMNIAS

INTRINSIC SLEEP DISORDERS

1. Psychophysiologic Insomnia (307.42-0)..........................28
2. Sleep State Misperception (307.49-1)...........................32
3. Idiopathic Insomnia (780.52-7)................................35
4. Narcolepsy (347)..38
5. Recurrent Hypersomnia (780.54-2)...............................43
6. Idiopathic Hypersomnia (780.54-7)..............................46
7. Posttraumatic Hypersomnia (780.54-8)...........................49
8. Obstructive Sleep Apnea Syndrome (780.53-0)....................52
9. Central Sleep Apnea Syndrome (780.51-0)........................58
10. Central Alveolar Hypoventilation Syndrome (780.51-1)..........61
11. Periodic Limb Movement Disorder (780.52-4)....................65
12. Restless Legs Syndrome (780.52-5).............................69
13. Intrinsic Sleep Disorder NOS (780.52-9)

Intrinsic Sleep Disorders

The intrinsic sleep disorders are primarily sleep disorders that either originate or develop within the body or that arise from causes within the body. This section contains only those disorders that are included in and defined by the group heading of dyssomnias. Some sleep disorders that are due to processes arising within the body are not listed in the intrinsic section but are listed in the sections of: parasomnia; sleep disorders associated with mental, neurologic, or other medical disorders; or proposed sleep disorders.

The list of intrinsic sleep disorders includes a varied group of disorders, some of which–such as psychophysiologic insomnia, sleep state misperception, restless legs syndrome, and idiopathic insomnia–are primarily disorders that produce insomnia. Narcolepsy, recurrent hypersomnia, idiopathic hypersomnia, and posttraumatic hypersomnia are primarily disorders of excessive sleepiness. Obstructive sleep apnea syndrome, central sleep apnea syndrome, central alveolar hypoventilation syndrome, and periodic limb movement disorder are disorders that can produce a complaint of either insomnia or excessive sleepiness. The term intrinsic implies that the primary cause of the disorder is an abnormality in physiology or pathology within the body. For some disorders, however, external factors are clearly important in either precipitating or exacerbating the disorder. The following examples are given to help explain the rationale in organizing the disorders under the group heading of intrinsic.

Post-traumatic hypersomnia is an example of an intrinsic disorder that could not exist without the occurrence of an external event that produced a head injury.

However, the primary cause of the hypersomnia is believed to be of central nervous system origin, and, because the disorder persists after the traumatic event has terminated, it is listed, in the intrinsic section. Obstructive sleep apnea syndrome can be induced by an external factor, such as alcohol ingestion, but the development of the syndrome would not be possible without the internal factor of upper airway obstruction; a predisposition to develop the disorder must also be present.

Some of the extrinsic sleep disorders may depend upon factors within the body important for the expression of the sleep disturbance; external factors are essential, however, for the continuation of the sleep disturbance and, if they are not present, the sleep disturbance does not occur. For example, although an adjustment sleep disorder is due to psychologically stressful factors and, therefore, could be considered to be internally generated, an external event is the cause and, if the factor is removed, the sleep disorder resolves. If the sleep disorder continues after removal of the external factor, an intrinsic sleep disorder, such as psychophysiologic insomnia, has developed.

Psychophysiologic Insomnia (307.42-0)

Synonyms and Key Words: Learned insomnia, conditioned insomnia, functionally autonomous insomnia, psychophysiologic arousal, chronic somatized tension, internal arousal without psychopathology.

Essential Features:

Psychophysiologic insomnia is a disorder of somatized tension and learned sleep-preventing associations that results in a complaint of insomnia and associated decreased functioning during wakefulness.

Psychophysiologic insomnia is an objectively verifiable insomnia that develops as a consequence of two mutually reinforcing factors: (a) somatized tension and (b) learned sleep-preventing associations.

Individuals who have psychophysiologic insomnia typically react to stress with somatized tension and agitation. The meaning of stressful events (other than insomnia) is typically denied and repressed but manifests itself as increased physiologic arousal (e.g., increased muscle tension, increased vasoconstriction, etc.).

Learned sleep-preventing associations not only exacerbate the state of high somatized tension but also directly interfere with sleep. These associations can be learned in response to either internal cognitions or external stimuli.

Learned internal associations consist mainly of a marked overconcern with the inability to sleep. A vicious cycle then develops: the more one strives to sleep, the more agitated one becomes, and the less able one is to fall asleep. Patients in whom this internal factor (trying too hard to sleep) is a driving force for insomnia often find that they fall asleep easily when not trying to do so (e.g., while watching television, reading, or driving). Conditioned external factors causing insomnia often develop from the continued association of sleeplessness with situations and behaviors that are related to sleep. Thus, simply lying in a bedroom in which one has frequently spent sleepless nights may cause conditioned arousal, as may behaviors that lead up to the frustration of not sleeping, such as brushing teeth or turning off the bedroom lights. Patients with externally conditioned arousal often report that they sleep better away from their own bedroom and away from their usual routines (e.g., in a motel, on the living room couch, or in the sleep laboratory). Because conditioning factors are not subjectively experienced, most patients with conditioned arousal have no idea why they sleep so poorly.

Both internal and external associations are frequently learned during a bout of insomnia caused by other precipitating factors, such as depression, pain, disturbed sleep environment, or shift work. Psychophysiologic insomnia then persists long after the precipitating factors have been removed. In other cases, however, the poor sleep develops gradually, "feeding on itself." In these latter cases, concerns about sleep quality grow progressively over months or years as sleep gradually deteriorates, until the desire to obtain a good night's sleep becomes the person's chief concern, while this same concern is in fact preventing sleep from occurring.

A hallmark of psychophysiologic insomnia, then, is the patient's focused absorption on the sleep problem (while the same patient typically minimizes other mental or emotional concerns). This heavy focus on insomnia continually interferes with good sleep. Consequently, this type of insomnia remains rather fixed over time, although occasional periods of better or worse sleep may occur either "out of the blue" or in response to life events such as vacations or stress.

The diagnosis of psychophysiologic insomnia is not made in persons who can be classified as having generalized anxiety syndromes, phobias, obsessive-compulsive neurosis, major depression, or other *DSM-III-R* diagnosable psychopathologies.

Associated Features: As in all insomnias, chronically poor sleepers tend to note decreased feelings of well-being during the day. There is a deterioration of mood and motivation; decreased attention, vigilance, energy, and concentration; and an increase in fatigue and malaise but no objective sleepiness.

Although patients with psychopathologic insomnia have little overt psychopathology, they tend to be guarded, with denial and repression often being their main defenses. They typically are sensation avoiders, claiming that they do not want to aggravate their insomnia by deviating from their daily routine. They do show an increased incidence of stress-related psychophysiologic problems, such as tension headaches or cold hands and feet.

Course: When not treated, psychophysiologic insomnia may last for years or decades. In some cases, it may gradually worsen over time because a vicious cycle of insomnia develops.

Predisposing Factors: Many patients were marginal, light sleepers even before developing psychophysiologic insomnia. One might speculate that in these patients an occasional, naturally occurring, poor night of sleep will reinforce the learned sleep-preventing associations so that the associations cannot be extinguished over time. In addition, parental overconcern with sleep may also be a predisposing factor, as may be anxious overconcern with one's general health and well-being or an increased sensitivity to the daytime effects of mild sleep deprivation.

Prevalence: In sleep disorders centers, about 15% of all insomniacs are diagnosed with psychophysiologic insomnia. The true incidence in the general population is unknown. Learned sleep-preventing associations, while paramount in psychophysiologic insomnia, also tend to play an important role in most other forms of chronic insomnia.

Age of Onset: Rare in childhood or adolescence, psychophysiologic insomnia typically starts in young adulthood (20s or 30s) and gradually exacerbates until help is sought typically in middle adulthood.

Sex Ratio: The complaint of insomnia leading to a diagnosis of psychophysiologic insomnia is more frequently found in females.

Familial Pattern: A predisposition toward light marginal sleep seems to "run in families" and may have a genetic basis. However, the concern with getting a good night's sleep and with issues of general health, emphasized in some households, is more likely to be learned.

Pathology: None known.

Complications: Frequently found are the excessive use of hypnotics or alcohol, plus either administration of tranquilizers during the day to combat the somatized tension, or excessive use of caffeine or abuse of stimulants to combat excessive fatigue. The chronic pattern of failure to attain good sleep may occasionally generalize to other areas of psychologic functions, leading to a passive, defeatist attitude.

Polysomnographic Features: The usual features indicating objective insomnia, such as increased sleep latency, increased wakefulness after sleep onset, and decreased sleep efficiency, are found. There is an increase of stage 1 sleep and, possibly, a decrease of delta sleep. There may be increased muscle tension and increased electroencephalographic alpha production. There may be a reverse first-night effect. If these patients sleep better in the laboratory than at home, they typically are aware of this circumstance and reveal embarrassment about it when interviewed after the polysomnographic evaluation.

Other Laboratory Test Features: Psychologic testing will show the profile described previously: malaise, guardedness, sensation avoidance, repression, and denial. Physiologic tests may show high arousal (e.g., increased muscle tension, cold hands and feet) or excessive physiologic reactivity to stress.

Differential Diagnosis: The diagnosis of psychophysiologic insomnia lies on a continuum with a number of other diagnostic categories.

Inadequate Sleep Hygiene: Inadequate sleep hygiene is the preferred diagnosis when negligence of good sleep hygiene is directly causing the insomnia, which resolves after correction of the sleep hygiene. Psychophysiologic insomnia is the preferred diagnosis to the extent that the insomnia has become independent of the precipitating factors (i.e., patients will still sleep poorly even after they have begun to maintain adequate sleep hygiene.

Affective Disorders: The issue is especially difficult in "masked" depression (i.e., when the patient does not consciously experience sadness, hopelessness, or helplessness). The discrimination, then, is often made on the basis of other "vegetative signs" of depression, such as loss of appetite, loss of libido, marked diurnal fluctuations in mood (morning being worst), digestive upsets (typically constipation), etc. Recent life events that are likely to lead to depression (e.g., a serious loss) may also be considered, as may biologic markers of depression, such as a short REM latency, dexamethasone nonsuppression, or early morning awakenings. Finally, it is important that the diagnostician sense that chronic depression, though covert, was a first event rather than a reaction to the frustrations of poor sleep and resulting fatigue. Psychophysiologic insomnia is also often confused with dysthymic-personality disease. Psychologic functioning before insomnia is often the key. In dysthymic personalities, depressive features are often seen before the insomnia develops.

Generalized Anxiety Disorder: Generalized anxiety disorder is the preferred diagnosis when symptoms of anxiety pervade all of waking life and to the extent that general adaptive functioning is significantly impaired. Psychophysiologic insomnia is the preferred diagnosis when the symptoms focus on insomnia, the consequences of which are present during wakefulness.

Although patients with psychophysiologic insomnia typically were marginal sleepers during childhood and adolescence, they typically "got by," except for occasional poor nights around especially exciting or stressful events. The patient with idiopathic insomnia, on the other hand, slept consistently poorly during childhood.

Other Psychiatric Diagnoses: Psychophysiologic insomnia should not be the main diagnosis if *DSM-III-R* diagnostic criteria are fulfilled for either an axis 1 or an axis 2 diagnosis.

Diagnostic Criteria: Psychophysiologic Insomnia (307.42-0)

A. A complaint of insomnia is present and is combined with a complaint of decreased functioning during wakefulness.
B. Indications of learned sleep-preventing associations are found and include the following:
   1. Trying too hard to sleep, suggested by an inability to fall asleep when desired, but ease of falling asleep during other relatively monotonous pursuits, such as watching television or reading.

2. Conditioned arousal to bedroom or sleep-related activities, indicated by sleeping poorly at home but sleeping better away from the home or when not carrying out bedtime routines.
C. There is evidence that the patient has increased somatized tension (e.g., agitation, muscle tension, or increased vasoconstriction)
D. Polysomnographic monitoring demonstrates all of the following:
   1. An increased sleep latency
   2. Reduced sleep efficiency
   3. An increased number and duration of awakenings
E. No other medical or mental disorders accounts for the sleep disturbance.
F. Other sleep disorders can coexist with the insomnia, e.g., inadequate sleep hygiene, obstructive sleep apnea syndrome, etc.

Minimal Criteria: A plus B.

Severity Criteria:

Mild: Mild insomnia, as defined on page 23.
Moderate: Moderate insomnia, as defined on page 23.
Severe: Severe insomnia, as defined on page 23.

Duration Criteria:

Acute: 4 weeks or less.
Subacute: More than 4 weeks but less than 6 months.
Chronic: 6 months or longer.

Bibliography:

Coleman RM. Diagnosis, treatment and follow-up of about 8,000 Sleep/Wake disorder patients. In: Guilleminault C, Lugaresi E, eds. Sleep/wake disorders: Natural history, epidemiology, and long-term evolution. New York: Raven Press, 1983; 87–97.
Hauri PJ. A cluster analysis of insomnia. Sleep 1983; 6(4): 326–338.
Hauri P, Fischer J. Persistent psychophysiologic (learned) insomnia. Sleep 1986; 9(1): 38–53.
Reynolds CF, Taska LS, Sewitch DE, et al. Persistent psychophysiologic insomnia: Preliminary research diagnostic criteria and EEG sleep data. Am J Psychiatry 1984; 141: 804–805.
Sugerman JL, Stern J, Walsh JK. Waking function in psychophysiological and subjective insomnia [abstract]. In: Chase MH, Webb WB, Wilder-Jones R, eds. Sleep research. Los Angeles, California: Brain Information Service/Brain Research Institute, 1984; 13: 169.
Walsh JK, Nau SD, Sugerman J. Multiple sleep latency test findings in five diagnostic categories of insomnia [abstract]. In: Chase MH, Webb WB, Wilder-Jones R, eds. Sleep research. Los Angeles, California: Brain Information Service/Brain Research Institute, 1984; 13: 173.

Sleep State Misperception (307.49-1)

Synonyms and Key Words: Pseudoinsomnia, subjective complaint of disorder of initiation and maintenance of sleep without objective findings, insomnia without objective findings, sleep hypochondriasis, subjective complaint.

Essential Features:

Sleep State misperception is a disorder in which a complaint of insomnia or excessive sleepiness occurs without objective evidence of sleep disturbance.

The complaint appears to be a convincing and honest complaint of "insomnia" made by an individual who lacks apparent psychopathology. Typically, the complaint is of an inability to fall asleep, inadequate sleep, or the inability to sleep at all. A marked discrepancy exists between the complaint and the objective polysomnographic findings. The patient will indicate that the primary symptom was present during the night of objective testing.

Some reasons for the disparity between subjective and objective findings and sleep state misperception have been advanced. Excessive mentation during sleep may contribute to the sensation of being awake. Physiologic abnormalities may exist in the sleep tracing that are too subtle to be detected by recording methods currently in use. Data exist that some of these patients are grossly inaccurate in their estimations of time spent asleep. Other patients may be obsessive about sleep processes, just as some persons are obsessionally hyperalert about certain somatic functions and systems. These symptoms may represent the sleep analogue of hypochondriasis or somatic delusion.

In some elderly patients, sleep state misperception may develop out of an inability to sleep as long as they were able to in former years. In their appraisal of adequate amount of current sleep, a distortion of total sleep time develops.

Associated Features: The patient may report that the insomnia will lead to impaired daytime functioning, which will improve upon resolution of the disorder.

Course: Not known, apparently long lasting.

Prevalence: Not known, but appears to comprise less than 5% of all patients presenting with insomnia.

Age of Onset: The disorder can occur at any age, but most commonly appears to occur in early to middle adulthood.

Sex Ratio: More common in women.

Familial Pattern: Not known.

Pathology: Not known.

Complications: This disorder may result in the development of anxiety and depression if it is not effectively treated. Patients may use hypnotic medications inappropriately and may even develop drug dependence.

Polysomnographic Features: Polysomnography demonstrates a normal sleep pattern, with sleep latencies of less than 15 to 20 minutes, and sleep durations in excess of 6½ hours. The number and duration of awakenings are normal, and other sleep disorders are not present. The patient indicates a marked discrepancy between subjective total sleep time and sleep quality compared with the objectively documented sleep.

Other Laboratory Test Features: Psychologic testing has not revealed any typical psychologic or cognitive disorder that is associated with sleep state misperception.

Differential Diagnosis: Sleep state misperception should be differentiated from other disorders producing difficulty in initiating and maintaining sleep, particularly psychophysiologic insomnia and insomnia related to mental disorders.

Patients with sleep state misperception also need to be differentiated from malingerers who claim inadequate nocturnal sleep in order to obtain drugs for other reasons or to receive medical attention.

Diagnostic Criteria: Sleep State Misperception (307.49-1)

A. The patient has a complaint of insomnia.
B. The sleep duration and quality are normal.
C. Polysomnographic monitoring demonstrates normal sleep latency, a normal number of arousals and awakenings, and normal sleep duration with or without a multiple sleep latency test that demonstrates a mean sleep latency of greater than 10 minutes.
D. No medical or mental disorder produces the complaint.
E. Other sleep disorders producing insomnia are not present to the degree that would explain the patient's complaint.

Minimal Criteria: A plus B.

Severity Criteria:

Mild: Usually associated with mild insomnia, as defined on page 23.
Moderate: Usually associated with moderate insomnia, as defined on page 23.
Severe: Usually associated with severe insomnia, as defined on page 23.

Duration Criteria:

Acute: 1 month or less.
Subacute: More than 1 month but less than 6 months.
Chronic: 6 months or longer.

Bibliography:

Beutler LE, Thornby JI, Karacan I. Psychological variables in the diagnosis of insomnia. In: Williams RL, Karacan I, eds. Sleep disorders: Diagnosis and treatment. New York: John Wiley & Sons, 1978; 61–100.

Carskadon MA, Dement WC, Mitler MM, Guilleminault C, Zarcone VP, Spiegel R. Self-reports versus sleep laboratory findings in 122 drug-free subjects with complaints of chronic insomnia. Am J Psychiatry 1976; 133: 1382–1388.

Spiegel R, Phillips R. REM arousal insomnia, a hypothesis. In: Levin P, Koella WP, eds. Sleep 1974. Basel: Karger, 1975; 464–467.

Idiopathic Insomnia (780.52-7)

Synonyms and Key Words: Childhood-onset insomnia, lifelong insomnia, insomnia associated with problems within the sleep-wake system, excessive arousal, inadequately developed sleep system.

Essential Features:

Idiopathic insomnia is a lifelong inability to obtain adequate sleep and is presumably due to an abnormality of the neurologic control of the sleep-wake system.

The disorder may be due to a neurochemical imbalance of either the arousal system (ascending reticular activating system) or the many sleep-inducing and sleep-maintaining systems (e.g., the raphe nuclei, medial forebrain area, etc.). Some patients with idiopathic insomnia may merely fall toward the extremely wakeful end of a normal distribution curve. In others, actual dysfunctions or lesions may exist within the sleep-wake system, be they neuroanatomic, neurophysiologic, or neurochemical. Theoretically, either hyperactivity within the arousal system or hypoactivity within the sleep system may cause idiopathic insomnia. In any case, the lifelong and serious insomnia of these patients cannot be explained by either psychologic trauma starting in early childhood or medical problems, such as pain or allergies, that originate outside of the sleep-wake system.

Associated Features: Chronically poor sleep in general leads to decreased feelings of well-being during the day. There is a deterioration of mood and motivation, decreased attention and vigilance, low levels of energy and concentration, and increased fatigue. In serious idiopathic insomnia, daytime functioning may be so severely disrupted that patients do not have the stamina to hold a job.

In most patients with idiopathic insomnia, psychologic functioning remains remarkably normal as long as the sleep disturbance is either mild or moderate. Such patients have adapted to the chronic sleep loss and have learned to not focus on their problem. If idiopathic insomnia is severe, the typical psychologic status of the patient is marked repression and denial of all emotional problems, occasionally bordering on paranoid-like suspiciousness. Depressive features, such as feelings of helplessness, pessimism, and resignation, may be prevalent.

During childhood and adolescence, idiopathic insomnia is often associated with soft neurologic signs, such as dyslexia or hyperkinesis. Many cases show notable but clinically nonsignificant abnormalities on the electroencephalogram, such as alpha waves that are "ragged" (i.e., not sinusoidal).

Course: Typically lifelong and relentless.

Predisposing Factors: Some forms of idiopathic insomnia seem to run in families. Also, exceptionally difficult births or prematurity are found more often in patients with idiopathic insomnia than are expected by chance.

Prevalence: Not known; in its pure form, the disorder is rare. Most sleep disturbances in childhood are associated with behavioral-psychologic issues, not with idiopathic insomnia.

Age of Onset: Typically starts at birth, although in some mild forms, childhood sleep is marginally adequate.

Sex Ratio: Not known.

Familial Pattern: There is evidence for a genetic disposition in some but not all patients with idiopathic insomnia.

Pathology: In some cases, biochemical abnormalities have been demonstrated, such as inadequate production of serotonin.

Complications: Patients often make excessive use of hypnotics or alcohol to induce sleep. Patients may use excessive caffeine and stimulants to maintain wakefulness after chronically inadequate sleep.

Polysomnographic Features: Idiopathic insomnia ranges from mild to severe, and includes some of the worst forms of insomnia ever recorded in a sleep laboratory. Sleep latencies are typically long, and sleep efficiency is often very poor. Somnograms are often difficult to score because sleep spindles may be poorly formed and the characteristics of different sleep stages may be intermixed. Typically, idiopathic insomniacs show long periods of rapid eye movement sleep that are devoid of any eye movements. Paradoxically, idiopathic insomniacs may show fewer body movements per unit of sleep time than do normal sleepers or other insomniacs. Many show a reversed first-night effect, sleeping best on the first night in the laboratory.

Other Laboratory Test Features: Patients with idiopathic insomnia may have nonspecific abnormalities on the electroencephalogram, rare biochemical abnormalities, etc., but these abnormalities are highly idiosyncratic.

Differential Diagnosis: Idiopathic insomnia is rarely seen in its pure form. It seems almost impossible to lead a life of chronic, serious insomnia without developing other factors complicating the insomnia, such as poor sleep hygiene, learned maladaptive associations aggravating insomnia, or mental disturbances. Idiopathic insomnia is diagnosed when the history of a serious sleep disturbance can be traced to early childhood, markedly predating the occurrence of other sleep-disturbing factors, and when, in the opinion of the diagnostician, the imbalances in the sleep-wake system play a paramount role.

Whereas the short sleeper awakens refreshed and shows no detrimental daytime effects secondary to short sleep, patients with idiopathic insomnia clearly need more sleep than they can obtain, leading them to develop strategies to increase daytime vigilance and deal with chronic fatigue.

The innate predisposition toward poor sleep that is often seen in patients with physiologic insomnia is less serious but clearly lies on a continuum with the sleep disturbances shown in idiopathic insomnia. Psychophysiologic insomnia is diagnosed if the inherent predisposition toward poor sleep is mild and needs the stress of maladaptive conditioning before bona fide insomnia develops, whereas idiopathic insomnia is relatively chronic and stable from early childhood on.

Psychologically, most patients with idiopathic insomnia are remarkably healthy, given their chronic lack of sleep. If mental abnormalities are found, they clearly develop after insomnia has been established for years, if not decades. Also, idiopathic insomnia is relentless, continuing almost unvaried through both poor and good periods of emotional adaptation.

Diagnostic Criteria: Idiopathic Insomnia (780.52-7)

A. A complaint of insomnia, combined with a complaint of decreased functioning during wakefulness, is present.
B. The insomnia is long-standing, typically beginning in early childhood, if not at birth.
C. The insomnia is relentless and does not vary through periods of both poor and good emotional adaptation.
D. Polysomnography demonstrates one or more of the following:
   1. An increased sleep latency
   2. Reduced sleep efficiency
   3. An increased number and duration of awakenings
   4. Often a reversed first night effect
E. No medical or mental disease can explain the early onset of insomnia.
F. Other sleep disorders producing insomnia can occur simultaneously (e.g., adjustment sleep disorder).

Minimal Criteria: A plus B plus E.

Severity Criteria:

Mild: Mild insomnia, as defined on page 23.
Moderate: Moderate insomnia, as defined on page 23.
Severe: Severe insomnia, as defined on page 23.

Duration Criteria:

Acute: Not applicable.
Subacute: Not applicable.
Chronic: 1 year or longer.

Bibliography:

Carey WB. Night waking and temperament in infancy. J Pediatr 1974; 84: 756–758.
Hauri PJ. A cluster analysis of insomnia. Sleep 1983; 6(4): 326–338.
Hauri P, Olmstead E. Childhood onset insomnia. Sleep 1980; 3(1): 59–65.
Monod N, Guidasci S. Sleep and brain malformation in the neonatal period. Neuropaediatrie 1976; 7: 229–249.
Regestein QR. Specific effects of sedative/hypnotic drugs in the treatment of incapacitating chronic insomnia. Am J Med 1987; 83: 909–916.
Regestein QR, Reich P. Incapacitating childhood-onset insomnia. Compr Psychiatry 1983; 24: 244–248.

Narcolepsy (347)

Synonyms and Key Words: Excessive sleepiness, abnormal rapid eye movement (REM) sleep, cataplexy, sleep paralysis, hypnagogic hallucinations, nocturnal sleep disruption, positive human leukocyte antigen (HLA) DR2 or DQ1, genetic component.

Essential Features:

Narcolepsy is a disorder of unknown etiology that is characterized by excessive sleepiness that typically is associated with cataplexy and other REM-sleep phenomena, such as sleep paralysis and hypnagogic hallucinations.

The excessive sleepiness of narcolepsy is characterized by repeated episodes of naps or lapses into sleep of short duration (usually less than one hour). The narcoleptic patient typically sleeps for 10 to 20 minutes and awakens refreshed but within the next two to three hours begins to feel sleepy again, and the pattern repeats itself. Sleep usually occurs in situations in which tiredness is common, such as traveling in transport; attending a monotonous meeting that requires no active participation; or listening to a play, concert, movie, or lecture. The patients often can tolerate the sleepiness if, with much effort and attention, they make a strong attempt to stay awake. Eventually, however, it is impossible to combat the recurrent daily sleepiness.

There may be sudden and irresistible sleep attacks in situations where sleep normally never occurs, including: during an examination; at interactive business talks; while eating, walking, or driving; and when actively conversing. Sleep attacks usually occur on a background of drowsiness that is a common daily feature.

A history of cataplexy is a characteristic and unique feature of narcolepsy. It is characterized by sudden loss of bilateral muscle tone provoked by strong emotion. Consciousness remains clear, memory is not impaired, and respiration is intact. The duration of cataplexy is usually short, ranging from a few seconds to several minutes, and recovery is immediate and complete. The loss of muscle tone varies in severity and ranges from a mild sensation of weakness with head droop, facial sagging, jaw drop, slurred speech, and buckling of the knees to complete postural collapse, with a fall to the ground. When mild, the weakness may not be noticeable to observers. Cataplexy is always precipitated by emotion that usually has a pleasant or exciting component, such as laughter, elation, pride, anger, or surprise. The body area affected by cataplexy can be localized or can include all skeletal-muscle groups. The waist, lower or upper limbs, neck, mouth, or eyelids may be regionally affected. Respiratory and oculomotor muscles are not affected. Sometimes strong emotion may provoke another episode of cataplexy in succession and is termed *status cataplecticus*. Episodes of status can last for many minutes or, rarely, even up to an hour. Sometimes cataplexy is immediately followed by sleep. The use of tricyclic antidepressant medications such as protriptyline hydrochloride or imipramine hydrochloride almost always ameliorates cataplexy.

The frequency of cataplexy shows wide interpersonal variation, from rare events during a year-long period in some patients, to countless attacks in a single day in others. Patients may learn to avoid conditions inducing cataplexy and may have a decrease in the frequency of cataplectic events over time.

Associated Features: Sleep paralysis, hypnagogic hallucinations, automatic behavior, and nocturnal sleep disruption commonly occur in patients with narcolepsy.

Hypnagogic hallucinations are vivid perceptual experiences occurring at sleep onset, often with realistic awareness of the presence of someone or something, and include visual, tactile, kinetic, and auditory phenomena. The accompanying affect is often fear or dread. Hallucinatory experiences, such as being caught in a fire, being about to be attacked, or flying through the air, are commonly reported. Hypnagogic hallucinations are experienced by most patients with narcolepsy.

Sleep paralysis is a transient, generalized inability to move or to speak during the transition between sleep and wakefulness. The patient usually regains muscular control within a short time (one to several minutes). Sleep paralysis is a frightening experience, particularly when initially experienced, and often is accompanied by a sensation of inability to breathe. Episodes often occur with hypnagogic hallucinations, and thus the frightful emotional experience is intensified. Sleep paralysis is experienced by most narcoleptic patients.

Both sleep paralysis and hypnagogic hallucinations almost always correspond with sleep-onset REM periods. These two symptoms are defined as auxiliary symptoms and, along with cataplexy and excessive sleepiness, comprise the narcolepsy tetrad.

Narcoleptic patients may report lapses of memory and automatic behavior without awareness of sleepiness, and show inappropriate activity and poor adjustment to abrupt environmental demands. Other symptoms include ptosis, blurred vision, and diplopia.

Nocturnal sleep disruption with frequent awakenings occurs in many patients.

Course: Cataplexy, hypnagogic hallucinations, and sleep paralysis decrease in frequency over time; however, excessive daytime sleepiness seems to be lifelong.

Although excessive sleepiness can show slight improvement over time, this may be due to increased coping abilities by the patients. In others, the excessive sleepiness can worsen over the years and may be associated with the development of periodic limb movement disorder or sleep apnea syndrome, both of which are more common in patients with narcolepsy than in the general population.

Prevalence: Narcolepsy is estimated to occur in 0.03% to 0.16% of the general population. Israeli studies suggest a much lower frequency in Israeli Jews.

Age of Onset: Narcolepsy most commonly begins in the second decade, with a peak incidence around 14 years of age. Excessive sleepiness is usually the first symptom to appear, with cataplexy appearing either simultaneously or with a delay of 1 to 30 years. Cataplexy rarely precedes the onset of sleepiness. Members of families with narcolepsy show similar ages of onset of symptoms.

Sex Ratio: No difference.

Familial Pattern: First-degree relatives of a narcoleptic proband are at about a 20-40 times greater risk of developing narcolepsy-cataplexy than are individuals in the general population.

Rarely, isolated cataplexy occurs on a familial basis.

Pathology: No positive brain histopathologic abnormalities on light microscopy have been reported.

Complications: Accidents due to sleepiness and cataplexy can occur in almost any situation but commonly occur while driving, operating dangerous equipment, in the home, or at regular employment. Serious social consequences can result because of the sleepiness and can lead to marital disharmony or loss of employment. Education difficulties commonly occur in adolescence, and advanced education opportunities may be lost.

Polysomnographic Features: Daytime polysomnography usually shows a reduced sleep latency of less than 10 minutes, and sleep-onset REM periods are characteristic findings. On all-night polysomnography, a short sleep latency of less than 10 minutes and a sleep-onset REM period (REM appearing within 20 minutes after sleep onset) also are frequent findings. Sleep-onset REM periods can be associated with reports of hypnagogic hallucinations or sleep paralysis. The all-night polysomnogram can demonstrate an increase in the amount of stage 1 sleep, and there may be a disruption of the normal sleep pattern, with frequent awakenings.

The multiple sleep latency test (MSLT) provides an objective measure of excessive sleepiness and demonstrates the presence of sleep-onset REM periods. Sleep latencies of less than 10 minutes, typically below 5 minutes, and two or more sleep-onset REM periods are found in most narcoleptic patients.

For the correct interpretation of polysomnographic findings, the recordings should be performed with the following conditions: patients must be free for at least 15 days of drugs that influence sleep (particularly REM sleep); the sleep-wake schedule must be previously standardized for at least 7 days; and nocturnal polysomnography must be performed on the night immediately preceding the MSLT to rule out other sleep disorders that could mimic the diagnostic features of narcolepsy, such as periodic limb movement disorder and central sleep apnea syndrome. Because other disorders can occur in patients with narcolepsy, their presence can make it difficult to confirm the diagnosis of narcolepsy.

Other Laboratory Test Features: Routine daytime electroencephalograms of patients with narcolepsy are characterized by persistent drowsiness, which the patient may be unaware of or deny. Eye opening can produce diffuse alpha activity that is called a paradoxical alpha response.

HLA typing of narcoleptic patients almost always shows the presence of HLA-DR2 and DQ1 (DR15 and DQ6 using a newer nomenclature). DR2-negative narcolepsy has been reported, particularly in black patients, whereas other ethnic patient groups, such as the Japanese, have a 100% association with DR2 positivity. The most specific HLA marker associated with narcolepsy across all ethnic groups is HLA DQB1*0602, a molecular subtype of DQ6. DQB1*0602-negative patients with cataplexy are very rare but have been reported in a familial context. DR2 and DQB1*0602 are also present in about 10% to 35% of the general population, although a lower percentage has been reported in certain ethnic groups (e.g., DR2 in Israeli Jews.) Therefore, DR2 or DQB1*0602 positivity does not directly indicate narcolepsy, but it instead indicates that a person has a genetic predisposition to developing the disease.

HLA typing is useful in assisting in making the diagnosis and in detecting high-risk subjects in the families of narcoleptic patients. The absence of HLA DQB1*0602 (or DR2 in Caucasians) should raise doubts regarding a potential diagnosis of narcolepsy.

Differential Diagnosis: Patients with recurrent daytime naps or lapses into sleep but without cataplexy need to be differentiated from those with narcolepsy. Many disorders, such as idiopathic hypersomnia, subwakefulness syndrome, obstructive sleep apnea syndrome, periodic limb movement disorder, insufficient-sleep syndrome, recurrent hypersomnia, etc., can produce excessive sleepiness. The presence of other sleep disorders, such as the sleep apnea syndromes or periodic limb movement disorder, however, does not preclude a diagnosis of narcolepsy if cataplexy is present.

Idiopathic hypersomnia is differentiated in part by the absence of REM-related features, such as cataplexy, sleep paralysis, hypnagogic hallucinations, and two or more REM periods on an MSLT.

The most difficult differential diagnosis concerns patients with daytime sleepiness, HLA-DR2 positivity, and two or more sleep-onset REM periods seen during a correctly performed MSLT. These patients can have hypnagogic hallucinations and sleep paralysis and have often been classified as having "narcolepsy" despite the absence of a history of cataplexy. Various terms, such as essential hypersomnia, primary hypersomnia, ambiguous narcolepsy, atypical narcolepsy, etc., have been used to classify these patients, who may be in the developing phase of narcolepsy.

Much less frequently, hypoglycemia, hypothyroidism, epilepsy, intracranial space-occupying lesions, myotonic dystrophy, Prader-Willi syndrome, alcoholism, fugue states, hysteria, and drug withdrawal (particularly from central stimulants) will lead to isolated sleepiness.

Cataplexy should be differentiated from hypotension, transient ischemic attacks, drop attacks, akinetic seizures, muscular disorders, vestibular disorders, psychologic or psychiatric disorders, and sleep paralysis. Some patients with sophisticated knowledge of narcolepsy may misperceive noncataplectic muscle weakness as cataplexy. The response to tricyclic antidepressant medications may aid in the diagnosis of cataplexy in some patients. Malingering has to be considered in any patients who try to mislead the clinician to obtain stimulant medications.

Diagnostic Criteria: Narcolepsy (347)

A. The patient has a complaint of excessive sleepiness or sudden muscle weakness.
B. Recurrent daytime naps or lapses into sleep occur almost daily for at least 3 months.
C. Sudden bilateral loss of postural muscle tone occurs in association with intense emotion (cataplexy).
D. Associated features include:
   1. Sleep paralysis
   2. Hypnagogic hallucinations
   3. Automatic behaviors
   4. Disrupted major sleep episode
E. Polysomnography demonstrates one or more of the following:
   1. Sleep latency less than 10 minutes
   2. REM sleep latency less than 20 minutes and
   3. An MSLT that demonstrates a mean sleep latency of less than 5 minutes and
   4. Two or more sleep-onset REM periods
F. HLA typing demonstrates DQB1*0602 or DR2 positivity.
G. No medical or mental disorder accounts for the symptoms.
H. Other sleep disorders (e.g., periodic limb movement disorder or central sleep apnea syndrome) may be present but are not the primary cause of the symptoms.

Minimal Criteria: B plus C, or A plus D plus E plus G.

Severity Criteria:

Mild: Mild sleepiness, as defined on page 23, or rare cataplexy (less than once per week).
Moderate: Moderate sleepiness, as defined on page 23, or infrequent cataplexy (less than daily).
Severe: Severe sleepiness, as defined on page 23, or severe cataplexy (daily).

Duration Criteria:

Acute: 6 months or less.
Subacute: More than 6 months but less than 12 months.
Chronic: 12 months or longer.

Bibliography:

Carskadon M, ed. Current perspectives on daytime sleepiness. Sleep 1982; 2(Suppl 5): S55–S202.
Guilleminault C. Narcolepsy. Sleep 1986; 9: 99–291.
Guilleminault C. Narcolepsy and its differential diagnosis. In: Guilleminault C, ed. Sleep and its disorders in children. New York: Raven Press, 1987; 181–194.
Guilleminault C, Passouant P, Dement WC, eds. Narcolepsy. New York: Spectrum, 1976.
Honda Y, Juji T, eds. HLA in narcolepsy. Berlin: Springer-Verlag, 1988.
Mitler MM, Nelson S, Hajdukovic R. Narcolepsy. Diagnosis, treatment, and management. Psychiatr Clin North Am 1987; 10: 593–606.
Roth B. Narcolepsy and hypersomnia. Basel: Karger, 1980.
van den Hoed J, Kraemer H, Guilleminault C, Zarcone VP Jr, Miles LE, Dement WC, Mitler MM. Disorders of excessive daytime somnolence: polygraphic and clinical data for 100 patients. Sleep 1981; 4: 23–37.

Recurrent Hypersomnia (780.54-2)

Synonyms and Key Words: Periodic hypersomnia, Kleine-Levin syndrome, binge eating, hypersexuality (excludes menstrual-associated sleep disorder).

Essential Features:

Recurrent hypersomnia is a disorder characterized by recurrent episodes of hypersomnia that typically occur weeks or months apart.

The best-known form of recurrent hypersomnia is the Kleine-Levin syndrome. Other forms of recurrent hypersomnia have the same pattern of sleepiness, but the associated features may be present in an incomplete form. Kleine-Levin syndrome is a disorder characterized by recurrent episodes of hypersomnia and binge eating (rapid consumption of a large amount of food), usually with onset in early adolescence in males but occasionally in later life and in women. A monosymptomatic form of the disorder with hypersomnia only can occur without binge eating or hypersexuality.

Typically, the episode lasts several days to several weeks and appears on average twice a year but can occur as many as 12 times a year. Patients may sleep as long as 18 to 20 hours of the day during somnolent episodes, waking only to eat and void. Urinary incontinence does not occur. Patients may respond verbally, but often unclearly, when aroused by a strong stimulus during the episodes. Body weight gain of 2 to 5 kg during an episode is common in the Kleine-Levin syndrome.

In the monosymptomatic type, however, weight loss may be observed. Disorientation, forgetfulness, depression, depersonalization, and occasional hallucinations are often observed. Transient behavior changes, such as irritability, aggression, and impulsive behaviors, can also occur during the episodes. Transient dysphoria, insomnia, elation, restlessness, or sexual hyperactivity may follow the period of somnolence. During intervals between episodes, patients sleep normally and are believed to be both medically and mentally healthy.

These constellations of clinical symptoms indicate the presence of very slight disturbance of consciousness, with disinhibited behaviors during the episode, and have been interpreted as being manifestations of hypothalamic dysfunction.

Associated Features: Social and occupational impairment during attacks is severe. Data on the long-term effects of recurrent hypersomnia on psychosocial adjustment are lacking.

Course: Unlike the course of most other disorders of excessive sleepiness, the course of recurrent hypersomnia is characterized by recurrent episodes of severe sleepiness, lasting up to several weeks, but with normal functioning between episodes. Long-term follow-up studies of patients with Kleine-Levin syndrome have not been performed, but anecdotal evidence suggests that the disorder has a benign course, with episodes lessening in duration, severity, and frequency over several years.

Predisposing Factors: The somnolent episodes are often precipitated by acute febrile episodes and severe somatic stresses.

Prevalence: Not known.

Age of Onset: Usually early adolescence, but occasionally in adulthood.

Sex Ratio: More commonly described in males, but true sex ratio is unknown.

Pathology: Hypersomnia, hyperphagia, hypersexuality, and mental status changes suggest a disorder of hypothalamic and limbic function, but no well-documented pathology has been described.

Familial Pattern: Rarely occurs in families.

Complications: Patients with recurrent hypersomnia can show disinhibited behaviors or depression. Data are not available on rates of accidental injury or psychosocial impairment.

Polysomnographic Features: During the somnolent episode, generalized low-voltage slow electroencephalographic activities or diffuse alpha patterns may be observed.

Results of few all-night polysomnographic or multiple sleep latency tests have been reported. All-night polysomnography has shown high sleep efficiencies, with reduced stage 3 and stage 4 sleep. Multiple sleep latency testing of patients with Kleine-Levin syndrome has demonstrated short sleep latencies and the onset of REM sleep in one or more naps.

The rarity of the disorder, together with differences in electrophysiologic methodology across studies, prevent confident generalization about electrophysiologic findings.

Other Laboratory Test Features: Neurologic tests such as brain imaging may be necessary to exclude some types of central nervous system pathology.

Differential Diagnosis: The differential diagnosis includes other disorders of excessive sleepiness, such as obstructive sleep apnea syndrome, narcolepsy, or periodic limb movement disorder. Unlike that noted in recurrent hypersomnia, the complaint of excessive sleepiness in these disorders is more persistent rather than recurrent or periodic. Patients with recurrent hypersomnia lack the other associated clinical features of narcolepsy (cataplexy) or sleep-disordered breathing (loud snoring). Recurring episodes of sleepiness can occur in association with the menstrual cycle and may be indicative of the menstrual-associated sleep disorder. There is no evidence that recurrent hypersomnia is a seizure disorder. In psychomotor epilepsy, prolonged seizures may mimic the sleepiness of Kleine-Levin syndrome.

Atypical depression with somnolence may mimic recurrent hypersomnia but can be differentiated by the predominance of depressive psychopathology and the absence of persistent somnolence over several days.

Diagnostic Criteria: Recurrent Hypersomnia (780.54-2)

A. The patient has a complaint of excessive sleepiness.
B. The episodes of somnolence last for at least 18 hours a day.
C. The excessive sleepiness recurs at least once or twice a year, lasting a minimum of 3 days and up to 3 weeks.
D. The disorder occurs predominantly in males, with an age of onset typically in adolescence.
E. Associated features during the episodes include at least one of the following:
  1. Voracious eating
  2. Hypersexuality
  3. Disinhibited behaviors, such as irritability, aggression, disorientation, confusion, and hallucinations
  4. Absence of urinary incontinence and presence of verbal responses on strong stimulation
F. Polysomnographic monitoring during an episode demonstrates all of the following:
  1. A high sleep efficiency
  2. Reduced stage 3 and stage 4 sleep
  3. Reduced sleep latency and REM latency
  4. An MSLT with a mean sleep latency of less than 10 minutes.
G. The hypersomnia is not associated with other medical or mental disorders, such as epilepsy or depression.
H. The symptom is not associated with other sleep disorders, such as narcolepsy, sleep apnea syndromes, or periodic limb movement disorder.

Note: If the disorder is solely one of recurrent episodes of hypersomnia, state and code as recurrent hypersomnia monosymptomatic type. If the disorder is associated with voracious eating or hypersexuality, state and code as recurrent hypersomnia Kleine-Levin type.

Minimal Criteria: A plus B plus C plus G plus H.

Severity Criteria:

Mild: Less than two episodes of prolonged sleep periods per year. The symptoms produce a minor impairment of social or occupational function.
Moderate: More than two episodes of prolonged sleep periods per year. The symptoms produce a moderate impairment of social or occupational function.
Severe: More than two episodes of prolonged sleep episodes per year. The symptoms produce a severe impairment of social or occupational function.

Duration Criteria:

Acute: 1 month or less.
Subacute: More than 1 month but less than 6 months.
Chronic: 6 months or longer.

Bibliography:

Critchley M, Hoffman HL. The syndrome of periodic somnolence and morbid hunger (Kleine-Levin syndrome). Br Med J 1942; 1: 137–139.
Gallicek A. Syndrome of episodes of hypersomnia, bulimia, and abnormal mental states. JAMA 1954; 154: 1081–1083.
Reynolds CF, Kupfer DJ, Christiansen CL, et al. Multiple sleep latency test findings in Kleine-Levin syndrome. J Nerv Ment Dis 1984; 172: 41–44.
Roth B. Narcolepsy and hypersomnia. Basel: Karger, 1980.
Takahashi Y. Clinical studies of periodic somnolence. Analysis of 28 personal cases. Psychiatr Neurol (Jpn) 1965; 853–889.
Takahashi Y. Periodic hypersomnia and sleep drunkenness. In: Shimazono Y, Hozaki H, Hishikawa Y, eds. Pathological aspects of sleep disorders. Psychiatr Mook (Jpn) 1988; 21: 233–247.

Idiopathic Hypersomnia (780.54-7)

Synonyms and Key Words: Dependent, idiopathic, or NREM (non-rapid eye movement) narcolepsy; idiopathic central nervous system (CNS) hypersomnia; functional, mixed, or harmonious hypersomnia. Idiopathic hypersomnia is the preferred term. This category does not include post-traumatic hypersomnia, which is described elsewhere.

Essential Features:

Idiopathic hypersomnia is a disorder of presumed CNS cause that is associated with a normal or prolonged major sleep episode and excessive sleepiness consisting of prolonged (1 to 2 hour) sleep episodes of NREM sleep.

Idiopathic hypersomnia is characterized by a complaint of constant or recurrent excessive daytime sleepiness, typically with sleep episodes lasting 1 or more hours in duration. It is enhanced in situations that allow sleepiness to become manifest, such as reading or watching television in the evening. The major sleep episode may be prolonged, lasting more than 8 hours. The capacity to arouse the subject may be normal, but some patients report great difficulty waking up and experience disorientation after awakening.

Associated Features: Some patients may complain of paroxysmal episodes of sleepiness culminating in sleep attacks, as in narcoleptic patients. Most often these attacks are preceded by long periods of drowsiness. Naps are usually longer than in narcolepsy or sleep apnea, and short naps are generally reported as being nonrefreshing. Often as disabling as narcolepsy, idiopathic hypersomnia has an unpredictable response to stimulants such as the amphetamines and methylphenidate hydrochloride. These patients often report more side effects, such as tachycardia or irritability, and the use of stimulants tend to exacerbate the associated symptoms of headache.

Associated symptoms suggesting dysfunction of the autonomic nervous system are not uncommon. They include headaches, which may be migrainous in quality; fainting episodes (syncope); orthostatic hypotension; and, most commonly, peripheral vascular complaints (Raynaud's-type phenomena with cold hands and feet).

Course: The disorder is initially progressive but often is stable by the time of diagnosis. It appears to be lifelong.

Prevalence: This syndrome is estimated to account for 5% to 10% of patients who bring a complaint of sleepiness to a sleep clinic. This estimate may vary considerably, depending on the criteria used to diagnose excessive sleepiness (see polysomnographic features).

Age of Onset: At the time of presentation, most patients have had the disorder for many years. Idiopathic hypersomnia usually becomes apparent during adolescence or the early twenties. Many changes, frequently those associated with stress or increased tension, may take place in the patient's life at that time. Consequently, the disorder is often difficult to diagnose at an early stage and may be confounded with other disorders of excessive sleepiness.

Sex Ratio: No difference

Familial Pattern: A familial manifestation of this disorder can be observed, but studies using standard diagnostic criteria and procedures are needed to estimate the ratio of familial to isolated cases, as well as to determine the mode of transmission.

Polysomnographic Features: Polysomnographic monitoring of nocturnal sleep usually demonstrates normal quantity and quality of sleep. Sleep at night is not disrupted as it is in narcolepsy. The sleep latency may be reduced in duration, and the sleep period tends to be of either normal or slightly greater than normal duration. Slow-wave sleep can be normal or slightly increased in amount and percentage.

Polysomnographic monitoring should rule out sleep-onset REM periods, pathologic apnea indexes, and periodic movements during sleep.

Sleep latencies are typically short in the daytime in idiopathic hypersomnia. The multiple sleep latency test (MSLT) usually demonstrates a sleep latency of less than 10 minutes. The clinical severity of idiopathic hypersomnia may not closely correlate with the MSLT results because latencies above 5 minutes are not uncommon in patients with clinically severe hypersomnia.

Other Laboratory Test Features: Human leukocyte antigen (HLA) determination may be helpful in the diagnosis. Most narcoleptic patients carry the HLA-DR2, whereas only HLA-Cw2 incidence is elevated in idiopathic hypersomnia, and the incidence of HLA-DR2 in this population is found to be either normal or even decreased.

Differential Diagnosis: Idiopathic hypersomnia must be differentiated from several other disorders of sleepiness, such as narcolepsy, sleep apnea syndromes, posttraumatic hypersomnia, periodic limb movement disorder, and sleepiness associated with affective disorders. The polygraphic features usually help to distinguish idiopathic hypersomnia from the sleep apnea syndromes, narcolepsy, and periodic limb movement disorder. Patients with idiopathic hypersomnia should be distinguished from long sleepers who do not have objective evidence of excessive sleepiness after a full major sleep episode.

The differential diagnosis of sleepiness associated with low-grade chronic depression may be more difficult. Although no systematic studies have been performed on the personality profile of patients with idiopathic hypersomnia, clinical experience reveals the presence of polymorphic psychologic disturbance in a large number of these patients. It is mainly polysomnographic features with short sleep latencies and normal sleep organization that can single out idiopathic hypersomnia. The diagnosis of sleepiness associated with dysthymia and related mood disorders relies primarily on the identification of depressive symptoms during the clinical evaluation, but psychometric tests may help in the diagnostic process. Patients with idiopathic hypersomnia often tend to deny subjective dysphoria, and depression should be inferred from restriction of interests, anhedonia, and observational signs of depression in facial expression or posture. A family history of mood disorder can also be helpful.

Two other syndromes of excessive sleepiness must be ruled out before diagnosing the primary form of idiopathic hypersomnia. First, sleepiness may be an early symptom of progressive hydrocephalus in children and adults. Other clinical features of hydrocephalus may be completely absent at that point. Computed tomography, skull radiography, and electroencephalography may be necessary to eliminate this diagnosis. Secondly, 6 to 18 months after receiving a head trauma, patients may gradually develop post-traumatic hypersomnia, showing all features of the primary form of idiopathic hypersomnia.

Diagnostic Criteria: Idiopathic Hypersomnia (780.54-7)

A. The patient has a complaint of prolonged sleep episodes, excessive sleepiness, or excessively deep sleep.

B. The patient has a prolonged nocturnal sleep period or frequent daily sleep episodes.

C. The onset is insidious and typically occurs before age 25.
D. The complaint is present for at least 6 months.
E. The onset does not occur within 18 months of head trauma.
F. Polysomnography demonstrates one or more of the following:
   1. A sleep period that is normal or prolonged in duration
   2. Sleep latency less than 10 minutes
   3. Normal REM sleep latency
   4. A less-than-10-minute sleep latency on MSLT
   5. Fewer than two sleep-onset REM periods.
G. No medical or mental disorder is present that could account for the symptom.
H. The symptoms do not meet the diagnostic criteria of any other sleep disorder causing excessive sleepiness (e.g., narcolepsy, obstructive sleep apnea syndrome, or post-traumatic hypersomnia).

Minimal Criteria: A plus B plus C plus D.

Severity Criteria:

Mild: Mild sleepiness, as defined on page 23.
Moderate: Moderate sleepiness, as defined on page 23.
Severe: Severe sleepiness, as defined on page 23.

Duration Criteria:

Acute: Not applicable.
Subacute: More than 6 months but less than 1 year.
Chronic: 1 year or longer.

Bibliography:

Guilleminault C. Disorders of excessive sleepiness. Ann Clin Res 1985; 17: 209–219.
Poirier G, Montplaisir J, Momege D, Decary F, Lebrun A. HLA antigens in narcolepsy and idiopathic CNS hypersomnolence. Sleep 1986; 9: 153–158.
Roth B. Narcolepsy and hypersomnia. Basel: Karger, 1980.

Post-traumatic Hypersomnia (780.54-8)

Synonyms and Key Words: Post-traumatic hypersomnia, secondary hypersomnolence.

Essential Features:

Post-traumatic hypersomnia is a disorder of excessive sleepiness that occurs as a result of a traumatic event involving the central nervous system.

This disorder clearly represents an alteration of the patient's pre-trauma sleep patterns. The hypersomnia is characterized by frequent daytime sleepiness, which may or may not be able to be resisted, with consequent sleep episodes. The duration of the major sleep episode may be prolonged compared with the prior sleep length.

Associated Features: The sleepiness is usually seen in the context of other posttraumatic encephalopathic symptoms, such as headaches, fatigue, difficulty concentrating, and memory impairment. Less commonly, an alteration in sleep patterns or alertness is the major complaint.

Course: Typically, the sleepiness is most evident in the immediate post-traumatic period and resolves over weeks to months.

Residual sleepiness and other sleep complaints may persist and even gradually worsen in the 6 to 18 months following an injury. Disabling degrees of sleepiness are more likely if the initial head trauma was severe (as judged by the presence of objective neurologic deficits, duration of initial coma, etc.).

Predisposing Factors: None, other than the head injury.

Prevalence: Not known.

Age of Onset: Can occur at any age.

Sex Ratio: No difference.

Familial Pattern: None known.

Pathology: The exact mechanism of the trauma is less important than is the actual neurologic site involved. Hypersomnia has been described following neurosurgical procedures for a variety of disorders, as well as following various types of trauma. The posterior hypothalamus, third ventricle (especially the pineal region), or posterior fossa (especially the midbrain and pons) are the most frequently implicated sites of injury leading to post-traumatic hypersomnia.

High cervical cord compression due to atlantoaxial dislocation has been described as a cause of sleep attacks, although the mechanism (e.g., direct compression and respiratory involvement vs. vascular compromise leading, perhaps, to more rostral ischemia) remains unclear. Many reports are solely clinical (i.e., without pathologic study) and often tend to equate narcolepsy and sleepiness but usually lack polysomnographic studies. Pathologic studies have demonstrated widespread lesions at autopsy, so that the specific anatomic substrate for the post-traumatic hypersomnia (as well as cataplexy, in a few cases) remains obscure.

With few exceptions, most of the spontaneous neurologic disorders reportedly associated with sleepiness or cataplexy (e.g., multiple sclerosis, neoplasms, encephalitis lethargica) have also had rather diffuse brain stem, diencephalic, and cortical lesions.

Complications: Not known.

Polysomnographic Features: Reported polysomnographic studies of this disorder are limited. Some patients, especially those with whiplash injury accompanying the head trauma, have demonstrable sleep-related respiratory abnormalities associated with the sleepiness. Many of these patients eventually improve in terms of both sleepiness and respiratory abnormalities.

Some patients have had objective sleepiness, as judged by polysomnography and the multiple sleep latency test (MSLT), but without the presence of sleep-onset REM periods.

Other patients show no objective features of sleepiness on polysomnographic studies, and some evidence suggests that patients with diffuse posttraumatic encephalopathy or mental disorders (e.g., depression) may be in this category. The possibility that some of these patients have repetitive daytime microsleeps that impair clear thinking may necessitate 24-hour polysomnographic investigation in some cases.

Other Laboratory Test Features: Neurologic studies, including brain imaging, are usually indicated. If a question of post-traumatic epilepsy is raised, multichannel electroencephalographic testing may be necessary.

Differential Diagnosis: A careful history is necessary to ensure that the symptom of hypersomnia did not antedate the head trauma. Preexisting conditions that may have contributed to the traumatic event (e.g., visual impairment from a tumor leading to a motor vehicle accident), as well as post-traumatic structural lesions that may be specifically treatable causes of sleepiness, should also be ruled out with appropriate studies.

Occult (preexisting or post-traumatic) hydrocephalus, atlantoaxial dislocation, subdural hematoma or hygroma, arachnoid cysts, seizure disorders (or side effects of anticonvulsant drugs used to treat posttraumatic seizures), and chronic meningitis need to be considered as causes of the sleepiness. These disorders especially need to be considered in those cases demonstrating a progressive course. Because traumatic events are often complicated by medicolegal issues, psychogenic factors (e.g., secondary gain) must also be considered.

Diagnostic Criteria: Posttraumatic Hypersomnia (780.54-8)

    A. The patient has a complaint of excessive sleepiness.
    B. Frequent daily sleep episodes occur.
    C. The onset of the sleepiness is temporally associated with head trauma.
    D. Polysomnography demonstrates all of the following:
        1. Normal timing, quality, and duration of sleep
        2. A mean sleep latency of less than 10 minutes on MSLT
        3. Fewer than two sleep-onset REM periods on MSLT
    E. No medical disorder is present that could account for the symptom.
    F. The symptoms do not meet the criteria of other sleep disorders that produce sleepiness (e.g., narcolepsy)

Minimal Criteria: A plus B plus C.

Severity Criteria:

Mild: Mild sleepiness, as defined on page 23.
Moderate: Moderate sleepiness, as defined on page 23.
Severe: Severe sleepiness, as defined on page 23.

Duration Criteria:

Acute: 1 month or less.
Subacute: More than 1 month but less than 6 months.
Chronic: 6 months or longer.

Bibliography:

Erlich SS, Itabashi HH. Narcolepsy: a neuropathologic study. Sleep 1986; 9: 126–132.
Guilleminault C, Faull KF, Miles L, van den Hoed J. Posttraumatic excessive daytime sleepiness: A review of 20 patients. Neurology 1983; 33: 1584–1589.
Hall CW, Danoff D. Sleep attacks–apparent relationship to atlantoaxial dislocation. Arch Neurology 1975; 32: 57–58.
Roth B. Narcolepsy and hypersomnia. Basel: Karger, 1980.

Obstructive Sleep Apnea Syndrome (780.53-0)

Synonyms and Key Words: Sleep apnea, obstructive apnea, upper airway apnea, mixed apnea, hypersomnia sleep apnea syndrome, obesity hypoventilation syndrome, adenoidal hypertrophy, cor pulmonale syndrome, Pickwickian syndrome. The terms *Pickwickian syndrome* and *obesity hypoventilation syndrome* are discouraged from use because they have been applied to several different sleep-related breathing disorders. (Excludes infant sleep apnea.)

Essential Features:

__Obstructive sleep apnea syndrome__ is characterized by repetitive episodes of upper airway obstruction that occur during sleep, usually associated with a reduction in blood oxygen saturation.

A characteristic snoring pattern is associated with this syndrome and consists of loud snores or brief gasps that alternate with episodes of silence that usually last 20 to 30 seconds. The loud snoring typically has been present for many years, often since childhood, and may have increased in loudness before the patient's presentation. The snoring is commonly so loud that it disturbs the sleep of bedpartners or others sleeping in close proximity. The patient occasionally will hear the snoring, but is usually not aware of the snoring intensity. The snoring may be exacerbated following the ingestion of alcohol before bedtime or following an increase in body weight.

Apneic episodes characterized by cessation of breathing may be noticed by an observer, but respiratory movements are usually maintained during the obstructive episodes, particularly in patients with apnea of mild severity. Patients with more-severe apnea can have prolonged episodes of absence of breathing that precede the resumption of respiratory movements. The cessation of breathing, sometimes associated with cyanosis, is usually of concern to a bedpartner and often leads to the patient's presentation. Typically the bedpartner will awaken the patient to reestablish breathing. The termination of the apneic event is often associated with loud snores and vocalizations that consist of gasps, moans, or mumblings. Whole-body movements usually occur at the time of the arousal and can be disturbing to a bedpartner; coupled with the loud snoring, these movements occasionally are the cause of the bedpartner moving to a separate bed or another room to sleep. The body movements can be violent, and patients with obstructive sleep apnea are often described as being restless sleepers. Rarely, severely affected patients will fall out of bed at these times. Patients are usually unaware of the loud snoring and breathing difficulty or of the frequent arousals and brief awakenings that occur throughout the night. Some patients, however, particularly the elderly, are intensely aware of the sleep disturbance and present with a complaint of insomnia due to the frequent awakenings, with a sensation of being unrefreshed in the morning. Patients may have nocturia that increases in frequency with the progression of symptoms.

Upon awakening, patients typically feel unrefreshed and may describe feelings of disorientation, grogginess, mental dullness, and incoordination. Severe dryness of the mouth is common and often leads the patient to get something to drink during the night or upon awakening in the morning. Morning headaches, characteristically dull and generalized, are often reported. The headaches last for 1 to 2 hours after awakening and may prompt the ingestion of analgesics.

Excessive sleepiness is a typical presenting complaint. The sleepiness usually is most evident when the patient is in a relaxing situation, such as when sitting reading or watching television. Inability to control the sleepiness can be evident in group meetings or while attending movies, theater performances, or concerts. With extreme sleepiness, the patient may fall asleep while actively conversing, eating, walking, or driving. Naps tend to be unrefreshing and may be accompanied by a dull headache upon awakening. The daytime sleepiness can be incapacitating, resulting in job loss, accidents, self-injury, marital and family problems, and poor school performance. Misdiagnosis can lead to patients being labeled as lazy or as having a primary mental disorder such as depression. The intensity of the sleepiness can vary considerably, however; some patients with severe obstructive sleep apnea syndrome present with minimal sleepiness, whereas other patients with relatively mild apnea can have severe sleepiness. Some patients will minimize the degree of impaired alertness, occasionally priding themselves on their ability to sleep anywhere at any time.

In the young child, the signs and symptoms of obstructive sleep apnea are more subtle than in the adult; therefore, the diagnosis is more difficult to make and should be confirmed by polysomnography. Snoring, which is characteristic of adult obstructive sleep apnea syndrome, may not be present. Young children with obstructive sleep apnea syndrome can exhibit loud habitual snoring, agitated arousals, and unusual sleep postures, such as sleeping on the hands and knees. Pectus excavatum and rib flaring can be seen. If the apnea is associated with adenotonsillar enlargement, children can have a typical "adenoidal face," with a dull expression, periorbital edema, and mouth breathing. Nocturnal enuresis is common, and the presence of enuresis should raise the possibility of obstructive sleep apnea syndrome if it occurs in a child who was previously dry at night. During wakefulness, children may manifest excessive sleepiness, although this is not as common or pronounced as it is in adults. Daytime mouth breathing, swallowing difficulty, and poor speech articulation are also common features in children with obstructive sleep apnea.

Associated Features: There can be sudden awakenings following the obstructive events and complaints of nocturnal chest discomfort, choking, or suffocation that are associated with intense anxiety. Gastroesophageal reflux can occur in association with the effort to reestablish breathing, particularly if the patient had eaten a large meal shortly before bedtime. Laryngospasm with stridor, and even cyanosis, may rarely occur as a result of the reflux.

Secondary depression, anxiety, irritability, and even profound despair are commonly associated with the obstructive sleep apnea syndrome. Patients can also have loss of both libido and erectile ability. Impotence is rarely the presenting complaint.

Most patients with the obstructive sleep apnea syndrome have an increase in the severity of symptoms with increasing body weight. Many patients, however, report that at a younger age their symptoms were less noticeable even though their body weight may have been greater. At the time of presentation, most patients with the obstructive sleep apnea syndrome are overweight. Weight reduction after the onset of the syndrome will occasionally lead to improvement of symptoms. Obstructive sleep apnea syndrome in patients of normal or below-normal body weight suggests upper airway obstruction due to a definable localized structural abnormality such as a maxillomandibular malformation or adenotonsillar enlargement.

Cardiac arrhythmias commonly occur during sleep in patients with the obstructive sleep apnea syndrome, and range from sinus arrhythmia to premature ventricular contractions, atrioventricular block, and sinus arrest. Bradytachycardia is most commonly seen in association with the apneic episodes. The bradycardia occurs during the apneic phase and alternates with tachycardia at the termination of the obstruction at the time of resumption of ventilation. Some patients, even those with severe obstructive sleep apnea syndrome, however, may not demonstrate bradytachycardia or other cardiac arrhythmias. The tachyarrhythmias most commonly occur during the time of reestablishing breathing following the apneic phase and may increase the risk of sudden death during sleep.

Mild hypertension with an elevated diastolic pressure is commonly associated with the obstructive sleep apnea syndrome.

Hypoxemia during sleep, sometimes with an oxygen saturation of less than 50%, is a typical feature of the disorder. Usually, the oxygen saturation returns to normal values following resumption of breathing. Some patients, however, particularly those with chronic obstructive pulmonary disease or alveolar hypoventilation, have continuously low oxygen saturation values during sleep and are predisposed to developing pulmonary hypertension and associated right-sided cardiac failure, hepatic congestion, and ankle edema.

"Blackouts," disorientation, and periods of automatic behavior with amnesia are occasionally reported.

In children, developmental delay, learning difficulties, decreased school performance, and behavioral disorders, including hyperactivity alternating with excessive sleepiness, are often seen, especially in older children.

Course: Spontaneous resolution has been reported in association with reduction of body weight, but the course usually is progressive and can ultimately lead to premature death. Profound functional impairment and life-threatening complications can occur. No information is available on the prognosis of obstructive sleep apnea syndrome of mild severity.

Predisposing Factors: Nasopharyngeal abnormalities that reduce the caliber of the upper airway are primarily responsible for the obstruction during sleep. In most adult patients, a generalized narrowing of the upper airway is a common finding; however, localized lesions, such as hypertrophied tonsils and adenoids, are often seen in children. A severe upper respiratory tract infection or chronic allergic rhinitis may produce transient obstructive sleep apnea syndrome, especially in young children.

Although obesity is often associated with obstructive sleep apnea syndrome, some patients with this disorder are not overweight; morbid obesity is present only in a minority of patients. In the absence of obesity, craniofacial abnormalities, such as micrognathia or retrognathia, are likely to be present.

Hypothyroidism and acromegaly can precipitate this disorder, as can neurologic disorders that lead to upper airway obstruction.

Prevalence: Obstructive sleep apnea syndrome is most common in middle-aged overweight men and women. The prevalence has been estimated to be 4% for men and 2% for women.

Age of Onset: Obstructive sleep apnea syndrome can occur at any age, from infancy to old age. Most patients present between the ages of 40 and 60. Women are more likely to develop obstructive sleep apnea after menopause.

Sex Ratio: In adults, the male to female ratio is about 2:1. The syndrome probably affects prepubertal males and females at equal rates.

Familial Pattern: A familial tendency for sleep apnea has been described. For most patients, the role of hereditary factors is unknown.

Pathology: Upper airway narrowing due to either excessive bulk of soft tissues or craniofacial abnormalities predisposes the patient to obstructive sleep apnea syndrome. An underlying abnormality of the neurologic control of the upper airway musculature or ventilation during sleep may be present. In some patients with neurologic disorders, a specific lesion affecting the control of pharyngeal muscles can be responsible for the development of obstructive sleep apnea syndrome.

Complications: In contrast to the adult, children with obstructive sleep apnea syndrome rarely have cardiac arrhythmias. In the adult, excessive sleepiness and cardiopulmonary abnormalities are the main complications (see associated features).

Polysomnographic Features: Studies of respiration during sleep demonstrate apneic episodes in the presence of respiratory muscle effort. Apneic episodes greater than 10 seconds in duration are considered clinically significant. The apneic episodes, as monitored by nasal and oral airflow, are typically 20 to 40 seconds in duration; rarely, episodes up to several minutes in duration can occur. The episodes usually occur during sleep stages 1 and 2, are rare during stages 3 and 4, and are more prevalent and can occur solely during rapid eye movement sleep. Many apneic episodes can have an initial central component followed by an obstructive component and are called *mixed apneas*. Central apneic episodes can also be seen. Some patients can have a predominance of partial obstructive respiratory events during sleep, called hypopneas. These hypopneas are characterized by a reduction of airflow of greater than 50%, which is associated with a reduction in the blood oxygen saturation levels.

Polysomnographic monitoring of obstructive sleep apnea syndrome should consist of monitoring of sleep by electroencephalography, electrooculography, electromyography, airflow, and respiratory muscle effort, and should also include measures of electrocardiographic rhythm and blood oxygen saturation. Changes in cardiac rhythm, particularly bradytachycardia, frequently occur with the apneic episodes. The arterial oxygen saturation level falls during the apneic episode and rises to baseline levels at the termination of the apneic episode. Due to a 10- to 20-second delay in detection of oxygen saturation by subcutaneous monitoring devices, a dissociation may occur between the respiratory patterns and the oxygen-saturation patterns seen on the polysomnogram. Carbon dioxide values in the blood are usually only transiently elevated, but sustained elevations can be seen in some patients. The obstructive apneic episodes can lead to gastroesophageal reflux in some patients; reflux can be detected during sleep by intraesophageal pH monitoring.

Sleep is disrupted by arousals that usually occur at the termination of the apneic events, resulting in excessive sleepiness, which may be detected by either the multiple sleep latency test (MSLT) or other tests of daytime alertness and sleepiness. Mean sleep latencies on the MSLT are often below 10 minutes and can be below 5 minutes (normal 10 to 20 minutes). Sleep-onset REM periods during the naps are not typical, but sleep-onset REM periods can occur on every nap.

Other Laboratory Test Features: Awake arterial blood gas measurements are usually normal, but some patients with severe obstructive sleep apnea syndrome can show abnormal values. Cephalometric radiographs, magnetic resonance imaging, computed tomographic scanning, or fiberoptic endoscopy can show obstruction of the upper airway. Cardiac testing may show evidence of impaired right ventricular function in some patients with severe obstructive sleep apnea syndrome. Hematologic studies may also show an elevated hemoglobin or hematocrit value, indicating polycythemia.

Differential Diagnosis: The most common presenting symptom in adults is excessive sleepiness; therefore, obstructive sleep apnea syndrome needs to be differentiated from other causes of sleepiness such as narcolepsy, idiopathic hypersomnia, insufficient sleep syndrome, or periodic limb movement disorder. Obstructive sleep apnea syndrome can be differentiated from narcolepsy by the absence of cataplexy and the presence of loud, characteristic snoring. Nocturnal polysomnography and multiple sleep latency testing will usually be required to confirm the diagnosis. Depressive episodes associated with excessive sleepiness should be differentiated by psychiatric interview and psychometric testing. Other disorders of sleepiness, such as insufficient sleep syndrome or periodic limb movement disorder, commonly can coexist with obstructive sleep apnea syndrome and may be the predominant cause of the symptoms.

Respiratory disturbance during sleep can also be due to central alveolar hypoventilation, central sleep apnea syndrome, primary snoring, paroxysmal nocturnal dyspnea, or asthma. Central alveolar hypoventilation and central sleep apnea syndromes can be differentiated from obstructive sleep apnea by the absence of respiratory effort and the presence of long episodes of reduced or absent tidal volume with oxygen desaturation on polysomnography. Cheyne-Stokes respiration and other disorders of ventilatory control can be mistaken for obstructive sleep apnea if not appropriately monitored during sleep. Such disorders can be aggravated or induced by sleep and also can be associated with mild to marked excessive sleepiness.

Occasionally, panic attacks, the sleep choking syndrome, and sleep-related laryngospasm can present with similar symptoms and need to be differentiated from obstructive sleep apnea syndrome. Sleep-related gastroesophageal reflux and sleep-related abnormal swallowing syndrome can also produce choking episodes.

All night polysomnographic testing with appropriate respiratory and cardiac monitoring is mandatory for characterization and documentation of the presence and severity of sleep apnea and should be performed along with multiple sleep latency testing, particularly in patients with excessive sleepiness.

Diagnostic Criteria: Obstructive Sleep Apnea Syndrome (780.53-0)

A. The patient has a complaint of excessive sleepiness or insomnia. Occasionally, the patient may be unaware of clinical features that are observed by others.
B. Frequent episodes of obstructed breathing occur during sleep.
C. Associated features include:
  1. Loud snoring
  2. Morning headaches
  3. A dry mouth upon awakening
  4. Chest retraction during sleep in young children
D. Polysomnographic monitoring demonstrates:
  1. More than five obstructive apneas, greater than 10 seconds in duration, per hour of sleep and one or more of the following:
    a. Frequent arousals from sleep associated with the apneas
    b. Bradytachycardia
    c. Arterial oxygen desaturation in association with the apneic episodes
  2. MSLT may or may not demonstrate a mean sleep latency of less than 10 minutes.
E. The symptoms can be associated with other medical disorders (e.g., tonsillar enlargement).
F. Other sleep disorders can be present (e.g., periodic limb movement disorder or narcolepsy).

Note: State and code obstructive sleep apnea syndrome on axis A and causative disorders on axis C (e.g., tonsillar enlargement).

Minimal Criteria: A plus B plus C.

Severity Criteria:

Mild: Associated with mild sleepiness or mild insomnia, as defined on page 23. Most of the habitual sleep period is free of respiratory disturbance. The apneic episodes are associated with mild oxygen desaturation or benign cardiac arrhythmias.

Moderate: Associated with moderate sleepiness or mild insomnia, as defined on page 23. The apneic episodes can be associated with moderate oxygen desaturation or mild cardiac arrhythmias.

Severe: Associated with severe sleepiness, as defined on page 23. Most of the habitual sleep period is associated with respiratory disturbance, with severe oxygen desaturation or moderate to severe cardiac arrhythmias. There can be evidence of associated cardiac or pulmonary failure.

Duration Criteria:

Acute: 2 weeks or less.
Subacute: More than 2 weeks but less than 6 months.
Chronic: 6 months or longer.

Bibliography:

Block AJ, Boysen PG, Wynne JW, Hunt LA. Sleep apnea, hypopnea and oxygen desaturation in normal subjects. A strong male predominance. N Engl J Med 1979; 300: 513–517.

Brouillette RT, Fernbach SK, Hunt CE. Obstructive sleep apnea in infants and children. J Pediatr 1982; 100: 31–40.

Guilleminault C. Clinical features and evaluation of obstructive sleep apnea. In: Kryger MH, Roth T, Dement WC, eds. Principles and practice of sleep medicine. Philadelphia: WB Saunders, 1989; 552–558.

Guilleminault C, Tilkian A, Dement WC. The sleep apnea syndromes. Ann Rev Med 1976; 27: 465–484.

Hudgel DW. Clinical manifestations of the sleep apnea syndrome: In: Fletcher EC, ed. Abnormalities of respiration during sleep. Orlando: Grune & Stratton, 1986; 21–37.

Sullivan CE, Issa FG. Obstructive sleep apnea. Clin Chest Med 1985; 6: 633–650.

Young T, Palta M, Dempsey J, Skatrud J, Weber S, Badr S. The occurrence of sleep-disordered breathing among middle-aged adults. N Engl J Med 1993;328:1230–1235.

Central Sleep Apnea Syndrome (780.51-0)

Synonyms and Key Words: Central apnea, nonobstructive sleep apnea, Cheyne-Stokes respiration

Essential Features:

Central sleep apnea syndrome is characterized by a cessation or decrease of ventilatory effort during sleep and is usually associated with oxygen desaturation.

This disorder is usually associated with a complaint of insomnia with an inability to maintain sleep; however, excessive sleepiness can also occur. Several awakenings during the course of the night usually occur, sometimes with a gasp for air and a sensation of choking. Patients can also be asymptomatic and may present for evaluation because of observations by a concerned bedpartner. Feelings of daytime tiredness, fatigue, and sleepiness are common.

Central sleep apnea syndrome may have a few associated obstructive apneas and episodes of hypoventilation; however, the predominant respiratory disturbance consists of central apneic episodes.

Associated Features: Snoring can occur but is not prominent. The hemodynamic complications of this syndrome include the development of systemic hypertension, cardiac arrhythmias, pulmonary hypertension, and cardiac failure. These hemodynamic findings may reflect a primary disorder of the cardiovascular system that leads to the development of the apnea.

Difficulties with memory and other cognitive functions may result from the excessive sleepiness. Headaches upon awakening are common in patients with severe alteration of blood gases during sleep. Patients occasionally complain of a loss of libido and erectile problems. Depressive reactions can occur.

Course: The severity of the central apneas and associated sleep disturbance may vary, being partially dependent on underlying contributing factors such as cerebrovascular disease and cardiac failure. Weight gain may exacerbate the disorder.

Predisposing Factors: Cerebrovascular or cardiac disease is often a contributing factor in patients with this disorder. Other predisposing factors include neurologic disorders that affect the central control of ventilation, such as lesions of the cerebral hemispheres, brain stem, or spinal cord.

Prevalence: Central sleep apnea can be asymptomatic; therefore, its exact prevalence is unknown. It is considered pathologic only when the events are sufficiently frequent to disturb sleep or result in hypoxemia or cardiac changes.

Age of Onset: Central sleep apnea is observed with increasing frequency in the general population as a function of age.

Sex Ratio: In adults, central apneic events appear to be more prevalent in men than in women. After menopause, this difference is less apparent.

Familial Pattern: Not known.

Pathology: Various central nervous system lesions affecting either the cerebral hemispheres or the brain stem have resulted in respiratory center failure. In most patients, however, specific anatomic abnormalities cannot be identified. The repetitive central sleep apneas appear to be related to the oscillations of a physiologic feedback loop from lung to brain.

Complications: The major complications are related to the cardiovascular effects such as hypertension and cardiac arrhythmias (see associated features).

Polysomnographic Features: Central apneas or hypopneas typically last from 10 to 30 seconds, followed by either gradual or abrupt resumption of respiratory effort. Often, a 10- to 60-second episode of hyperventilation follows the central apnea, with a gradual decrease in tidal volume that leads to the cessation of air flow. Nightly variations in the number of central apneic events are observed, often associated with use of sedating drugs or alcohol. Central apneas are most prevalent in the transition from wake to sleep and when the patient is in the supine position.

The central events are associated with variable degrees of hypoxemia or cardiac disturbances.

Central apneic pauses may be difficult to differentiate from obstructive episodes, particularly if the means of demonstrating respiratory effort do not include a measure of intrathoracic pressure, such as by esophageal manometry.

A multiple sleep latency test (MSLT) may show excessive sleepiness, depending upon the severity of the sleep disruption.

Other Laboratory Test Features: A Holter monitor can show sleep-related cardiac arrhythmias. Awake arterial blood-gas values can be impaired in severe cases. Neurologic tests may demonstrate central nervous system lesions. Cardiac function and pulmonary function tests can show abnormalities, depending upon the underlying predisposing disorder.

Differential Diagnosis: Obstructive sleep apnea syndrome can have similar presenting features and may be mistaken for central sleep apnea. Patients with obstructive sleep apnea syndrome will often have respiratory events during sleep that consist of both a central and an obstructive component and is called a "mixed apnea." The presence of mixed apneas is an important feature that distinguishes obstructive sleep apnea syndrome from central sleep apnea syndrome. Choking episodes during sleep can be associated with obstructive sleep apnea syndrome, central alveolar hypoventilation syndrome, sleep choking syndrome, or sleep-related laryngospasm. Patients with narcolepsy have an increased prevalence of central apneic events. Insufficient-sleep syndrome or idiopathic hypersomnia and other disorders of excessive sleepiness must be considered in patients presenting with excessive sleepiness due to central sleep apnea syndrome. Causes of insomnia, such as psychophysiologic insomnia and periodic limb movement disorder, also need to be considered in the differential diagnosis.

Diagnostic Criteria: Central Sleep Apnea Syndrome (780.51-0)

A. The patient has a complaint of either insomnia or excessive sleepiness. Occasionally, the patient may be unaware of clinical features observed by others.
B. The patient has frequent episodes of shallow or absent breathing during sleep.
C. Associated features include at least one of the following:

1. Gasps, grunts, or choking during sleep
2. Frequent body movements
3. Cyanosis during sleep
D. Polysomnographic monitoring demonstrates:
    1. Central apneic pauses greater than 10 seconds (20 seconds in infancy) in duration, and one or more of the following:
        a. Frequent arousals from sleep associated with the apneas
        b. Bradytachycardia
        c. Oxygen desaturation in association with the apneic episodes
    2. An MSLT may or may not demonstrate a mean sleep latency of less than 10 minutes.
E. Other sleep disorders can be present (e.g., periodic limb movement disorder, obstructive sleep apnea syndrome, or central alveolar hypoventilation syndrome).

Minimal Criteria: A plus B plus D.

Severity Criteria:

Mild: Usually associated with mild sleepiness or mild insomnia, as defined on page 23. Most of the habitual sleep period is free of respiratory disturbance and can be associated with mild oxygen desaturation or benign cardiac arrhythmias.

Moderate: Usually associated with moderate sleepiness or mild insomnia, as defined on page 23. Moderate oxygen desaturation or mild cardiac arrhythmias are usually present.

Severe: Usually associated with severe sleepiness, as defined on page 23. Most of the habitual sleep period is associated with respiratory disturbance, with severe oxygen desaturation or cardiac arrhythmias.

Duration Criteria:

Acute: 7 days or less.
Subacute: More than 7 days but less than 3 months.
Chronic: 3 months or longer.

Bibliography:

Bradley TD, McNicholas WT, Rutherford R, Popkin J, Zamel N, Phillipson EA. Clinical and physiologic heterogeneity of the central sleep apnea syndrome. Am Rev Respir Dis 1986; 134: 217–221.
Cherniack NS. Respiratory dysrhythmias during sleep. N Engl J Med 1981; 305: 325–330.
Guilleminault C, Eldridge FL, Dement WC. Insomnia with sleep apnea: a new syndrome. Science 1973; 181: 856–858.
Guilleminault C, Quera-Salva MA, Nino-Murcia G, Partinen M. Central sleep apnea and partial obstruction of the upper airway. Ann Neurol 1987; 21: 465–469.
Issa FG, Sullivan CE. Reversal of central sleep apnea using nasal CPAP. Chest 1986; 90: 165–171.

Central Alveolar Hypoventilation Syndrome (780.51-1)

Synonyms and Key Words: Central alveolar hypoventilation, primary alveolar hypoventilation, idiopathic alveolar hypoventilation, nonapneic alveolar hypoventilation. Central alveolar hypoventilation syndrome is the preferred term for the disorder.

Essential Features:

Central alveolar hypoventilation syndrome is characterized by ventilatory impairment, resulting in sleep-related arterial oxygen desaturation that occurs in patients with normal mechanical properties of the lung.

During sleep, patients with central alveolar hypoventilation syndrome have a decreased tidal volume, and hypercapnia and hypoxemia usually occur. The episodes of hypoventilation are associated with arousals that cause a transition to a lighter sleep stage or result in awakenings. These sleep effects may lead to insomnia or, if the arousals and awakenings are frequent enough, result in excessive sleepiness. During stage-REM sleep, hypoventilation is more pronounced, with aggravation of the hypoxemia and hypercapnia. Occasionally, patients can have severe oxygen desaturation during sleep, with few arousals and therefore, few, if any, sleep complaints. Headaches upon awakening are not infrequent and may be related to the blood-gas changes during sleep.

Cardiac arrhythmias, particularly bradytachycardia, can be associated with the respiratory disturbance. The episodes of oxygen desaturation, which are usually of longer duration than those seen in other forms of sleep-related respiratory impairments (e.g., obstructive or central sleep apnea syndrome) can be associated with the development of pulmonary hypertension and heart failure.

Alveolar hypoventilation can be caused by severe lung dysfunction and respiratory-muscle impairment. In the absence of these peripheral impairments, the chronic disorder is referred to as central alveolar hypoventilation syndrome. This syndrome has been called the obesity hypoventilation syndrome when associated with severe obesity. In nonobese patients, the syndrome can be considered to be idiopathic, and a primary disorder of respiratory control can be inferred.

Associated Features: Obstructive or central sleep apneas may occur intermittently or repetitively on the episodes of hypoventilation but do not form the predominant respiratory pattern during sleep. Pulmonary hypertension and heart failure can develop. In adults, there may be impaired psychosocial or work functioning. The clinical signs of hypoxia can be quite subtle in children, who may not look distressed. Children do not develop inspiratory retractions, nasal flaring, or other signs of increased respiratory effort in response to the hypoxia. As a result, hypoxia may progress for quite some time without notice until the child appears to deteriorate suddenly, with a cardiopulmonary arrest or severe decompensation.

Course: The course of central alveolar hypoventilation can be variable but often is slowly progressive, eventually leading to severe respiratory impairment and cardiac failure. Children who initially present with hypoventilation during both sleep and wakefulness often will be able to sustain adequate spontaneous ventilation during wakefulness later in life.

Predisposing Factors: The use of central nervous system depressants, such as alcohol, anxiolytics, and hypnotics, may further worsen or precipitate central alveolar hypoventilation during sleep. Neurologic lesions, such as infection, infarction, or demyelination, may result in the acquired form of the disorder.

Prevalence: Not known, but the idiopathic form is quite rare.

Age of Onset: Variable. The idiopathic type often presents in adolescence or early adulthood. The acquired form can develop at any age.

Sex Ratio: The idiopathic form appears to be more common in males.

Familial Patterns: None known.

Pathology: Ventilatory studies reveal reduced responsiveness to hypercapnia or hypoxia during wakefulness and sleep. Spirometric studies and other pulmonary tests usually demonstrate normal lung functioning. A lesion of the medullary chemoreceptors controlling ventilation is postulated in the idiopathic form. A central nervous system lesion affecting brain-stem function, such as poliomyelitis or brain-stem infarction, may be found in patients with the acquired form.

Complications: Severe hypoxemia and hypercapnia may result in the development of cardiac arrhythmias. Pulmonary hypertension and, eventually, heart failure and death can occur.

Polysomnographic Features: Periods of decreased tidal volume lasting up to several minutes, with sustained arterial oxygen desaturation, are usually observed. These episodes are often worse during REM sleep. Obstructive sleep apneas may also contribute to the arterial oxygen desaturation. Carbon-dioxide levels show an increase during the episodes of hypoventilation, with some improvement following the termination of the respiratory event.

Sleep may be characterized by frequent awakenings and arousals associated with body movements.

Other Laboratory Test Features: Patients with normal awake pulmonary function tests may demonstrate a marked decrease in ventilatory response to inhalation of carbon dioxide. Daytime arterial blood gases may be normal or impaired.

Brain imaging may be necessary to detect structural lesions that can account for the impaired respiratory control. No associated lesions are present in the idiopathic form of alveolar hypoventilation syndrome. Rarely, phrenic-nerve conduction tests and electromyography, or muscle biopsy of the respiratory musculature, may be indicated. Electrocardiography, chest radiography, and echocardiography may show evidence of pulmonary hypertension. Elevated hematocrit and hemoglobin levels indicate polycythemia from chronic hypoxia.

Differential Diagnosis: Patients with central alveolar hypoventilation syndrome must be distinguished from patients with peripheral neurologic, muscular, skeletal, orthopedic, or pulmonary lesions. Cardiac disease and hypothyroidism need to be considered in the differential diagnosis.

Diagnostic Criteria: Central Alveolar Hypoventilation Syndrome (780.51-1)

A. The patient can have a complaint of either insomnia or excessive sleepiness. The patient is usually unaware of the clinical features observed by others such as hypoventilation during sleep.
B. Frequent episodes of shallow breathing occur during sleep.
C. No primary lung disease, skeletal malformations, or peripheral neuromuscular disorders that affect ventilation are present.
D. Polysomnographic monitoring demonstrates:
   1. Episodes of shallow breathing greater than 10 seconds in duration associated with arterial oxygen desaturation, and one or more of the following:
      a. Frequent arousals from sleep associated with the breathing disturbances
      b. Bradytachycardia
      c. A mean sleep latency of less than 10 minutes on an MSLT
E. The disorder can be associated with neurologic disorders that affect the central nervous system's control of breathing.
F. Other sleep disorders can be present (e.g., periodic limb movement disorder, central sleep apnea syndrome, or obstructive sleep apnea syndrome).

Note: If the disorder is of unknown origin, state and code as central alveolar hypoventilation syndrome–idiopathic type. If the disorder is of known etiology (e.g., poliomyelitis), state and code as central alveolar hypoventilation syndrome on axis A and the cause on axis C.

Minimal Criteria: A plus B plus C plus D.

Severity Criteria:

Mild: Usually associated with mild sleepiness or mild insomnia, as defined on page 23. Most of the major sleep episode is free of respiratory disturbance but it can be associated with mild oxygen desaturation or mild cardiac arrhythmias.
Moderate: Usually associated with moderate sleepiness or mild insomnia, as defined on page 23. There may be moderate oxygen desaturation, cardiac arrhythmias, and evidence of pulmonary hypertension.
Severe: Usually associated with severe sleepiness, as defined on page 23. Most of the habitual sleep period is associated with respiratory disturbance, with severe oxygen desaturation or severe cardiac arrhythmias. Pulmonary hypertension with cor pulmonale is usually present.

Duration Criteria:

Acute: 6 months or less.
Subacute: More than 6 months but less than 1 year.
Chronic: 1 year or longer.

Bibliography:

Mellins RB, Balfour HH Jr, Turino GM, Winters RW. Failure of automatic control of ventilation (Ondines curse). Report of an infant born with this syndrome and review of the literature. Medicine 1970; 49: 487–504.

Plum F, Leigh RJ. Abnormalities of central mechanisms. In: Hornbein TF, ed. Regulation of breathing. Part II. Lung biology in health and disease, Volume 17. New York: Marcel Dekker, 1981; 989–1067.

Rochester DF, Enson Y. Current concepts in the pathogenesis of the obesity-hypoventilation syndrome. Mechanical and circulatory factors. Am J Med 1974; 57: 402–420.

Sullivan CE, Issa FG, Berthon-Jones M, Saunders NA. Pathophysiology of sleep apnea. In: Saunders NA, Sullivan CE, eds. Sleep and breathing. Lung biology in health and disease. New York: Marcel Dekker, 1984; 21: 299–364.

Periodic Limb Movement Disorder (780.52-4)

Synonyms and Key Words: Periodic leg movements (PLMs), nocturnal myoclonus, periodic movements in sleep (PMS), leg jerks. The term periodic limb movement disorder is preferred because the movements can occur in the upper limbs.

Essential Features:

Periodic limb movement disorder is characterized by periodic episodes of repetitive and highly stereotyped limb movements that occur during sleep.

The movements usually occur in the legs and consist of extension of the big toe in combination with partial flexion of the ankle, knee, and sometimes hip. Similar movements can occur in the upper limbs. The movements are often associated with a partial arousal or awakening; however, the patient is usually unaware of the limb movements or the frequent sleep disruption. Between the episodes, the legs are still. There can be marked nightly variability in the number of movements.

There may be a history of frequent nocturnal awakenings and unrefreshing sleep. Patients who are unaware of the sleep interruptions may have symptoms of excessive sleepiness. It is probable that the nature of the patient's complaint is affected by the frequency of the movement as well as the associated awakenings.

The clinical significance of the movements needs to be decided on an individual basis. Periodic limb movements may be an incidental finding, and medication that reduces the number of limb movements can produce little or no change in sleep duration or sleep efficiency.

It is possible that a centrally mediated event can give rise to both the periodic movements and the related sleep disturbance. It is necessary to integrate the clinical history and the polysomnographic findings to assess the role of this phenomenon in a sleep disorder.

Associated Features: The disorder can produce anxiety and depression related to the chronicity of the sleep disturbance.

Course: The natural history is not known. Periodic limb movement disorder appears to increase in prevalence with advancing age.

Predisposing Factors: Individuals with restless legs syndrome usually have periodic leg movements detected during polysomnographic monitoring. Periodic limb movements can accompany narcolepsy and the obstructive sleep apnea syndrome.

Periodic limb movement disorder can be associated with, or evoked by, a variety of medical conditions. Episodes of limb movements can develop in patients with chronic uremia and other metabolic disorders. The use of tricyclic antidepressants and monoamine oxidase inhibitors can induce or aggravate this disorder, as does withdrawal from a variety of drugs, such as anticonvulsants, benzodiazepines, barbiturates, and other hypnotic agents. Limb movements associated with ingestion or withdrawal from drugs should be distinguished from the disorder in the drug-free patient.

Prevalence: Not known. It appears to be rare in children and progresses with advancing age to become a common finding in up to 34% of patients over the age of 60 years. It has been reported to occur in 1% to 15% of patients with insomnia.

Age of Onset: Appears to be most prevalent in middle adulthood and is rarely seen in children.

Sex Ratio: No difference.

Familial Pattern: A familial pattern may exist.

Pathology: None known.

Complications: Periodic limb movement disorder can result in fragmented, restless sleep and complaints of insomnia or excessive sleepiness. The limb movements can disrupt the sleep of a bedpartner. Some patients with severe periodic limb movement disorder can also have the movements during wakefulness.

Polysomnographic Features: Periodic limb movements can appear immediately with the onset of non-REM stage-1 sleep, are frequent during stage 2 sleep, and decrease in frequency in stage 3 and stage 4 sleep. The periodic limb movements are usually absent during REM sleep.

Typically, both lower limbs are monitored for the presence of the limb movements; however, movement of the upper limbs may be sampled if clinically indicated. The anterior tibialis electromyogram (EMG) shows repetitive contractions, each lasting 0.5 to 5 seconds (mean duration, 1.5 to 2.5 seconds). The movement may begin with a leg jerk, followed by a short interval (milliseconds) and a tonic contraction. There may often be repeated myoclonic jerks occurring at the beginning of each movement. The movements may affect one or both of the lower limbs, although usually both extremities are involved, but not necessarily in a symmetric or simultaneous pattern. The events may show some alternations from leg to leg. The interval between movements is typically 20 to 40 seconds; movements that are separated by an interval of less than 5 or more than 90 seconds are not counted when determining the total number of movements or movement indexes. Four or more consecutive movements are required for minimal analysis. Contractions occurring during drowsiness, before the onset of stage 1 sleep, are not counted as part of the sleep disorder.

The periodic leg movements may be associated with a K-complex with an electroencephalographic arousal or an awakening. An increase in heart rate and blood pressure can accompany the movements. Periodic limb movements can occur in discrete episodes that last from a few minutes to several hours or may be present throughout the entire recording.

The movements are often reported as an index of total sleep time called the periodic limb movement index (PLM index). The PLM index is the number of movements per hour of total sleep time, as determined by polysomnography of the major sleep episode; an index of 5 or more is regarded as abnormal. Only movements occurring during sleep are counted for the index. The numbers of movements that occur in each leg are added together, as long as they occur in episodes of at least four movements; isolated movements are not counted. Simultaneous movements in both legs are counted as one movement. The periodic limb movement–arousal index (PLM–arousal index) is the number of periodic limb movements associated with an arousal, expressed per hour of total sleep time.

Differential Diagnosis: Sleep starts may need to be differentiated from periodic limb movements; the appearance of sleep starts during drowsiness, prior to sleep onset, is the main distinguishing feature. Sleep starts do not recur during sleep stages nor do they occur with a regular periodicity. Leg movements seen in association with disorders that produce frequent sleep fragmentations, such as sleep apnea, may resemble periodic limb movements but disappear upon treatment of the primary condition. A patient may have both disorders, however.

Periodic limb movement disorder must be differentiated from movements associated with nocturnal epileptic seizures and myoclonic epilepsy and from a number of forms of waking myoclonus, such as that seen in the Lance-Adams syndrome (and tension myoclonus), Alzheimer's disease, Creutzfeldt-Jakob disease, and other neuropathologic conditions.

Diagnostic Criteria: Periodic Limb Movement Disorder (780.52-4)

A. The patient has a complaint of insomnia or excessive sleepiness. The patient occasionally will be asymptomatic, and the movements are noticed by an observer.
B. Repetitive highly stereotyped limb muscle movements are present; in the leg, these movements are characterized by extension of the big toe in combination with partial flexion of the ankle, knee, and sometimes hip.
C. Polysomnographic monitoring demonstrates:
   1. Repetitive episodes of muscle contraction (0.5 to 5 seconds in duration) separated by an interval of typically 20 to 40 seconds
   2. Arousal or awakenings may be associated with the movements
D. The patient has no evidence of a medical or mental disorder that can account for the primary complaint.

E. Other sleep disorders (e.g., obstructive sleep apnea syndrome) may be present but do not account for the movements.

Note: If periodic limb movement disorder is due to a medication effect or due to drug withdrawal, state and code on axis A as periodic limb movement disorder: medication-induced type or periodic limb movement disorder: drug-withdrawal type, respectively. If associated with an underlying medical disorder, the disorder should be stated and coded on axis C (e.g., uremia).

Minimal Criteria: A plus B.

Severity Criteria:

Mild: Mild insomnia or mild sleepiness, as defined on page 23, and typically associated with a PLM index of 5 or more but less than 25.
Moderate: Moderate insomnia or moderate sleepiness, as defined on page 23, and typically associated with a PLM index of 25 or more but less than 50.
Severe: Severe insomnia or severe sleepiness, as defined on page 23, and typically associated with a PLM index of 50 or more or a PLM–arousal index of greater than 25.

Duration Criteria:

Acute: 1 month or less.
Subacute: More than 1 month but less than 6 months.
Chronic: 6 months or longer.

Bibliography:

Coleman RM. Periodic movements in sleep (nocturnal myoclonus) and restless legs syndrome. In: Guilleminault C, ed. Sleeping and waking disorders: Indications and techniques. Menlo Park, California: Addison-Wesley, 1982; 265–295.

Lugaresi E, Cirignotta F, Coccagna G, Montagna P. Nocturnal myoclonus and restless legs syndrome. Advances in neurology. In: Fahn S et al., eds. Myoclonus. New York: Raven Press, 1986; 295–306.

Lugaresi E, Coccagna G, Berti-Ceroni G, Ambrosetto C. Restless legs syndrome and nocturnal myoclonus. In: Gastaut H, Lugaresi E, Berti-Ceroni G, Coccagna G, eds. The abnormalities of sleep in man; proceedings of the 15th European meeting on electroencephalography. Bologna: Auto Gaggi Editore, 1968; 285–294.

Restless Legs Syndrome (780.52-5)

Synonyms and Key Words: Restless legs syndrome (RLS), disagreeable sensations in legs.

Essential Features:

Restless legs syndrome is a disorder characterized by disagreeable leg sensations that usually occur prior to sleep onset and that cause an almost irresistible urge to move the legs.

The most characteristic feature is the partial or complete relief of the sensation with leg motion and the return of the symptoms upon cessation of leg movements. The sensations and associated leg movements usually interfere with sleep onset. A variety of words may be used to describe the sensations, usually including "ache," "discomfort," "creeping," "crawling," "pulling," "prickling," "tingling," or "itching."

The patient usually feels the sensations between the ankle and the knee but may experience the sensations in the thighs or feet and, rarely, in the arms. Although usually bilateral, the symptoms can be asymmetric in severity and frequency and rarely occur unilaterally. They typically are present only at rest and just prior to the patient's sleep period; they can occur at other times of the day, however, particularly when the patient sits for prolonged periods (e.g., when driving). The symptoms may last for a few minutes or several hours; however, even the most severely affected patients will usually be able to sleep for several hours.

Associated Features: The disorder can be associated with pregnancy, anemia, and uremia. When associated with pregnancy, restless legs syndrome usually appears after the 20th week of the pregnancy.

Most, if not all, patients with restless legs syndrome show periodic leg movements during sleep. Unlike patients with only periodic limb movements, patients with both syndromes may show involuntary limb movements even while awake.

Patients may experience features of intense anxiety and depression in association with restless legs syndrome. In some patients, the emotional distress may be severe and associated with psychosocial dysfunction.

Course: Restless legs syndrome may be of many years' duration, with waxing and waning of symptoms. Restless legs syndrome may improve during times of fever and may worsen with sleep disruption. Severe cases may improve with time.

Predisposing Factors: Predisposing factors include pregnancy, anemia, and rheumatoid arthritis.

Prevalence: Definitive data are not available. Symptoms of restless legs syndrome have been identified in 5% to 15% of normal subjects, 11% of pregnant women, 15% to 20% of uremic patients, and up to 30% of patients with rheumatoid arthritis.

Age of Onset: Restless legs syndrome has rarely been reported to begin in infancy and may be seen for the first time in advanced old age. The peak onset is usually in middle age.

Sex Ratio: Appears to be more common in females.

Familial Pattern: Restless legs syndrome is most often seen as an isolated case, but a definitive familial pattern has been reported. An autosomal dominant transmission in some families has been proposed but is not yet established.

Pathology: None known.

Complications: Severe insomnia, psychologic disturbance, and depression, sometimes producing severe social dysfunction.

Differential Diagnosis: Chronic myelopathy, peripheral neuropathy, akathisia, painful legs and moving toes syndrome should be ruled out by history and clinical examination. Erythromelalgia, muscular pain fasciculation syndromes, myokymia, and leg compartment syndromes may all have some similarities to restless legs syndrome. Caffeinism, uremia, and anemia should also be considered as causes of leg discomfort.

Diagnostic Criteria: Restless Legs Syndrome (780.52-5)

A. The patient has a complaint of an unpleasant sensation in the legs at night or difficulty in initiating sleep.
B. Disagreeable sensations of "creeping" inside the calves are present and are often associated with general aches and pains in the legs.
C. The discomfort is relieved by movement of the limbs.
D. Polysomnographic monitoring demonstrates limb movements at sleep onset.
E. There is no evidence of any medical or mental disorders that account for the movements.
F. Other sleep disorders may be present but do not account for the symptom.

Minimal Criteria: A plus B plus C.

Severity Criteria:

Mild: Occurs episodically, with no more than a mild disruption of sleep onset that does not cause the patient significant distress.
Moderate: Occurs less than twice a week, with significant delay of sleep onset, moderate disruption of sleep, and mild impairment of daytime function.
Severe: Episodes occur three or more times a week, with severe disruption of nighttime sleep patterns and marked daytime symptoms.

Duration Criteria:

Acute: 2 weeks or less.
Subacute: More than 2 weeks but less than 3 months.
Chronic: 3 months or longer.

Bibliography:

Ekbom KA. Restless legs syndrome. Neurology 1960; 10: 868–873.
Lugaresi E, Cirignotta F, Coccagna G, Montagna P. Nocturnal myoclonus and restless legs syndrome. Adv Neurol 1986; 43: 295–307.

DYSSOMNIAS

EXTRINSIC SLEEP DISORDERS

1. Inadequate Sleep Hygiene (307.41-1) 73
2. Environmental Sleep Disorder (780.52-6) 77
3. Altitude Insomnia (289.0) 80
4. Adjustment Sleep Disorder (307.41-0) 83
5. Insufficient Sleep Syndrome (307.49-4) 87
6. Limit-Setting Sleep Disorder (307.42-4) 90
7. Sleep-Onset Association Disorder (307.42-5) 94
8. Food Allergy Insomnia (780.52-2) 98
9. Nocturnal Eating (Drinking) Syndrome (780.52-8) 100
10. Hypnotic-Dependent Sleep Disorder (780.52-0) 104
11. Stimulant-Dependent Sleep Disorder (780.52-1) 107
12. Alcohol-Dependent Sleep Disorder (780.52-3) 111
13. Toxin-Induced Sleep Disorder (780.54-6) 114
14. Extrinsic Sleep Disorder NOS (780.52-9)

Extrinsic Sleep Disorders

The extrinsic sleep disorders include those disorders that originate or develop from causes outside of the body. External factors are integral in producing these sleep disorders, and removal of the external factors leads to resolution of the sleep disorder. This is not to say that internal factors are not important in the development or maintenance of the sleep disorder, just as external factors can be important in the development or maintenance of an intrinsic sleep disorder. However, the internal factors would not, by themselves, have produced the sleep disorder without presence of an external factor.

Many of the extrinsic sleep disorders listed here were not previously described in the *Diagnostic Classification of Sleep and Arousal Disorders.* Although there appears to be overlap between some disorders (e.g., alcohol-dependent sleep disorder, environmental sleep disorder, and inadequate sleep hygiene), the text and diagnostic criteria highlight the differences. Further explanation may also be helpful.

Inadequate sleep hygiene applies to a sleep disorder that develops out of normal behavioral practices that for another person usually would not cause a sleep disturbance. For example, an irregular bedtime or waketime that might not be important in one person may be instrumental in producing insomnia in another. Although environmental factors can produce a disorder of inadequate sleep hygiene, the diagnosis of an environmental sleep disorder is only made when the environmental factors are particularly abnormal (e.g., excessive noise or extreme lighting effects that would produce sleep disturbance in most people). Caffeine ingestion in the form of coffee or sodas can produce a disorder of inadequate sleep hygiene if the intake is normal and within the limits of common use, whereas stimulant ingestion that is considered excessive by normal standards can lead to a diagnosis of a stimulant-dependent sleep disorder. Similarly, sleep that is disrupted by alcohol ingestion that would be considered socially normal can lead to a diagnosis of inadequate sleep hygiene, whereas sleep that is disrupted by alcohol ingestion that is considered by most people to be abnormal can lead to a diagnosis of alcohol-dependent sleep disorder.

Altitude insomnia is a sleep disturbance that is due to acute mountain sickness. The term acute mountain sickness is not used because it can apply to physiologic disturbances that may be unrelated to an effect upon sleep. Additional information to help differentiate the extrinsic sleep disorders is contained within the texts.

Inadequate Sleep Hygiene (307.41-1)

Synonyms and Key Words: Sleep hygiene abuse, bad sleep habits, irregular sleep habits, excessive napping, sleep-incompatible behaviors. Inadequate sleep hygiene is the preferred diagnostic term because it suggests various habits and activities of daily living that may promote a sleep difficulty.

Essential Features:

Inadequate sleep hygiene is a sleep disorder due to the performance of daily living activities that are inconsistent with the maintenance of good-quality sleep and full daytime alertness.

A common element in the diverse presentations that make up this condition is the deleterious effect on sleep of practices that are under the individual's behavioral control. Although an exhaustive list of these practices is not feasible, the specific behaviors can be classified into two general categories: practices that produce increased arousal and practices that are inconsistent with the principles of sleep organization.

Arousal may be produced by commonly used substances such as caffeine and cigarettes. Alcohol ingestion may also interfere with sleep by producing arousal during the sleep period, which results in sleep-maintenance difficulties. Stress and excitement, such as vigorous exercise close to bedtime, intense mental work late at night, party-going in the evening, and watching the clock during an awakening in the middle of the night, may also lead to arousal. Arousal due to environmental factors may result from the neglect of caretaking activities, such as not regulating ambient temperature within a comfortable range, allowing nocturnal prodding by pets, and failing to prevent early morning light in the bedroom.

Due to the complementarity and interdependence of sleep and waking, practices that interfere with the regular timing and duration of the sleep and wakeful periods may disturb the stability and amounts of the two processes. Sleep may become disrupted or variable when too much time is spent in bed; when there is excessive daily variation in bedtime, arising time, and amount of sleep; and when naps are taken during the day. Although clinicians usually have no trouble identifying grossly excessive time in bed and nightly variability of retiring and arising times, the influence of more subtle changes may go undetected. For example, just as the daily quota of sleep varies in noncomplaining individuals, so too does time in bed. Therefore, 7.5 hours in bed may be sufficient for individuals who sleep 7 hours per night and excessive for those who habitually sleep 6 hours. Because a single regular daytime nap does not necessarily interfere with nocturnal sleep, judgment is required to determine if the frequency, duration, proximity to nocturnal sleep, or variable timing of naps suggests an impact on sleep.

Associated Features: Inadequate sleep hygiene shares daytime symptoms (e.g., mood and motivational disturbance; reduced attention, vigilance, and concentration; and daytime fatigue and sleepiness) with the other conditions that produce sleep disturbance. Preoccupation with the sleep difficulty is also common.

Course: Inadequate sleep hygiene practices may produce and perpetuate insomnia. When sufficiently strong or habitual, these inadequate sleep hygiene practices may precipitate insomnia. For example, consuming excessive amounts of caffeine or taking naps at different times of the day becomes part of the behavioral repertoire over time. Although adaptation to these changes is possible at first, with time and increasing intensity of these practices, they begin to have an effect on sleep.

The importance of assessing the contribution of inadequate sleep hygiene in maintaining a preexisting sleep disturbance cannot be overemphasized. Once insomnia is present, individuals attempt to cope by taking such actions as going to sleep earlier, staying in bed later, napping, lying down to rest during the day, and drinking coffee. These strategies are attempts to obtain more sleep or minimize the fatigue, performance decrements, and sleepiness that result from insomnia. Although these alterations may lead to increased sleep and reduced daytime decrements, they also lead to increased variability of the timing of sleep and weaken the self-sustaining properties of a regular sleep-wake cycle. Therefore, sleep hygiene should be evaluated in the context of every insomnia to determine how much of a contribution it is making to sustaining the sleep disturbance.

Predisposing Factors: Individuals who are intolerant of any debilitating daytime consequences of sleep loss will resort more quickly to practices that defy good sleep hygiene principles. For example, those people who accept the sleep loss and compromised performance and mood that result from a night or two of poor sleep can ride out the sleep disturbance without restructuring their sleep schedule, taking naps, or increasing daytime caffeine or nighttime alcohol consumption. On the other hand, those individuals who are so distressed by fatigue, sleepiness, moodiness, and reduced performance that they will not put up with a period of incapacity due to sleep loss will institute countermeasures designed to limit these problems. Although these measures may, in the short run, increase alertness and buoy mood, they contribute toward instability of sleep and waking, thus establishing features that contribute to insomnia.

Prevalence: The prevalence of this disorder in the general population is not known, although it is believed to be a fairly common primary cause or contributing factor of sleep disturbance. It is the rare case of insomnia that does not necessitate some attention to shaping the sleep schedule or prescribing certain arousing practices. Inadequate sleep hygiene may not reach sufficient salience to independently produce insomnia; however, these practices may produce nightly variability, lower the threshold to arousal, and have other effects that render the individual more susceptible to developing insomnia as a result of some other factor. In many cases, it is a confluence of factors that produce a clinically significant insomnia. For example, a habitual sleep-wake schedule and level of coffee consumption in and of themselves may have caused no sleep problem, but the addition of other factors to these preexisting conditions could produce an insomnia. At this stage, each factor may be understood as making an independent contribution to the sleep disturbance.

Age of Onset: Inadequate sleep hygiene is not diagnosed in prepubescent individuals because some independence from caretakers and responsibility for one's own sleep pattern is assumed in the diagnosis.

Sex Ratio: Not known.

Familial Pattern: Not known.

Pathology: Mental status examination and psychologic testing reveal little or no psychopathology. Physical examination uncovers no medical explanation for the sleep disturbance.

Complications: Caffeine addiction, alcoholism, and conditioned insomnia are all complications of inadequate sleep hygiene. In addition, chronic sleep loss and frequent or irregular timing of daytime naps may produce excessive sleepiness and the need for daytime naps.

Polysomnographic Features: The usual polysomnographic features associated with sleep disturbance, such as prolonged sleep latency, fragmented sleep, early morning awakening, and reduced sleep efficiency, are present.

Recording in the sleep laboratory environment may correct some inadequate sleep hygiene practices; therefore, there may be some attenuation of the severity of the problem.

Other Laboratory Test Features: None.

Differential Diagnosis: Psychophysiologic insomnia, environmental sleep disorder, mental disorders, hypnotic-dependent sleep disorder, alcohol-dependent sleep disorder, central sleep apnea syndrome, short sleeper, delayed sleep-phase syndrome, irregular sleep-wake pattern, restless legs syndrome, periodic limb movement disorder, limit-setting sleep disorder, and sleep-onset association disorder.

Diagnostic Criteria: Inadequate Sleep Hygiene (307.41-1)

A. The patient has a complaint of either insomnia or excessive sleepiness.
B. At least one of the following is present
   1. Daytime napping at least two times each week
   2. Variable wake-up times or bedtimes
   3. Frequent periods (two to three times per week) of extended amounts of time spent in bed
   4. Routine use of products containing alcohol, tobacco, or caffeine in the period preceding bedtime
   5. Scheduling exercise too close to bedtime
   6. Engaging in exciting or emotionally upsetting activities too close to bedtime
   7. Frequent use of the bed for non-sleep-related activities (e.g., television watching, reading, studying, snacking, etc.)
   8. Sleeping on an uncomfortable bed (poor mattress, inadequate blankets, etc.)
   9. Allowing the bedroom to be too bright, too stuffy, too cluttered, too hot, too cold, or in some way not conducive to sleep
   10. Performing activities demanding high levels of concentration shortly before bed
   11. Allowing mental activities, such as thinking, planning, reminiscing, etc., to occur in bed
C. Polysomnography demonstrates one or more of the following:
   1. Increased sleep latency
   2. Reduced sleep efficiency
   3. Frequent arousals
   4. Early morning awakening
   5. Excessive sleepiness on a multiple sleep latency test
D. No evidence of a medical or mental disorder accounts for the sleep disturbance.
E. No other sleep disorder either produces difficulty in initiating or maintaining sleep or causes excessive sleepiness.

Minimal Criteria: A plus B.

Severity Criteria:

Mild: Mild insomnia or mild sleepiness, as defined on page 23.
Moderate: Moderate insomnia or moderate sleepiness, as defined on page 23.
Severe: Severe insomnia or severe sleepiness, as defined on page 23.

Duration Criteria:

Acute: 7 days or less.
Subacute: More than 7 days but less than 3 months.
Chronic: 3 months or longer.

Bibliography:

Bootzin RR, Nicassio PM. Behavioral treatments for insomnia. In: Hersen M, Eisler RM, Miller PM, eds. Progress in behavior modification, Volume 6. New York: Academic Press, 1978; 1–45.
Spielman AJ. Assessment of insomnia. Clin Psychol Rev 1986; 6: 11–25.
Spielman AJ, Saskin P, Thorpy MJ. Treatment of chronic insomnia by restriction of time in bed. Sleep 1987; 10(1): 45–56.

Environmental Sleep Disorder (780.52-6)

Synonyms and Key Words: Environmental insomnia, environment-induced somnolence, environment-induced sleep disorder, noise-induced sleep disturbance, temperature-induced sleep disturbance, bedpartner-related sleep disorder, hospital-induced sleep disorder, sleep disorder associated with forced vigilance. Environmental sleep disorder is the preferred term because it may connote either an insomnia or excessive sleepiness that may arise from a variety of environmental factors.

Essential Features:

Environmental sleep disorder is a sleep disturbance due to a disturbing environmental factor that causes a complaint of either insomnia or excessive sleepiness.

This category covers those environmental conditions that invariably result in a disorder of either insomnia or excessive sleepiness. The onset, time course, and termination of the sleep complaint are tied directly to a causative environmental condition. Amelioration or removal of the environmental condition brings about either an immediate or gradual reduction of the sleep problem.

A variety of physically measurable environmental factors can result in insomnia or excessive sleepiness. Sleep-disturbing circumstances include heat, cold, noise, light, movements of a bedpartner, and the necessity of remaining alert in a situation of danger or when having to provide attention to an infant or invalid. A variety of medical procedures and an imposed abnormal sleep-wake schedule often associated with hospitalization also may result in a sleep disorder. The sensitivity of the patient to such environmental circumstances is often more critical than is the level of noxious stimulation. Sensitivity to environmental disturbances in nocturnal sleepers increases toward morning. Older individuals are generally more sensitive to environmental factors than are younger ones, although substantial variability in sensitivity may be noted within a particular age group.

Three conditions must be present to make a diagnosis of environmental sleep disorder: (1) the sleep problem is temporally associated with the introduction of a physically measurable stimulus or definable set of environmental circumstances, (2) the physical rather than the psychologic properties of the environmental factors are the critical causative elements, and (3) removal of the responsible factors results in an immediate or gradual return to normal sleep and wakefulness.

Mental status examination and psychologic evaluation reveal no psychiatric explanation for the sleep complaint. Physical examination reveals no underlying medical cause.

Associated Features: Depending upon the chronicity and extent of sleep disturbance resulting from the environmental cause, secondary symptoms (including deficits in concentration, attention, and cognitive performance; reduced vigilance; daytime fatigue; malaise; depressed mood; and irritability) may result. Also, certain environmental factors that have been shown to reduce slow-wave sleep (e.g., noise, high ambient temperatures, bedpartner movements) may result in muscle aches, social withdrawal, and somatic preoccupation.

Course: In the early stages of insomnia resulting from environmental factors, mild mood disturbance, daytime fatigue, concentration problems, irritability, and preoccupation with sleep loss may develop. If the insomnia is untreated, symptoms typical of chronic sleep deprivation, including depressed mood, reduced work performance, malaise, chronic daytime sleepiness, and lethargy, result. In patients presenting primarily with excessive sleepiness, more prominent features may be depressed mood, daytime fatigue, and a compelling sense of sleepiness. In either case, the patient may develop disruptive habits that further contribute to the sleep problem.

Predisposing Factors: Residence near a busy airport or highway, a sleeping environment that is poorly heated in cold seasons of the year or inadequately air-conditioned in warm months, subjection to a physically dangerous environment, a bedpartner who snores or is restless, and responsibility for a newborn infant are all predisposing factors for environmental sleep disorder with insomnia. Routine and monotonous vocations, social isolation, and physical confinement are predisposing factors for environmental sleep disorder with excessive sleepiness. Hospitalization that results in imposed abnormal sleep-wake schedules or discomfort from drainage tubes, hemodialysis, etc., may contribute to environmental sleep disorder.

Prevalence: Although the prevalence of environmental sleep disorder is not known, transient sleep disturbances of this nature are likely to be very common. The percentage of the general population with chronic environment-induced sleep disorders has not been determined. Somewhat less than 5% of patients seen at sleep disorders centers receive this diagnosis.

Age of Onset: May occur at any age, although the elderly are more at risk for this condition.

Sex Ratio: Not known.

Familial Pattern: None known.

Pathology: None.

Complications: See associated features above.

Polysomnographic Features: Laboratory polysomnography, particularly in those patients with an insomnia complaint, should reveal a total sleep time that is longer than is reported as typical for the home environment. Sleep architecture is similar to that of the normal sleeper.

Ambulatory polysomnography that allows the patient to sleep in the usual sleeping environment is likely to reveal a reduced total sleep time, such as that seen in the laboratory, as well as reduced slow-wave sleep, lowered sleep efficiency, and, depending upon the nature of the environmental disturbance, a reduction in REM sleep percentage.

Patients with environment-induced excessive sleepiness show mild to moderate sleepiness during a scheduled series of polysomnographically monitored daytime naps (multiple sleep latency test).

Polysomnography reveals no evidence of other sleep disorders such as periodic limb movement disorder or sleep-related breathing disorder.

Other Laboratory Test Features: Twenty-four-hour temperature recordings reveal no circadian rhythm disturbance. Other laboratory tests, such as blood tests, urinalysis, etc., suggest no medical basis for the sleep disorder.

Differential Diagnosis: Inadequate sleep hygiene, insufficient sleep syndrome, psychophysiologic insomnia, psychiatric sleep disorders, irregular sleep-wake pattern, obstructive sleep apnea syndrome, central sleep apnea syndrome, narcolepsy, idiopathic hypersomnia, delayed sleep-phase syndrome.

Diagnostic Criteria: Environmental Sleep Disorder (780.52-6)

A. The patient complains of insomnia or excessive sleepiness.
B. The complaint is temporally associated with the introduction of a physically measurable stimulus or environmental circumstance that disturbs sleep.
C. The physical properties of the environmental factor account for the sleep complaint; the psychologic meaning of the environmental factor does not account for the complaint.
D. Removal of the causative environmental factor results in an immediate or gradual restoration of normal sleep.
E. The disorder has been present for more than 3 weeks.
F. Polysomnographic monitoring demonstrates normal sleep efficiency and duration.
G. No evidence of significant underlying mental or medical disorder accounts for the complaint.
H. The patient's symptoms do not meet the diagnostic criteria for any other sleep disorder causing a complaint of insomnia or excessive sleepiness (e.g., toxin-induced sleep disorder).

Note: If the disorder has been present for less than 3 weeks, specify and code under adjustment sleep disorder.

Minimal Criteria: A plus B plus C plus D plus E.

Severity Criteria:

Mild: Mild insomnia or mild sleepiness, as defined on page 23.
Moderate: Moderate insomnia or moderate sleepiness, as defined on page 23.
Severe: Severe insomnia or severe sleepiness, as defined on page 23.

Duration Criteria:

Acute: 3 months or less.
Subacute: More than 3 months but less than 6 months.
Chronic: 6 months or longer.

Bibliography:

Cantrell RW. Prolonged exposure to intermittent noise: audiometric, biochemical, motor, psychological and sleep effects. Laryngoscope 1974; 84: 1–55.
Coleman RM, Roffwarg HP, Kennedy SJ, et al. Sleep-wake disorders based on polysomnographic diagnosis. A national cooperative study. JAMA 1982; 247: 997–1003.
Haskell EH, Palca JW, Walker JM, Berger RJ, Heller HC. The effects of high and low ambient temperatures on human sleep stages. Electroencephalogr Clin Neurophysiol 1981; 51: 494–501.
Roth T, Kramer M, Trinder J. The effect of noise during sleep on the sleep patterns of different age groups. Can Psychiatr Assoc J 1972; 17: SS197–SS201.
Thiessen GJ, Lapointe AC. Effect of continuous traffic noise on percentage of deep sleep, waking, and sleep latency. J Acoust Soc Am 1983; 73: 225–229.

Altitude Insomnia (289.0)

Synonyms and Key Words: Acute mountain sickness (289.0), Acosta's disease. (Includes Andes disease [993.2], Alpine sickness [993.2], hypobaropathy [993.2])

Essential Features:

***Altitude insomnia** is an acute insomnia, usually accompanied by headaches, loss of appetite, and fatigue, that occurs following ascent to high altitudes.*

This is a common complaint of mountain climbers or other individuals who sleep in high-altitude environments. Symptoms typically occur within 72 hours of exposure. A disturbance of respiration that appears to be directly related to lack of inspired oxygen is associated with the difficulty in initiating and maintaining sleep. Patients may awaken and be aware of the fact that they are apneic.

The disturbance to sleep usually develops when sleeping at elevations greater than 4,000 meters. Medications such as acetazolamide, which can increase ventilation and reduce hypoxemia during sleep, have been reported to improve sleep quality. However, administration of oxygen, which can abolish periodic breathing during sleep, does not necessarily improve the sleep symptoms. Not only hypoxemia, but also the effects of the hypocapnia, may therefore cause altitude insomnia.

In addition to the direct effects of respiratory disturbances during sleep, other internal or environmental factors, such as stress and increased vigilance, the cold, an uncomfortable sleeping surface, and varied exposure to light, may also play a part in the development of insomnia related to altitude in mountaineers.

Associated Features: Altitude insomnia can be associated with other symptoms of acute mountain sickness such as headache, anorexia, tachycardia, and fatigue.

Course: Mountain sickness and altitude insomnia become progressively more severe as higher altitudes are reached. Pulmonary edema, coma, and even death may rarely occur at high altitudes. The disorder may improve spontaneously with increasing duration spent at high altitudes due to acclimatization to the lower levels of inspired oxygen. When the person returns to lower altitudes, the sleep disturbance usually reverses spontaneously.

Predisposing Factors: Primary lung disease, as well as anemia or impaired cardiac function, is thought to predispose an individual to developing altitude insomnia.

Prevalence: Altitude insomnia occurs in most individuals who ascend to high altitudes (greater than 4,000 meters) in the absence of administered oxygen. Twenty-five percent of individuals who ascend from sea level to 2,000 meters will have some symptoms.

Age of Onset: Altitude insomnia can occur in an individual of any age.

Sex Ratio: No evidence of any sex predominance.

Familial Pattern: None known.

Pathology: Physiologic control of respiration in the presence of low inspired oxygen leads to a pattern of periodic breathing. This breathing pattern can induce arousals during sleep that are associated with the hyperpneic phase of ventilation.

The changes in body chemistry are believed to be due to hypoxia, which stimulates respiration and leads to a hypocapnic alkalosis. Over a few days, renal compensation leads to increased urinary bicarbonate excretion and the gradual correction of the alkalosis.

Complications: For reasons that are unclear, some individuals may develop pulmonary edema even at low altitudes. Cerebral edema and death can sometimes occur. Changes in protein permeability of the lung may lead to edema as a result of an idiosyncratic reaction or as a manifestation of central nervous system effects (neurogenic edema).

82 EXTRINSIC SLEEP DISORDERS

Polysomnographic Features: At levels above 2,000 meters but below 4,000 meters, the predominant change in sleep is a slight reduction in sleep efficiency; awake activity during sleep may increase and total sleep time may decrease. At altitudes higher than 4,000 meters, sleep is markedly disturbed, with reduced duration and efficiency of sleep, a prolonged sleep-onset latency, and increased movement during sleep. The amount of REM sleep is also reduced.

A pattern of periodic breathing with central apneic episodes occurs. The arousals may be associated with the hyperventilatory portion of the periodic breathing. The usual pattern is one of alternating hyperpnea and hypopnea, the latter often associated with brief nonobstructive apneas. Arousals or awakenings may occur at the end of apneic episodes. The cycles are associated with periodic fluctuations of oxygen-saturation values.

Reports of multiple sleep latency testing performed at high altitude have not been published.

Other Laboratory Test Features: Arterial blood gases measured during the awake or sleep state will show a reduction in both oxygen and carbon dioxide levels and a respiratory alkalosis with varying degrees of metabolic compensation.

Differential Diagnosis: The association of the sleep disturbance with a change in altitude helps differentiate this form of insomnia from other causes. Patients with obstructive sleep apnea syndrome or central sleep apnea syndrome may have their disorders exacerbated by the reduced arterial-oxygen tension at high altitude. Other causes of difficulty in initiating and maintaining sleep, such as an environmental sleep disorder due to factors other than altitude, insomnia associated with psychiatric disorders, and psychophysiologic insomnia, may need to be differentiated from altitude insomnia, particularly in individuals living at high altitude for prolonged periods.

Diagnostic Criteria: Altitude Insomnia (289.0)

A. The patient has a complaint of insomnia.
B. The complaint is related temporally to ascent to a high altitude (typically above 4,000 meters).
C. Polysomnographic monitoring demonstrates:
   1. Reduced total sleep duration, decreased sleep efficiency with an increased sleep latency, and increased arousals and awake time
   2. A pattern of periodic breathing during sleep
   3. Oxygen desaturation during sleep
D. Other mental or medical disorders can be present but are not the cause of the primary complaint.
E. The complaint is not caused by other sleep disorders such as obstructive sleep apnea syndrome, central sleep apnea syndrome, or other causes of insomnia.

Minimal Criteria: A plus B.

Severity Criteria:

Mild: Usually associated with mild insomnia, as defined on page 23.
Moderate: Usually associated with moderate insomnia, as defined on page 23.
Severe: Usually associated with severe insomnia, as defined on page 23.

Duration Criteria:

Acute: 7 days or less.
Subacute: More than 7 days but less than 1 month.
Chronic: 1 month or longer.

Bibliography:

Miller JC, Horvath SM. Sleep at altitude. Aviat Space Environ Med 1977; 48: 615-620.
Montgomery AB, Mills J, Luce JM. Incidence of acute mountain sickness at intermediate altitude. JAMA 1989; 261: 732–734.
Nicholson AN, Smith PA, Stone BM, Bradwell AR, Coote JH. Altitude insomnia: Studies during an expedition to the Himalayas. Sleep 1988; 11(4): 354–361.
Reite M, Jackson D, Cahoon RL, Weil JV. Sleep physiology at high altitude. Electroencephalogr Clin Neurophysiol 1975; 38: 463–471.
Weil JV. Sleep at high altitude. In: Kryger MH, Roth T, Dement WC, eds. Principles and practice of sleep medicine. Philadelphia: WB Saunders, 1989; 269–275.
Weil JV, Kryger MH, Scoggin CH. Sleep and breathing at high altitude. In: Guilleminault C, Dement WC, eds. Sleep apnea syndromes. New York: Alan R. Liss, 1978; 119–136.

Adjustment Sleep Disorder (307.41-0)

Synonyms and Key Words: Transient psychophysiologic insomnia; transient insomnia; short-term insomnia; acute stress; emotional shock; acute emotional arousal; acute anxiety; loss or threat of loss, conflict, situational, episodic, seasonal, or maladaptive reaction; unfamiliar sleep environment.

Essential Features:

Adjustment sleep disorder represents sleep disturbance temporally related to acute stress, conflict, or environmental change that causes emotional arousal.

The reaction to stress is an essential feature of this disorder and may develop during the course of "normal" developmental events, such as an insomnia in the week preceding the first day of school for a child, before examinations, or in reaction to job- or family-related problems.

To be diagnosed as adjustment sleep disorder, the sleep disturbance must represent a clear change from the patient's norm. Symptoms must develop in association with the identified stressor and remit if either the stressor is removed or the level of adaptation is increased. In most cases, the disturbance is brief and sleep returns quickly to baseline levels. A person may present with a history of repeated episodes of adjustment sleep disorder. Only if clear periods of remission (normal sleep) are present between episodes should an adjustment sleep disorder be diagnosed; without remissions, a diagnosis of psychophysiologic or idiopathic insomnia should be considered.

Adjustment sleep disorder represents a classic form of the effect of psychologic factors on sleep. With resolution of the emotional reaction, sleep returns to normal.

Associated Features: Most adjustment sleep disorders are triggered by an emotional shock or immediate fear of threat to one's security, such as the death of a close person, divorce, change of job, or an examination. Occasionally, the sleep disturbance is related to anticipation of, or response to, intense positive emotions, such as the exhilaration felt in response to a marriage proposal or an upcoming vacation. Another common source of temporary changes in sleep patterns is related to the poor sleep experienced in an unfamiliar sleep environment.

Individuals may present with complaints of either insomnia or sleepiness. The insomnia may involve prolonged sleep onset or premature awakenings. The sleepiness may involve specific times of the day or may be a constant state of sleepiness. Mild or moderate cases may present with irritability, anxiety, lethargy, or tearfulness. Social, occupational, or educational dysfunction may be found in moderate to severe cases. In addition to having the previously mentioned symptoms, patients with severe cases may present with a depressive reaction or acute psychotic behavior; however, a diagnosis of adjustment sleep disorder implies that the symptoms of affective or thought disorder are secondary to the sleep disturbance and that the symptoms will remit or return to baseline with resolution of the sleep disturbance.

In most cases, the person is clearly aware of and able to identify the source of his/her stress. On rare occasions, persons with limited psychologic awareness may not have made the connection with a life event. Yet, these persons are, with rare exception, able to identify a significant psychosocial event and recognize its effect on sleep during the course of a thorough diagnostic interview.

Course: Adjustment sleep disorder generally has a short course. Within 3 months of the identified stressor taking place, the sleep disturbance usually will remit when the stress is removed or the level of adaptation increases. If the stress is an acute event, such as a car accident or being fired from a job, the onset of the adjustment sleep disorder is usually within a few days, and its duration is brief. If the stressor persists or represents an enduring condition, as in chronic physical illness or death of a spouse, it may take longer to achieve a new level of adaptation. In rare instances, generally involving severe cases, the sleep disturbance may persist longer than 6 months. Ruling out the development of psychiatric or medical complications is important when the sleep disturbance persists beyond 6 months.

Predisposing Factors: Systematic data are unavailable; however, it appears that individuals who are insecure and have a low threshold for emotional arousal are most vulnerable.

Prevalence: All people are subjected to situational episodes of insomnia, and many people may experience episodes of excessive sleepiness throughout the course of their lifetime. Some epidemiologic studies suggest that one third of all adults experience brief episodes of poor sleep each year. Systematically obtained data are insufficient to indicate the number of people who experience transient periods of sleepiness.

Age of Onset: Adjustment sleep disorder may occur at any age. Children with this disorder apparently are more likely to present with insomnia than daytime sleepiness.

Sex Ratio: Some studies suggest that adjustment sleep disorder may be more common among adult women than adult men; it also appears that women are more likely to seek treatment for their sleep disturbance. Systematically obtained data regarding sex differences among children and adolescents currently are insufficient.

Familial Pattern: Not known.

Pathology: None.

Complications: Serious complications are generally absent due to the short duration of most disturbances. A possibility exists that negative associations with the bedroom environment or changes in self-perception as a sleeper, which could result in the development of a long-term maladaptive reaction, will occur if the condition goes untreated. Occasionally, a sharp increase in alcohol intake or non-prescription sleeping aids and stimulants may be reported; however, serious medical or psychologic complications are rare unless the adjustment sleep disorder is superimposed on a preexisting mental or medical condition.

Polysomnographic Features: The nature of the sleep disturbance related to this disorder varies widely from person to person. Polysomnography may demonstrate normal architecture and timing of sleep, prolonged sleep onset, premature awakenings, or slightly longer than normal sleep time. Similarly, mean sleep latencies on the multiple sleep latency test may be normal or demonstrate mild to severe sleepiness. In most cases, concordance exists between the presenting complaint and polysomnographic findings. Persons exhibiting discordance between the presenting complaint and polysomnographic findings may represent a distinct subclassification of adjustment sleep disorder; however, no systematically obtained data exist on this issue. An example would be patients who complain of acute insomnia after learning that they have cancer, yet sleep normally when evaluated in the sleep center.

Other Laboratory Features None.

Differential Diagnosis: Due to the wide variability in polysomnographic features present in this disorder, a thorough diagnostic interview and psychologic assessment are imperative and probably reveal the most important data when ruling out adjustment sleep disorder. Sudden and sharp episodes of insomnia or sleepiness are more likely to represent adjustment sleep disorder than any other condition; however, a prolonged course of the sleep disturbance may prompt a retrospective opinion that the commencement was the onset of a persistent and serious psychiatric disturbance, which occasionally may be precipitated by identifiable disturbing life events (see sleep disorders associated with mental, neurologic, or other medical disorders).

Adjustment sleep disorder may be a proper diagnosis even when a preexisting psychiatric disorder is present but is not contributory to the current sleep disturbance. For example, a previously sound-sleeping psychotic patient may exhibit brief insomnia upon learning that his or her mother has died. In this case, the sleep disturbance should be diagnosed as adjustment sleep disorder rather than a sleep disorder associated with psychosis.

Temporary sleep disturbance may also be related to medical, toxic, or environmental conditions (see extrinsic sleep disorders). Bedtime rituals and caretaker-child interactions are sometimes related to sleep disturbances; bedtime behaviors should be closely examined to rule out sleep-onset association disorder and limit-setting sleep disorder.

A sleep disturbance commonly occurs during a time of change in environments such as hospitalization or staying in a hotel room for a short period of time; the most typical presenting complaint is insomnia. Adjustment sleep disorder is an appropriate diagnosis if the sleep disturbance solely reflects the apprehension related to being removed from a "safe" home environment. Adjustment sleep disorder is also appropriately diagnosed when a medical condition is not accompanied with discomfort, or the sleep disturbance begins only after the diagnosis of a medical condition is revealed (without change in medical status).

A central distinction between psychophysiologic insomnia and adjustment sleep disorder is the presence of a clearly identifiable stressor. The absence of a stressor would also support consideration of a sleep disorder associated with mental, neurologic, or other medical disorder.

Diagnostic Criteria: Adjustment Sleep Disorder (307.41-0)

A. The patient has a complaint of insomnia or excessive sleepiness.
B. The complaint is a temporally associated reaction to an identifiable stressor.
C. The disorder is expected to remit if the stress is reduced or the level of adaptation is increased.
D. Associated features include one or more of the following:
   1. Fatigue, lethargy, or tiredness
   2. Excessive time spent in bed
   3. Anxiety, irritability
   4. Somatic symptoms such as aches, pains, sore eyes, or headaches
   5. Sad or depressed emotional reactions
E. Polysomnographic monitoring demonstrates at least one of the following:
   1. An increased sleep latency, reduced sleep efficiency, or increased number and duration of awakenings
   2. A slightly prolonged total sleep time
   3. A reduced mean sleep latency on the multiple sleep latency test.

F. No other mental or medical disorder accounts for the symptom.
G. The symptoms do not meet the diagnostic criteria for other sleep disorders that produce insomnia or excessive sleepiness (e.g., psychophysiologic insomnia or environmental sleep disorder).

Minimal Criteria: A plus B plus C.

Severity Criteria:

Mild: Mild insomnia or mild sleepiness, as defined on page 23.
Moderate: Moderate insomnia or moderate sleepiness, as defined on page 23.
Severe: Severe insomnia or severe sleepiness, as defined on page 23.

Duration Criteria:

Acute (transient): 7 days or less.
Subacute (short-term): More than 7 days but less than 3 months.
Chronic: 3 months or longer.

Bibliography:

Agnew HJ Jr, Webb WW, Williams RL. The first night effect: An EEG study of sleep. Psychophysiology 1966; 7: 263–266.
Beutler LE, Thornby JI, Karacan I. Psychological variables in the diagnosis of insomnia. In: Williams RL, Karacan I, eds. Sleep disorders. Diagnosis and treatment. New York: John Wiley & Sons, 1978; 61–100.
Kales A, Kales JD. Evaluation and treatment of insomnia. New York: Oxford University Press, 1984.
Karacan I, Thornby J, Williams RL. Sleep disturbance: A community survey. In: Guilleminault C, Lugaresi E, eds. Sleep/wake disorders: natural history, epidemiology, and long-term evolution. New York: Raven Press, 1983; 37–60.
Welstein L, Dement W, Redington D, Guilleminault C, Mitler M. Insomina in the San Francisco Bay area: A telephone survey. In: Guilleminault C, Lugaresi E, eds. Sleep/wake disorders: natural history, epidemiology, and long-term evolution. New York: Raven Press, 1983; 73–86.

Insufficient Sleep Syndrome (307.49-4)

Synonyms and Key Words: Insufficient nocturnal sleep, sleep curtailment, sleep reduction, sleep restriction, inadequate sleep. Insufficient nocturnal sleep is the preferred term because it connotes a voluntary, albeit unintentional, sleep deprivation without the presence of neuropathologic sleep disturbance or abnormal sleep quality. Sleep curtailment, reduction, and restriction are typically used to refer to experimental procedures and treatment.

Essential Features:

Insufficient sleep syndrome is a disorder that occurs in an individual who persistently fails to obtain sufficient nocturnal sleep required to support normally alert wakefulness.

The individual engages in voluntary, albeit unintentional, chronic sleep deprivation. Examination reveals unimpaired or above-average ability to initiate and maintain sleep. Mental status examination and psychologic evaluation reveal little or no psychopathology, and physical examination reveals no medical explanation for the patient's sleepiness.

A clear, detailed history of the current sleep pattern in relation to the amounts of sleep routinely obtained in the past, currently desired, possible to achieve, and actually obtained is revealing. The disparity between the need for sleep and the amount actually obtained is substantial, and its significance is unappreciated by the patient. An extended sleep time on weekend nights as compared to weekday nights is also suggestive of this disorder. A therapeutic trial of a longer major sleep episode can reverse the symptoms.

Associated Features: Depending upon chronicity and extent of sleep loss, individuals with this condition may develop secondary symptoms, including irritability, concentration and attention deficits, reduced vigilance, distractability, reduced motivation, anergia, dysphoria, fatigue, restlessness, incoordination, malaise, loss of appetite, gastrointestinal disturbance, muscle pain, diplopia, and dry mouth. Secondary symptoms may become a primary focus of the patient, serving to obscure the primary cause of the difficulties and resulting in apprehension or depression in regard to health status.

Sleep loss in the absence of depression, anxiety, or use of stimulant agents inevitably results in sleepiness. Psychologically and somatically normal individuals who obtain less sleep than they physiologically require typically experience sleepiness during waking hours. This phenomenon is reinforced by experience in most normal individuals and is taken for granted. Situational factors, such as battlefield combat, preparation for school examinations, writing deadlines, political campaigning, etc., may obviate adequate sleep. Individuals who are sleep deprived as a result of such factors should not be classified here unless they are not aware that more sleep would be recuperative and seek intervention for their symptoms.

Course: In its early stages, this condition results in increased daytime sleepiness, concentration problems, lowered energy level, and malaise. If unchecked, insufficient sleep syndrome may cause depression and other psychologic difficulties, with poor work performance and withdrawal from family and social activities occurring.

Predisposing Factors: Low intellectual capacity, cultural factors, and psychologic denial may dispose the individual to search for causes other than the obvious one. A day-shift work schedule that requires the individual to be at work at an early hour, coupled with perceived family or social demands that lead the individual to delay bedtime and thus reduce total sleep time, may also be contributory.

Prevalence: The prevalence of this disorder in the general population is not known. Insufficient sleep syndrome is diagnosed in about 2% of those patients who present to sleep disorders centers.

Age of Onset: Insufficient sleep syndrome usually has its onset between the middle and the end of the third decade of life. It is not uncommon, however, for the condition to go undiagnosed until the individual is over 40 years of age.

Sex Ratio: A slightly greater number of men are affected than women.

Familial Pattern: Not known.

Pathology: None.

Complications: Chronic mood disturbance, documented work-performance deficits, disruption of social functioning, and marital discord may be due to this disorder. Traffic accidents or injury at work may result from loss of normal vigilance.

Polysomnographic Features: All-night polysomnographic evaluation reveals a reduced sleep-onset latency, an atypically high (>85%) sleep efficiency, and a prolonged sleep time (longer than the reported sleep time for a weekday night at home). The distribution of REM and NREM sleep stages is like that of normal sleepers (individuals without sleep complaints or documented central nervous system-related sleep pathology).

The multiple sleep latency test (MSLT) reveals excessive sleepiness, with stage 1 sleep occurring in most (99%) naps and an average latency to stage-1 sleep of 5 to 8 minutes. Stage 2 sleep occurs in a large percentage (>80%) of MSLT naps.

Measures of sleep-onset latency and the disparity between reported sleep at home (for a weekday night) and observed total sleep time in the sleep laboratory are the most sensitive and specific measures. Other polysomnographic measures obtained during all-night recording or during the MSLT have high sensitivity but low to moderate specificity.

Other Laboratory Test Features: Twenty-four-hour temperature recordings reveal no circadian rhythm disturbance. Other laboratory tests, blood tests, urinalysis, etc., suggest no physical basis for the excessive sleepiness.

Differential Diagnosis: Environmental sleep disorder, psychophysiologic insomnia, affective disorder, obstructive sleep apnea syndrome, central sleep apnea syndrome, narcolepsy, idiopathic hypersomnia, posttraumatic hypersomnia, short sleeper, shift work sleep disorder, delayed sleep-phase syndrome, periodic limb movement disorder.

Diagnostic Criteria: Insufficient Sleep Syndrome (307.49-4)

A. The patient has a complaint of excessive sleepiness or, in prepubertal children, of difficulty in initiating sleep.
B. The patient's habitual sleep episode is shorter in duration than is expected for his or her age.

C. When the habitual sleep schedule is not maintained (e.g., weekends or vacation time, patients will have a sleep episode that is greater in duration than the habitual sleep episode and will awaken spontaneously).
D. The abnormal sleep pattern is present for at least 3 months.
E. A therapeutic trial of a longer sleep episode eliminates the symptoms.
F. Polysomnographic monitoring performed over the patient's habitual sleep period demonstrates:
   1. Sleep latency less than 15 minutes, a sleep efficiency greater than 85%, and a final awakening of less than 10 minutes
   2. An MSLT demonstrates excessive sleepiness
G. No significant underlying medical or mental disorder accounts for the symptoms.
H. The patient's symptoms do not meet the criteria for any other sleep disorder producing either insomnia or excessive sleepiness.

Minimal Criteria: A plus B plus C plus G plus H.

Severity Criteria:

Mild: Mild sleepiness or, in prepubertal children, mild insomnia, as defined on page 23.
Moderate: Moderate sleepiness or, in prepubertal children, moderate insomnia, as defined on page 23.
Severe: Severe sleepiness, as defined on page 23.

Duration Criteria:

Acute: 6 months or less.
Subacute: More than 6 months but less than 1 year.
Chronic: 1 year or longer.

Bibliography:

Carskadon MA, Dement WC. Effects of total sleep loss on sleep tendency. Percept Mot Skills 1979; 48: 495–506.
Carskadon M, Dement W. Sleepiness during sleep restriction. Sleep Res 1979; 8: 254.
Roehrs T, Zorick F, Sicklesteel J, Wittig R, Roth T. Excessive daytime sleepiness associated with insufficient sleep. Sleep 1983; 6: 319–325.
Zorick F, Roehrs T, Koshorek G, et al. Patterns of sleepiness in various disorders of excessive daytime somnolence. Sleep 1982; 5: S165–S174.

Limit-Setting Sleep Disorder (307.42-4)

Synonyms and Key Words: Childhood insomnia, limit-setting, caretaker.

Essential Features:

Limit-setting sleep disorder is primarily a childhood disorder that is characterized by the inadequate enforcement of bedtimes by a caretaker, with the patient then stalling or refusing to go to bed at an appropriate time.

Stalling or refusing to go to sleep, which usually occurs at bedtime but occasionally occurs after nighttime wakings, characterizes limit-setting sleep disorder. If and when limits are enforced by a caretaker, sleep comes quickly; otherwise, sleep onset may be delayed.

This is both a childhood disorder and a caretaker complaint. The child does not go to sleep when the caretaker desires, and the child usually wants to stay up later. Once patients are old enough (typically in adolescence) to make such decisions for themselves, to be aware of and responsible for the consequences, and to be willing to allow the caretakers to sleep, the complaints may stop. If the patients then do not set appropriate limits for themselves, shortened sleep may still occur, but it is by their own choice, which now is the main concern. Struggles between the caretaker and the patient cease, and the problem becomes one of poor sleep hygiene, irregular scheduling, and insufficient sleep.

Setting limits usually does not become a problem until children can climb out of crib or have been moved to a bed. The limits provided by the bars of the crib are lost. If parents give in to requests made by a child in the crib, however, this problem may be seen earlier.

Requests are typically for an extra drink, to make a trip to the bathroom, to be tucked in again, to have a light turned on or off, to have another story, to watch television, or to have help dealing with fear. "Fears" in this setting either are not true fears or are only mild ones exacerbated by the caretakers' inability to be firm and convincingly protective. The most common request is one that the child finds the caretakers are most likely to respond to (bathroom, monsters). Caretakers, on the other hand, often do not want to remain close to the child's room at night to enable a prompt and consistent response. Frequently, the caretakers are in another part of the house or apartment, often on a different floor, eating, doing chores, visiting, or watching television.

Limits may not be set at all. In this case, the child decides when to go to sleep and often will fall asleep in the living room with the television on and adults nearby. An older child may even remain in his or her room watching television. Limits may be set but only very inconsistently and in an unpredictable manner. Often when a certain level of exacerbation is reached, caretakers do enforce limits, and the child stays in bed and goes to sleep. This historic point is of much diagnostic significance.

Associated Features: Caretaker and interactional factors are most important. Some caretakers simply do not know how to set limits, and so they may keep sending their child back to bed but never enforce it. They may not recognize the importance of limits. They copy the overly permissive way, or react to the overly stern way, in which they were raised. Increased problems are seen not only in children of overly solicitous parents but also in poorly nurtured children. Here, the nighttime struggles seem to allow for some interaction, albeit negative.

Some caretakers have significant problems of their own (depression, alcoholism, drug addiction, long work hours, illness), making it difficult to focus on their child at night in an organized fashion. Marital disputes at night may cause a child to get out of bed to intervene, even at the risk of punishment. Parents may receive secondary gains from their child's stalling tactics, perhaps to avoid their own issues or perhaps because they actually enjoy the company.

Guilt may even be important, particularly to parents of a child: born with medical problems, anomalies, or handicaps; who required an operation at a young age; or who was born prematurely and required prolonged hospitalization. Standing up to such a child's requests may be difficult indeed. Sometimes, limits are difficult to set because of the environmental setting (e.g., several children and a parent sharing a single room). Or, lack of structure and imposed limits may be the pattern in the family's social milieu.

Course: The course of limit-setting sleep disorder is variable, dependent upon the reasons limits are not set. When limit-setting factors are resolved, sleep usually improves. As the child grows, privacy becomes more important, and nighttime struggles with the caretaker may not be desired. With the demands of school and increased maturity in the child, recognition of the need for enough sleep may eliminate staying up later as a goal in and of itself. On the other hand, with increased age may come the desire for increased independence, particularly as adolescence approaches. Children may want to take on full responsibility for their own schedules, even though they may not be yet mature enough to do so alone.

Predisposing Factors: Inherent factors are probably relevant but have not yet been carefully studied. Thus, those children fitting the description of "owls" will be more likely to try to stay up late if allowed to, whereas "larks" may be less likely to test limits and would go to sleep on time whether or not limits are set.

Prevalence: The prevalence of limit-setting sleep disorder is estimated at approximately 5% to 10% of the childhood population.

Age of Onset: Limit-setting sleep disorder is usually not seen before the child is capable of verbal demands and interchange (i.e., at age two years). The disorder is more common when the child is able to climb out of the crib or is moved into a bed, typically about age three years. Depending upon social circumstances, however, this may occur at any point from late infancy through adolescence.

Sex Ratio: There is either no sex prevalence or a slightly increased incidence in males.

Familial Pattern: No pattern in terms of inborn characteristics is known. However, patterns of childrearing in which limits are not set may easily be passed along generation lines.

Pathology: None.

Complications: The major complications would be those of insufficient sleep, with irritability, decreased attention, decreased school performance, and increased family tensions.

Polysomnographic Features: When appropriate limits are set in the laboratory, polysomnographically monitored sleep is normal.

Other Laboratory Test Features: Psychologic testing occasionally is helpful in sorting out patient factors from caretaker factors.

Differential Diagnosis: Any of several disorders causing delayed sleep initiation in childhood must be considered. Most important are a delayed sleep phase, a normal sleep phase (sometimes with a short sleep requirement) but a bedtime set inappropriately early, and anxiety with bedtime fears. The first two of these diagnoses can be distinguished from a problem in limit setting by the fact that sleep onset tends to occur at the same time each night regardless of bedtime and regardless of the degree to which limits are set. A truly anxious child at night is really asking for someone's presence, and if one stays with the child, sleep will come quickly without continued demands. An irregular sleep schedule or medication effects may lead to bedtime stalling, but here too sleep will be slow to come even if limits are firmly set.

Diagnostic Criteria: Limit-Setting Sleep Disorder (307.42-4)

A. The patient has difficulty in initiating sleep.
B. The patient stalls or refuses to go to bed at an appropriate time.
C. Once the sleep period is initiated, sleep is of normal quality and duration.
D. Polysomnographic monitoring demonstrates normal timing, quality, and duration of the sleep period.
E. No significant underlying mental or medical disorder accounts for the complaint.
F. The symptoms do not meet criteria for any other sleep disorder causing difficulty in initiating sleep (e.g., sleep-onset association disorder).

Minimal Criteria: B plus C.

Severity Criteria:

Mild: The major sleep episode is reduced by less than one hour, with up to three episodes per night of stalling, calling out, or leaving the bedroom.
Moderate: The major sleep episode is reduced by one to two hours, with three to four episodes per night of stalling, calling out, or leaving the bedroom.
Severe: The major sleep episode is reduced by at least two hours, with five or more episodes per night of stalling, calling out, or leaving the bedroom.

Duration Criteria:

Acute: 7 days or less.
Subacute: More than 7 days but less than 3 months.
Chronic: 3 months or longer.

Bibliography:

Ferber R. The sleepless child. In: Guilleminault C, ed. Sleep and its disorders in children. New York: Raven Press, 1987; 141–163.

Ferber R. Sleeplessness in the child. In: Kryger MH, Roth T, Dement WC, eds. Principles and practice of sleep medicine. Philadelphia: WB Saunders, 1989; 633–639.

Sleep-Onset Association Disorder (307.42-5)

Synonyms and Key Words: Inappropriate sleep-onset associations.

Essential Features:

Sleep-onset association disorder *occurs when sleep onset is impaired by the absence of a certain object or set of circumstances.*

Sleep-onset association disorder is mainly a disorder of childhood. Sleep is normal when certain conditions are present; when they are not, transitions to sleep, both at bedtime and after nighttime wakings, are delayed. Adults may have the disorder, affecting only initial sleep onset at the beginning of the night. In children, the number of nighttime wakings may seem excessive to caretakers, but their actual frequency is normal. When the required conditions are reestablished, return to sleep is rapid; however, the sleep-onset-associated conditions usually require involvement of, or participation by, the caretakers.

Associated Features: Typically, the child falls asleep under a certain set of conditions (e.g., using a bottle or sucking on a pacifier). The child often is not even in the crib or bed and may well not be in the bedroom. For an adult, the associations may include television, radio, lights, or outside noise.

When the child is transferred to the bed or crib (or the adult's television or radio is turned off), waking may occur unless sleep is deep enough. Nighttime wakings are actually normal, typically occurring every one to four hours. In the sleep-onset association disorder, return to sleep is difficult unless the conditions associated with sleep onset are reestablished. This means rocking, nursing, sucking a pacifier, or watching television. When these conditions are reestablished, return to sleep is usually rapid.

When the condition associated with sleep also provides stimulation or interest, such as occurs with watching the television or participating in conversations, sleep onset may be delayed. Sleep transitions may also be prolonged if the associated condition is difficult to maintain, such as the caretaker having to continuously rub the child's back with constant rhythm and pressure or the child continuously sucking on a pacifier without letting it fall out of his or her mouth.

Often no wakings occur for the first few hours of the night when delta sleep is present. The early morning hours, at least in children, also tend to be associated with more continuous sleep, presumably because of the early-morning return of delta sleep typical of that age.

Sleep-onset association disorder is mainly a disorder of early childhood, when the conditions associated with sleep require a caretaker's assistance to become established. Later on (barring physical or mental handicap), the associations come under more independent control of the person with the disorder. At times of waking, even if the conditions associated with falling asleep are not present, older patients can usually reestablish the conditions rapidly themselves (e.g., replacing the pillow, pulling up the blanket, walking from the living room to bedroom, turning on the radio). For this reason, this form of insomnia becomes progressively uncommon with increased age.

Course: Untreated, the course is variable. In infants, spontaneous resolution may occur at any time. Often, however, symptoms persist until age three or four, when nursing, sucking on bottles or pacifiers, rocking, and holding decrease markedly. Bedtime rituals also change (e.g., with story reading replacing rocking). Occasionally, symptoms may persist into middle childhood, especially if a child and parent share a bed, at least during the transition from crib to bed sleeping. Although there is no suggestion that children with this problem are more likely to develop another form of insomnia as an adult, the occurrence of this finding is not known. Similarly, it is not known if treatment in childhood alters the frequency of adult sleep difficulties.

Predisposing Factors: Predisposing factors can include any transient or chronic sleep disruption, including scheduling abnormalities, social upheaval, or a period of illness and pain requiring caretaker attention and interaction at sleep times. Sleep-onset associations may form as caretakers become more involved with the sleep-transition process as the caretakers try to help the child with sleep difficulties. The child may have been a colicky infant with the need to be carried about and rocked much of the evening. Alternatively, the child may have had feeding difficulties, which required the encouragement of nighttime feedings, or the child may have had ongoing recurrent ear infections with pain, which necessitated frequent holding during much of the night. Various associations to sleep onset may arise during these difficult periods. Once learned, these associations may persist even after the initial difficulties, illness, and pain disappear.

Inherent factors are probably important as well (i.e., some normal children seem better able to calm themselves and fall asleep rapidly than do others). For this reason, they seem more resistant to developing persistent unhelpful sleep-onset associations during a transient sleep disruption and, thus, are less likely to have a chronic problem emerge. These hypotheses remain to be proven.

Perinatal factors, including prematurity, do not seem to affect waking frequency. Parents of a child who suffered medical problems and was hospitalized at a young age may feel overprotective, however, and may be quicker to become and stay intimately involved in the child's sleep-transition process. Severe perinatal anoxia may be followed by increased irritability and wakings and may set the stage for the formation of caretaker-involved associations. Parents who feel they were mistreated as children may overcompensate with their own children. Parental inexperience may predispose a first child to this disorder.

Prevalence: In children aged six months to three years, the prevalence appears to be approximately 15% to 20%. After age three, the prevalence decreases markedly. The disorder is relatively uncommon in adults.

Age of Onset: Sleep-onset associations of an older infant or young toddler often can be traced without interruption back to the child's first days of life. Because children are not expected to sleep through the night with regularity until they are three to six months of age, six months is a reasonable age to first consider this disorder, unless the sleeplessness is very marked. Frequently, sleep improves significantly during the period of three to six months, only to regress during the second half year of the child's life. The disorder may have its onset at any time during late infancy and the toddler years.

The disorder may begin at any age in the adult.

Sex Ratio: Studies vary, suggesting either no sex difference or a slightly increased incidence in males.

Familial Pattern: There is little evidence for any familial tendency. Symptoms commonly exist in only one of a group of siblings. When several siblings are involved, parental factors often seem more important than do the children's inherent factors. The appearance of this disorder in successive generations is not known, and even if it were, separation of familial childhood practices from inherited tendencies would be difficult.

Pathology: None.

Complications: Caretakers' loss of sleep, with subsequent anger and frustration, may lead to marital difficulties and altered parent-child interaction, with less warmth and decreased nurturance. Also, when these children do not get satisfactory amounts of sleep, the consequent sleep deprivation may be associated with irritability and tantrums. Parents may form negative feelings about their children, and these feelings may be difficult to reverse. Long-term consequences remain speculative.

An adult may develop obsessive behavior related to the sleep-onset association; the behavior then prevents the person from being able to sleep in certain environments if the association is not present.

Polysomnographic Features: Sleep is essentially normal. If the caretaker is present in the patient's laboratory bedroom to respond rapidly and in the usual manner to the nighttime wakings, then those wakings are brief and incomplete, and the recording is completely normal.

Polysomnographic studies in adults show an increased sleep latency when the association is not present and an increase in frequency and duration of awakenings after sleep onset.

Other Laboratory Test Features: None.

Differential Diagnosis: In the child, other causes of childhood sleeplessness must be considered. Problems such as poor limit setting, a delayed sleep phase, or an inappropriately early bedtime will usually only present as a bedtime problem. Pain (such as occurs with otitis or esophageal reflux), social stresses (and a poorly nurtured child), an irregular sleep-wake schedule, and even the stress of inadequate sleep may present with multiple wakings as well, but in these cases, rapid parental intervention does not ensure rapid return to sleep regardless of what conditions are reestablished.

In the adult, the primary diagnostic consideration is differentiation from psychophysiologic insomnia. Conditioned factors are relevant in both disorders; in psychophysiologic insomnia, however, it is the presence of conditions negatively associated with sleep (typically the bed and bedroom) that cause arousal and fear of insomnia. In sleep-onset association disorder, fear of insomnia (except by the caretakers) is not an issue. Although arousal may still be triggered, in this case it is because of the absence of those conditions positively associated with sleep. There is no direct stimulation by any negative association, and sleep onset is not a concern when the positive associations are present. If the disorder has been present for less than three weeks, the differentiation must be made from adjustment sleep disorder.

Diagnostic Criteria: Sleep-Onset Association Disorder (307.42-5)

A. The patient has a complaint of insomnia.
B. The complaint is temporally associated with absence of certain conditions (e.g., being held, rocked, or nursed at the breast; listening to the radio; or watching television; etc).
C. The disorder has been present for at least three weeks.
D. With the particular association present, sleep is normal in onset, duration, and quality.
E. Polysomnographic monitoring demonstrates:
   1. Normal timing, duration, and quality of the sleep period when the associations are present
   2. Sleep latency and the duration or number of awakenings can be increased when the associations are absent.
F. No significant underlying mental or medical disorder accounts for the complaint.
G. The symptoms do not meet the criteria for any other sleep disorder causing difficulty in initiating sleep (e.g., limit-setting sleep disorder).

Note: If the disorder has been present less than three weeks, specify and code under adjustment sleep disorder.

Minimal Criteria: A plus B plus D plus F plus G.

Severity Criteria:

Mild: Mild insomnia, as defined on page 23. In infants, the criteria are a prolonged sleep latency and two or three wakings, each lasting less than 5 minutes, or one waking lasting less than 10 minutes. The awakenings occur at least 5 nights per week.

Moderate: Moderate insomnia, as defined on page 23. In infants, the criteria are a prolonged sleep latency and two or three wakings, each lasting 5 to 10 minutes, or one waking lasting 10 to 15 minutes. The awakenings occur at least 5 nights per week.

Severe: Severe insomnia, as defined on page 23. In infants, the criteria are a prolonged sleep latency and more than three nightly wakings; or two or three wakings, each lasting over 10 minutes; or one waking lasting over 15 minutes. The awakenings occur at least 5 nights per week.

Duration Criteria:

Acute: 3 months or less.
Subacute: More than 3 months but less than 6 months.
Chronic: 6 months or longer.

Bibliography:

Ferber R. Sleeplessness in the child. In: Kryger MH, Roth T, Dement WC, eds. Principles and practice of sleep medicine. Philadelphia: WB Saunders, 1989; 633–639.

Ferber R. The sleepless child. In: Guilleminault C, ed. Sleep and its disorders in children. New York: Raven Press, 1987; 141–163.

Largo RH, Hunziker UA. A developmental approach to the management of children with sleep disturbances in the first three years of life. Eur J Pediatr 1984; 142: 170–173.

Richman N. A community survey of characteristics of one- to two- year-olds with sleep disruptions. J Am Acad Child Psychiatry 1981; 20: 281–291.

Food Allergy Insomnia (780.52-2)

Synonyms and Key Words: Cow's milk allergy, food intolerance.

Essential Features:

Food allergy insomnia *is a disorder of initiating and maintaining sleep due to an allergic response to food allergens.*

The sleep disturbance is typically one of difficulty initiating sleep and of frequent arousals and awakenings. Additional symptoms include frequent arousals and crying, psychomotor agitation, and daytime lethargy.

Associated Features: Other symptoms of allergy may accompany the sleep disturbance (e.g., skin irritation, respiratory difficulties, or gastrointestinal upset).

Course: Food allergy insomnia usually begins in infancy and resolves spontaneously by age two to four years. The duration to onset of symptoms after the exposure to the allergen is not known. Adults may suffer food allergy insomnia due to various allergens (e.g., eggs, fish, etc.).

Predisposing Factors: A family history of food allergy may increase the risk in offspring.

Prevalence: The prevalence is unknown, but the disorder appears to be common.

Age of Onset: The onset of symptoms can occur from birth or from the introduction of cow's milk into the diet, usually within the first two years of life. In adults, a change of diet may precipitate the first symptoms.

Sex Ratio: Not known.

Familial Pattern: None known.

Pathology: None known.

Complications: Allergic phenomena may produce their own sequelae, such as skin irritation or respiratory distress, but the stress usually is limited to the caretakers. The use of sedative medications may induce adverse reactions.

Polysomnographic Features: Frequent arousals occur from any sleep stage and are not preceded by gastrointestinal acid reflux or electroencephalographic or cardiorespiratory abnormalities.

Other Laboratory Test Features: Elevated levels of serum antibodies may be detected against the allergen (e.g., IgG against β-lactoglobulin). Allergen testing can be negative in children under one year of age. IgE, total eosinophils, and skin reactivity tests may be normal.

Differential Diagnosis: Within the first three months, the main differential includes infantile colic. Gastroesophageal reflux, infantile spasms, and respiratory irregularity during sleep may need to be excluded.

Diagnostic Criteria: Food Allergy insomnia (780.52-2)

A. The patient has a complaint of insomnia.
B. The complaint is temporally associated with the introduction of a particular food or drink.
C. Removal of the agent results in restoration of normal sleep and wakefulness, either immediately or within four weeks. Daytime behavior may improve before the sleep pattern improves.
D. Two or more of the following symptoms are present
   1. Psychomotor agitation
   2. Daytime lethargy
   3. Respiratory difficulties
   4. Skin irritation
   5. Gastrointestinal upset

E. Disturbed sleep and altered daytime behavior reoccur when the suspected allergen is reintroduced into the diet.
F. Levels of serum antibodies against the allergen are elevated.
G. Polysomnographic monitoring demonstrates frequent arousals from any sleep stage.
H. No other medical disorder accounts for the symptoms.
I. The symptoms do not meet the diagnostic criteria for any other sleep disorder producing insomnia (e.g., sleep-onset association disorder, noctural eating [drinking] syndrome, limit-setting sleep disorder, etc).

Note: If an associated allergic response is prominent, state and code the associated response on axis C (e.g., dermatitis due to food allergy 693.1).

Minimal Criteria: A plus B plus C, or A plus B plus E.

Severity Criteria:

Mild: Occasional arousals, crying, psychomotor agitation, and daytime lethargy; mild or no evidence of gastrointestinal upset, skin irritation, or respiratory difficulties.
Moderate: Frequent arousals, crying, psychomotor agitation, and daytime lethargy; moderate evidence of gastrointestinal upset, skin irritation, or respiratory difficulties (in children under three years of age, physical symptoms of allergy can be absent).
Severe: Frequent and severe arousals, crying, psychomotor agitation, and daytime lethargy; severe evidence of gastrointestinal upset, skin irritation, or respiratory difficulties (in children under three years of age, physical symptoms of allergy can be absent).

Duration Criteria:

Acute: 7 days or less.
Subacute: More than 7 days but less than 3 months.
Chronic: 3 months or longer.

Bibliography:

Kahn A, Mozin MJ, Casimir G, Montauk L, Blum D. Insomnia and cow's milk allergy in infants. Pediatrics 1985; 76: 880–884.
Kahn A, , Rebuffat E, Blum D, Casimir G, Duchateau J, Mozin MJ. Difficulty in initiating and maintaining sleep associated with cow's milk allergy in infants. Sleep 1987; 10: 116–121.

Nocturnal Eating (Drinking) Syndrome (780.52-8)

Synonyms and Key Words: Excessive nighttime fluid intake, nighttime hunger, nocturnal eating syndrome, night eating syndrome.

Essential Features:

Nocturnal eating (drinking) syndrome is characterized by recurrent awakenings, with the inability to return to sleep without eating or drinking.

This condition is primarily a problem of infancy and early childhood, with intake of large volumes by nursing or bottle feeding at times of waking; however, it is also seen in adults. After the patient consumes the expected amount of food or liquid, return to sleep is rapid.

In the childhood form of the disorder, the child is usually nursed (breast or bottle) to sleep and then again repeatedly during the night. The association of nursing (and possibly holding and rocking) with sleep onset is thus important, but the large number of wakings (typically three to eight) is usually greater than is seen when only the learned sleep-onset associations represent the problem. The child seems hungry at most of the wakings and takes milk or juice eagerly. Large amounts are consumed, usually 4 to 8 ounces or more each time and 12 to 32 ounces across the night. Wetting is also excessive, requiring at least one nighttime diaper change, and may be the cause of some of the wakings.

True hunger signals (probably sufficient to wake the child or to prevent return to sleep after a normal waking) are presumed to be present by the way the child takes the feeding, but the timing of these signals seems learned rather than representative of a true nutrition requirement. Full-term, normally growing, healthy infants of six months of age or more should have the ability to sleep through the night without requiring feedings.

In adults, nighttime waking can also become conditioned to hunger and eating, with several wakings a night for a sandwich or other food. This behavior may have several origins; regardless of the origin, however, once the behavior is learned, the wakings with hunger may continue even when the underlying cause is treated. Occasionally, the eating behavior becomes obsessional, with the patient exhibiting dramatic attempts to obtain food at any time of night or when sleeping in any environment.

Associated Features: Circadian effects are also presumed to have an impact on the nocturnal eating (drinking) syndrome. Repeated nutrition intake across the sleep episode directly affects digestive and endocrine rhythms and indirectly affects the control of the sleep-wake cycle. The child remains on a pattern more typical of early infancy, with broken sleep and frequent feedings occurring across the night. Sleep consolidation at night, which usually takes place between three and six months of age, is disrupted.

Course: The course is variable. Some children seem to stop waking even though the feedings are never withheld, whereas others continue until the caretakers establish a limit. Those children in the latter category may continue waking until they are weaned completely. This usually is achieved by age three to four years. Occasionally, a youngster being weaned will be allowed to continue to consume the milk or juice (or even solid food) during the night but receives the nourishment from a cup. In this case, the wakings may persist. In adults, the behavior may remit spontaneously or respond to behavior modification techniques.

Predisposing Factors: Because not all children offered the breast or bottle at bedtime and at all nighttime wakings fail to consolidate their nighttime sleep, inherent factors are suspected.

Caretaker factors are very important. This disorder is more likely to occur if the caretaker believes that feedings should be continued until no longer "demanded" by the child. Caretakers often have difficulty distinguishing a child's true need from habit and, because the child seems hungry at night, conclude that the child should be fed. At times, the caretaker derives secondary gains from the nursing process; the behavior serves the needs of the caretaker and not those of the child. It may be the only time the caretaker feels important and needed. A parent working long hours may find that the night is one of the few times spent with the child, and the feeding process provides rewards as well as reduces feelings of guilt. The child who is given no opportunity during the day to learn to deal with any upset, but instead is always brought to the breast or given a bottle (whether or not there is any hunger), may find it difficult to deal with nighttime wakings in any other way.

Adults may be predisposed to developing this disorder if: they already maintain poor sleep hygiene; have varied daily, meal, and work schedules (including night or rotating shifts); live in an environment where there is much nighttime activity, including eating; are already obese and lack normal recognition of hunger signals; or suffer from discomfort caused by gastritis, an ulcer, or reflux that is relieved by eating.

Prevalence: Precise values are not known. Estimate is approximately 5% of the population aged six months to three years, with a marked decrease after weaning. Prevalence in adults is not known.

Age of Onset: Although this syndrome may be present soon after birth, it should not require treatment until the child is about six months of age, when sleeping through the night is expected. It may be diagnosed earlier when wakings and feedings are clearly excessive for age (e.g., a three-month-old fed hourly). The adult form can begin at any age but appears to be less common in the elderly.

Sex Ratio: None known.

Familial Pattern: No known familial pattern of inherent tendencies, but child-rearing habits may be passed along for several generations.

Pathology: None.

Complications: Infants who nurse excessively at night, particularly when supine, may have an increased incidence of dental disease and ear infections. Increased feedings at night may not be compensated for by decreased feeding during the day, and therefore obesity may occur, with possible long-term significance. Although the infant's sleep is broken, total nighttime sleep is usually not significantly shortened. Caretakers may lose significant sleep, however, causing anger, frustration, and altered interactions with the child. Frequent nursing may cause the mother to have breast tenderness.

Excessive weight gain may be a major concern and cause for presentation in the adult group.

Polysomnographic Features: The major sleep period is normal, except for an increased number of awakenings.

Other Laboratory Test Features: None.

Differential Diagnosis: All other causes of nighttime wakings in young children should be considered. The excessive food or fluid intake must not represent a "binge" in a bulimic patient. Anorexia nervosa and bulimia should be excluded. Vomiting is not a feature of the nocturnal eating (drinking) syndrome.

Diagnostic Criteria: Nocturnal Eating (Drinking) Syndrome (780.52-8)

A. The patient has a complaint of difficulty maintaining sleep.
B. The patient frequently and recurrently awakens to eat or drink.
C. Sleep onset is normal following ingestion of the desired food or drink.
D. Polysomnographic monitoring demonstrates an increase in the number or duration of awakenings.
E. No medical or mental disorder accounts for the complaint (e.g., hypoglycemia, bulimia).
F. No other sleep disorder produces the difficulty in maintaining sleep.

Note: If the disorder is predominantly one of eating at night, then state and code the disorder as nocturnal eating syndrome; if predominantly one of drinking at night, nocturnal drinking syndrome.

Minimal Criteria: B plus C.

Severity Criteria:

Mild: Awakenings to eat or drink occur no more than four times per week. Children usually awaken and require feeding fewer than 3 times per night; the wakings are associated with an intake of less than 12 ounces during the night.
Moderate: Awakenings to eat or drink occur almost nightly. Children usually awaken and require feeding 3 to 5 times per night; the wakings are associated with an intake of 12 to 20 ounces during the night.
Severe: Awakenings to eat or drink occur more than once per night. Children usually awaken and require feeding more than 5 times per night; the wakings are associated with an intake of over 20 ounces during the night (including bedtime).

Duration Criteria:

Acute: 7 days or less.
Subacute: More than 7 days but less than 3 months.
Chronic: 3 months or longer.

Bibliography:

Ferber R. The sleepless child. In: Guilleminault C, ed. Sleep and its disorders in children. New York: Raven Press, 1987; 141–163.
Stunkard AJ, Grace WJ, Wolfe HG. The night eating syndrome. Am J Med 1955; 7: 78–86.

Hypnotic-Dependent Sleep Disorder (780.52-0)

Synonyms and Key Words: Hypnotic-dependency insomnia, sleeping-pill withdrawal, hypnotic-drug-rebound insomnia, hypnotic-induced dyssomnia.
The classes of agents that are implicated in this syndrome include, but are not limited to, benzodiazepines and barbiturates.

Essential Features:

Hypnotic-dependent sleep disorder is characterized by insomnia or excessive sleepiness that is associated with tolerance to or withdrawal from hypnotic medications.

Acute use of hypnotics for several days may result in sleeplessness upon withdrawal, which leads to continued use of the medication. Sustained use of hypnotics induces tolerance, with a decrease of the sleep-inducing effects, often leading to an increase in dosage. Partial withdrawal of medication can lead to the development of a secondary, drug-related sleep disturbance. With abrupt termination of drug therapy, severe sleeplessness can occur.

Associated Features: Many patients are apprehensive about the need to use hypnotics in order to sleep, particularly when the initial therapeutically beneficial effects start to wane. As dosages are increased to offset tolerance, daytime carryover effects can increase and may include excessive sleepiness, sluggishness, poor coordination, ataxia, slurred speech, visual-motor problems, and late-afternoon restlessness and nervousness.

Patients can become focused on the efficacy of the hypnotic, convinced that many daytime symptoms are related to how poorly they slept the previous night. Patients may consult many doctors, receive prescriptions from several physicians, and try a variety of sleep-inducing compounds.

Upon cessation of the medication, the drug blood levels can remain elevated for several days or even weeks. Sleep architecture rapidly regresses to predrug baseline values. The subjective estimate of sleep quality and quantity, however, will often be considered worse than before hypnotic therapy commenced. Daytime symptoms similar to general central nervous system-depressant withdrawal may be observed if large doses of medication have been used for a prolonged time. Abstinence from medication can induce nausea, muscle tension, aches, irritability, restlessness, and nervousness. The 24-hour withdrawal symptoms following termination or reduction of hypnotic intake predispose the patient toward perpetuation of hypnotic use in an attempt to normalize sleep and improve daytime function.

Course: In a patient who is predisposed to having insomnia, sleeplessness may be precipitated by a variety of stressful events. Hypnotic drugs used to treat the initial insomnia can perpetuate the insomnia. Increasing the hypnotic dose often provides temporary relief, but the development of tolerance may offset advantages gained. Daytime sleepiness and functional impairment can result from the increased drug dosage, and withdrawal leads to regression of objective sleep measures to the predrug baseline state. The subjective perception of rebound insomnia is considered much worse than before commencement of hypnotic therapy and often leads the patient to resume ingesting the hypnotic drug.

Predisposing Factors: A predisposition to having chronic insomnia is likely to be common in patients who develop hypnotic-induced sleep disorder. The use of hypnotics can sometimes act to aggravate or perpetuate other forms of sleep disturbance. Many patients manifest symptoms of tension, anxiety, or depression that may predispose them to the development of this sleep disorder.

Patients may be first introduced to the use of hypnotics during a hospitalization for other causes. Hypnotic use for a transient insomnia may lead to automatic renewal of the prescription even though the acute symptoms and complaints have subsided.

Prevalence: Not known.

Age of Onset: Hypnotic-dependent sleep disorder is more commonly observed in elderly patients but can begin at any age, whenever hypnotic drug use is instituted.

Sex Ratio: Hypnotic use is more common in females than in males.

Familial Pattern: None known.

Pathology: Not known.

Complications: Excessive sleepiness or profound insomnia, anxiety, nervousness, and depression may result from hypnotic-dependent sleep disorder, especially during drug withdrawal. The use of hypnotics, particularly in combination with alcohol, may lead to severe central nervous system depression. Sleep-related breathing disorders may be exacerbated by hypnotic use.

Polysomnographic Features: Polysomnographic recordings in patients using hypnotic medications chronically show disrupted sleep architecture, which can include decreased sleep stages 1, 3, and 4 and REM sleep; increased stage 2 sleep; and fragmented NREM and REM sleep, with frequent sleep-stage transitions. Electroencephalographic waveform alterations have also been noted, including decreased K complexes, decreased delta waves, increased 14- to 18-Hz "pseudospindles," and increased alpha and beta activity. REM-sleep eye movements can be reduced in number.

Upon drug withdrawal, sleep-stage measures will quickly regress to the abnormal pre-drug values. Some features, in particular waveform changes, may persist until blood levels of the drug have diminished.

The multiple sleep latency test may demonstrate increased sleepiness with chronic long-acting hypnotic use.

Other Laboratory Test Features: Blood assays can indicate persistently elevated drug levels, even during withdrawal. Daytime performance on psychomotor testing may be impaired.

Differential Diagnosis: Hypnotic-dependent sleep disorder must be differentiated from drug abuse. A mental and medical history and a detailed inquiry into the initiation and subsequent pattern of drug use are helpful for differentiating patients with hypnotic-dependent sleep disorder from malingerers, who can present with chronic tension, somatic disturbance, and a complaint of various disorders of sleep.

After withdrawal from the hypnotic medication, the patient may find that sleep returns to normal. More commonly, however, the sleep disturbance will persist. In such cases, attempts should be made to determine the etiology and to treat the sleep disorder that provoked the drug use. Hypnotic-dependent sleep disorder often occurs along with borderline personality disorder, chronic tension anxiety, or depression. Hypnotic-dependent sleep disorder then must be differentiated from psychophysiologic insomnia or a sleep disorder associated with mental disorders.

Polysomnographic monitoring will help differentiate sleep disorders due to sleep apnea syndromes, periodic limb movement disorder, or sleep-related gastroesophageal reflux. Myoclonic activity during hypnotic withdrawal must be differentiated from periodic limb movements and fragmentary myoclonus.

Diagnostic Criteria: Hypnotic-Dependent Sleep Disorder (780.52-0)

A. The patient has a complaint of insomnia or excessive sleepiness.
B. The history includes nearly daily use of a hypnotic agent for at least 3 weeks.
C. Hypnotic withdrawal is associated with exacerbation of the primary complaint, which is often judged to be worse than the original sleep problem.
D. Daytime symptoms of nausea, muscle tension, aches, restlessness, and nervousness occur during drug withdrawal.
E. Polysomnographic monitoring demonstrates either of the following:
   1. While on medication, the patient's sleep architecture is normal
   2. During withdrawal of medication, sleep latency is increased total sleep time and sleep efficiency are reduced, with reduced stages 3, 4, and REM sleep; and stage 1 and stage 2 sleep are increased
F. Other mental or medical disorders, e.g., mood disorders, cannot account for the primary symptom.
G. Other sleep disorders can be present but do not account for the primary symptom.

Minimal Criteria: A plus B plus C.

Severity Criteria:

Mild: Mild insomnia or mild excessive sleepiness, as defined on page 23.
Moderate: Moderate insomnia or moderate excessive sleepiness, as defined on page 23. Withdrawal is marked by a rebound in the subjective complaint, which is often worse than the complaint that occurred before hypnotic use.
Severe: Severe insomnia or severe excessive sleepiness, as defined on page 23. Other features of central-nervous-system-drug ingestion or withdrawal may be seen, such as performance deficits, severe anxiety, and incoordination or ataxia.

Duration Criteria:

Acute: 3 months or less.
Subacute: Longer than 3 months but less than 1 year.
Chronic: 1 year or longer.

Bibliography:

Adam K, Adamson L, Brezinova V, Hunter WM. Nitrazepam: Lastingly effective but trouble on withdrawal. Br Med J 1976; 1: 1558–1560.
Gillin JC, Spinwebber CL, Johnson LC. Rebound insomnia: A critical review. J Clin Psychopharmacol 1989; 9: 161–172.
Kales A, Bixler EO, Tan TL, Scharf MB, Kales JD. Chronic hypnotic-drug use. Ineffectiveness, drug-withdrawal insomnia, and dependence. JAMA 1974; 227: 513–517.
Kales A, Malinstrom EJ, Scharf MB, Rubin RT. Psychophysiological and biochemical changes following use and withdrawal of hypnotics. In: Kales A, ed. Sleep, physiology and pathology. Philadelphia: JB Lippincott, 1969; 331–343.
Kales A, Scharf MB, Kales JD. Rebound insomnia: A new clinical syndrome. Science 1978; 201: 1039–1041.
Kales A, Soldatos CR, Bixler EO, Kales JD. Rebound insomnia and rebound anxiety: A review. Pharmacology 1983; 26: 121–137.
Roehrs T, Kribbs N, Zorick F, Roth T. Hypnotic residual effects of benzodiazepines with repeated administration. Sleep 1986; 9: 309–316.

Stimulant-Dependent Sleep Disorder (780.52-1)

Synonyms and Key Words: Stimulant sleep suppression, drug-induced sleep disturbance, substance abuse, withdrawal syndromes, amphetamine, phenylethylamine, cocaine, stimulants.

Essential Features:

Stimulant-dependent sleep disorder *is characterized by a reduction of sleepiness or suppression of sleep by central stimulants and resultant alterations in wakefulness following drug abstinence.*

The characteristic features of the various clinical syndromes encountered are primarily dictated by whether the behavior effect is an unwanted or unrecognized effect of the drug, when the drug is employed for purposes other than the maintenance of vigilance or whether the pharmacologic agent is employed solely as a means of maintaining alertness or maintaining a drug-mediated sense of well-being.

Central stimulants encompass a wide variety of drugs, including phenylethylamines (ephedrine, amphetamines), cocaine, thyroid hormones, and various xanthine derivatives (caffeine, theophylline). Many stimulants are used for their peripheral sympathomimetic effects (decongestants, bronchodilators, antihypotensives). Others are employed for appetite suppression or for the treatment of attention-deficit disorders. Complaints of difficulty in initiating sleep are encountered when treatment is started, when dosage is increased, or when administration times are moved closer to the customary bedtime. The sleep disturbance usually ceases after chronic administration of a fixed dose of medication, with the development of cross tolerance to other agents in the same class. The cessation of chronic high-dosage administration of these agents may be associated with withdrawal symptoms (which are short lived) such as sleepiness, irritability, or lassitude. Occasionally, a clinical presentation of cyclic difficulty in initiating and maintaining sleep may be reported when administration is intermittent (as in the case of decongestants for seasonal allergy). Individuals with these forms of stimulant-induced sleep disturbance routinely call medical attention to the disorder themselves.

Individuals who self-administer or abuse central stimulants are often called to medical attention by their families or peers; because drug administration is self-directed, the behavior consequences are usually not viewed as problematic. Sustained periods of total sleep suppression are followed by periods of deep somnolence. Periods of drug administration are often associated with garrulousness and increased behavior activity but may progress to states of hypomania, paranoid ideation, and repetitive behavior (stereotypy). As tolerance to the alerting effect of the stimulant occurs, higher doses are employed and intravenous routes of administration may be used to maximize initial euphoriant effects of the drug. In the case of cocaine, generalized convulsions may occur following administration, a feature not seen with amphetamines. Ultimately, periods of high-dosage drug administration are interrupted only by periods of somnolence, which occur when exhaustion interrupts a prolonged period of total sleep suppression.

Although physiologic dependence to stimulants does occur, psychologic dependence is characteristic, and severe depression, often with suicidal ideation, may be observed following drug detoxification. Whereas tolerance to the alerting and euphoriant effects of stimulants is typical, tolerance to the mental side effects of stimulants does not occur, and paranoid ideation, stereotypic behavior, and auditory and tactile hallucinosis tend to occur at progressively lower dosages while administration is maintained.

Diagnosis is based on identification of a stimulant medication in association with a clinical disorder of sleep initiation or a cyclic pattern of total sleep suppression and excessive somnolence. A positive drug history or positive results of urine screening for drug metabolites is required for diagnosis.

Associated Features: Mental symptoms are predominant in the chronic stimulant abuser. During the period of drug administration, symptoms may closely mimic those of paranoid schizophrenia. Neurologic findings can include dilated pupils and a variety of motor disorders, with hyperactivity; tremor; and, rarely, choreiform movements. A history of repetitive behaviors (i.e., compulsive disassembly of machinery, repetitive cleaning tasks, ritualistic behaviors) with no discernible goal is often reported. Because of the frequent use of intravenous routes of administration, infectious hepatitis, acquired immunodeficiency syndrome, and systemic arteritis, particularly from intravenous amphetamine abuse, may complicate the clinical picture.

Course: During the administration of stimulants for nonalerting effects, sleep-related symptoms persist until tolerance develops or until the offending agent is discontinued. Sustained high-dosage stimulant administration is associated with social disability and antisocial behavior. Infections (especially human immunodeficiency virus), medical complications, or overdosage are typical risks in abusers of intravenously administered stimulants. Acute toxicity may result in death from cardiac arrhythmia; intracerebral hemorrhage; or, in the case of cocaine, convulsions and respiratory arrest.

Predisposing Factors: Sleep-disrupting effects of stimulants are highly individual and not entirely dose dependent. Abuse of central stimulants has no known predisposing factors. Preexistent mental illness (specifically schizophrenia and mania) are reported to enhance the probability of adverse mental reactions to stimulants.

Age of Onset: Abuse is more prevalent in adolescents and young adults.

Sex Ratio: Not known.

Familial Pattern: None known.

Pathology: None reported.

Polysomnographic Features: Stimulants increase sleep latency, decrease total sleep time, and increase spontaneous awakenings. REM latency is prolonged, and total REM time is decreased. For a given individual, the effects are dose dependent. On withdrawal, sleep latency is reduced, total sleep time is increased, and REM rebound is observed; however, the increase in REM percentage may not be observed until the second recovery night. REM latency during recovery may be markedly reduced, with associated increases in total REM time. Chronic withdrawal has not been associated with specific polysomnographic abnormalities.

The results of the multiple sleep latency test (MSLT) during withdrawal may be suggestive of narcolepsy, and drug screening may be necessary to obtain an accurate diagnosis. Patients with a prior history of stimulant treatment should not be evaluated polysomnographically for possible narcolepsy and other disorders of excessive sleepiness until a one-week period of documented drug abstinence is established.

Other Laboratory Test Features: Drug screening of body fluids reveals metabolites of phenylethylamines or cocaine. Frequently, metabolites of sedatives or anxiolytics concomitantly administered to offset untoward stimulant side effects are also present.

Differential Diagnosis: In its mild form, this disorder may be misdiagnosed as anxiety-related sleep initiation insomnia. In chronic stimulant abuse, the differential diagnosis includes schizophrenia or mania. Because stimulant abusers may attempt to obtain drugs from physicians, they may offer a history compatible with narcolepsy.

Diagnostic Criteria: Stimulant-Dependent Sleep Disorder (780.52-1)

A. The patient has a complaint of insomnia or excessive sleepiness.
B. The complaint is temporally associated with the use or withdrawal of a stimulant medication.
C. The use of stimulant medication leads to disruption of the habitual sleep period, or more than one attempt to withdraw from the stimulant leads to the development of symptoms of excessive sleepiness.
D. Polysomnographic monitoring during stimulant ingestion demonstrates:
  1. Sleep disruption with reduced sleep efficiency and an increased number and duration of awakenings
  2. Upon withdrawal of the stimulant, the MSLT demonstrates a mean sleep latency of less than 10 minutes
E. Other mental or medical disorders producing insomnia or excessive sleepiness may coexist.
F. The symptoms do not meet the criteria for other sleep disorders that produce a primary complaint of insomnia or excessive sleepiness.

Note: If the clinical features are indicative thereof, a diagnosis of psychoactive-substance dependence or abuse should be additionally stated and coded on axis C (e.g., amphetamine abuse, and the following code numbers should be used: amphetamine or similarly acting sympathomimetic abuse, 305.70; amphetamine or similarly acting sympathomimetic dependence, 304.40).

Minimal Criteria: A plus B plus C.

Severity Criteria:

Mild: Mild insomnia or mild excessive sleepiness, as defined on page 23. Few if any symptoms in excess of those required to make the diagnosis.
Moderate: Moderate insomnia or moderate excessive sleepiness, as defined on page 23. Additional non-sleep-related symptoms of stimulant use may be present, causing mild to moderate impairment.
Severe: Severe insomnia or severe excessive sleepiness, as defined on page 23. Stimulant use produces non-sleep-related symptoms that markedly interfere with occupational or social functioning.

Duration Criteria:

Acute: 3 weeks or less.
Subacute: More than 3 weeks and less than 6 months.
Chronic: 6 months or longer.

Bibliography:

Connell PH. Amphetamine psychosis. Maudsley Monograph No. 5. London: Chapman and Hall, 1958.
Ellinwood E. Amphetamine psychosis: A multidimensional process. Semin Psychiatry 1969; 1: 208–226.
Kalant OJ. Amphetamines: toxicity and addiction. Springfield, Illinois: CC Thomas 1966.
Nausieda PA. Central stimulant toxicity. In: Vinken PJ, Bruyn GW, eds. Handbook of clinical neurology. Amsterdam: Elsevier-North Holland, 1979; 37: 223–297.
Oswald I. Sleep and dependence on amphetamine and other drugs. In: Kales A, ed. Sleep: physiology and pathology. Philadelphia: Lippincott, 1969; 317–330.
Watson R, Hartmann E, Schildkraut JJ. Amphetamine withdrawal: affective state, sleep patterns, and MHPG excretion. Am J Psychiatry 1972; 129: 263–269.

Alcohol-Dependent Sleep Disorder (780.52-3)

Synonyms and Key Words: Bedtime use of alcohol, tolerance, dependence, withdrawal, overdosage, alcohol-dependency insomnia, REM sleep rebound, alcohol-induced sleep maintenance complaint. (Excludes alcoholism [303].)

Essential Features:

Alcohol-dependent sleep disorder is characterized by the sustained ingestion of ethanol for its hypnotic effect.

Ethanol-related sleep disorders are caused by the self-prescribed use of ethanol as a sedative. The patient may have underlying syndromes that cause the complaint of sleep-initiation difficulty for which the ethanol is self-prescribed. The use of ethanol begins in the late evening 3 to 4 hours before bedtime. The patient usually consumes the equivalent of 6 to 8 drinks of an alcoholic beverage (e.g., 8 ounces of 100-proof whiskey). The condition is not associated with alcoholic patterns of drinking (i.e., drinking in the waking hours) and does not cause problems for the patient in terms of socio-occupational adjustment, physical health, or family relationships.

Sustained use of ethanol as a sedative results in tolerance and a decrease of sleep-inducing effects. In addition, unrecognized periods of partial and relative withdrawal occur, which contribute to the development of a secondary ethanol-related sleep maintenance complaint. The patient often will complain of sudden arousals from dreams with sweating, headache, and a dry mouth, indicating a mild dehydration and a mild withdrawal state. If the patient discontinues the use of ethanol suddenly, severe sleeplessness that is usually not accompanied by any other general features of a drug-withdrawal syndrome can supervene.

For this condition to be diagnosed, the patient must have used ethanol on a daily basis as a bedtime hypnotic agent for a minimum of 30 days. During the period of chronic use of ethanol, the patient's nocturnal sleep is marked by frequent awakenings, each lasting several minutes.

Associated Features: Many patients with this syndrome seem to have a psychologic dependence on ethanol without marked physiologic tolerance or dependence. Some patients will report that they have little or no sleep disturbance as long as they continue to take the ethanol nightly.

Course: Patients commonly complicate their difficulties by increasing the dose or by the addition of other sedatives. It is particularly important to determine if the patient has added benzodiazepines to the nightly use of ethanol because of the obvious dangers of the combination. The severity is usually mild to moderate; the patient responds to counseling.

Predisposing Factors: Predisposing factors include the presence of any other disorder that can lead to a sleep-initiation complaint, such as restless legs syndrome, psychophysiologic insomnia, or depression.

Prevalence: Rare.

Age of Onset: Particularly frequent after the age of 40.

Sex Ratio: Not known.

Familial Pattern: Not known.

Pathology: Not known.

Complications: The condition can be life threatening if the underlying cause of the self-prescription of ethanol is a sleep apnea syndrome. Complications include the development of chronic alcoholism, although that development seems to be rare.

Polysomnographic Features: Polygraphic recordings in chronic ethanol users at these dosages will show: increases in sleep stages 3 and 4 and REM fragmentation; some increase in REM activity; and frequent awakenings and sleep-stage transitions, particularly in the latter part of the sleep period as the ethanol blood level declines.

Other Laboratory Test Features: Screening of body fluids or expired air can reveal alcohol. Liver function tests may present evidence of alcohol hepatitis in severe cases.

Differential Diagnosis: The condition has to be distinguished from chronic alcoholism. Insomnia due to other causes may be present in a patient who takes alcohol in the evening but who does not have alcohol-dependent sleep disorder.

Diagnostic Criteria: Alcohol-Dependent Sleep Disorder (780.52-3)

A. The patient has a complaint of insomnia.
B. The complaint is temporally associated with more than one attempt to withdraw from bedtime alcohol ingestion.

C. The alcohol must have been taken daily as a bedtime sleep aid for at least 30 days.
D. Polysomnographic monitoring during alcohol ingestion demonstrates both of the following:
   1. Frequent awakenings, particularly during REM sleep in the latter half of the night, when the alcohol blood level declines
   2. Increased percentage of slow-wave sleep
   3. Upon withdrawal of alcohol, more marked sleep disruption occurs, with an increased number and duration of awakenings
E. No mental or medical disorder produces the insomnia. This disorder must be distinguished from alcoholism.
F. The symptoms do not meet the criteria for other sleep disorders that produce a primary complaint of insomnia.

Minimal Criteria: A plus B plus E.

Severity Criteria:

Mild: Mild insomnia, as defined on page 23; the patient has few if any symptoms in excess of those required to make the diagnosis.
Moderate: Moderate insomnia, as defined on page 23; additional non-sleep-related symptoms of alcohol use may be present, causing mild to moderate psychosocial impairment.
Severe: Severe insomnia, as defined on page 23. Alcohol use produces non-sleep-related symptoms that markedly interfere with occupational or social functioning.

Duration Criteria:

Acute: Less than 3 months.
Subacute: More than 3 months and less than 12 months.
Chronic: 12 months or longer.

Bibliography:

Gross MM, Goodenough DR, Hasty J, Lewis E. Experimental study of sleep in chronic alcoholics before, during, and after four days of heavy drinking, with a nondrinking comparison. Ann NY Acad Sci 1973; 215: 254–265.
Johnson LC, Burdick JA, Smith J. Sleep during alcohol intake and withdrawal in the chronic alcoholic. Arch Gen Psychiatry 1970; 22: 406–418.
Pokorny AD. Sleep disturbances, alcohol, and alcoholism: A review. In: Williams RL, Karacan I, eds. Sleep disorders. Diagnosis and treatment. New York: John Wiley & Sons, 1978; 233–260.
Rundell OH, Williams HL, Lester BK. Sleep in alcoholic patients: Longitudinal findings. In: Gross MM, ed. Alcohol intoxication and withdrawal. IIIb. Studies in alcohol dependence. New York: Plenum Press, 1977; 389–402.
Williams HL, Salamy A. Alcohol and sleep. In: Kissin B, Begleiter H, eds. The biology of alcoholism. New York: Plenum Press, 1972; 435–483.
Zarcone VP. Sleep and alcoholism. In: Chase M, Weitzman ED, eds. Sleep disorders: Basic and clinical research. Advances in sleep research. New York: Spectrum, 1983; 6: 319–333.

114   EXTRINSIC SLEEP DISORDERS

Toxin-Induced Sleep Disorder (780.54-6)

Synonyms and Key Words: Toxins, heavy metals, organic toxins, poisoning, chemicals.

Essential Features:

Toxin-induced sleep disorder is characterized by either insomnia or excessive sleepiness produced by poisoning with heavy metals or organic toxins.

Substances that can produce toxin-induced sleep disorder include mercury, lead, arsenic, and copper. Chronic poisoning may result from repeated exposure to low concentrations of these substances, which can also produce sleep disturbance. Insomnia is likely to accompany generalized agitation that results from central nervous system excitation. Alternatively, central nervous system depression may cause somnolence or even coma. Both excitation and depression may be seen as consecutive phases in the same episode of poisoning.

Associated Features: The central nervous system dysfunction that causes the sleep symptoms is likely to be evidenced by other symptoms such as memory loss and changes in mental status or cardiac and respiratory function. Gastrointestinal inflammation may cause nausea, vomiting, and diarrhea. Compromise of renal, liver, and cardiac function may also occur, depending on the severity and nature of the toxicity.

Course: The course is variable, depending on the chronicity and severity of exposure to the toxin and whether consequent long-term abnormalities develop.

Predisposing Factors: Individuals working in industrial settings who routinely use toxic chemicals and substance abusers, such as glue sniffers, are most at risk. Also, children are likely to ingest certain toxic substances and can be exposed to exhaust fumes from leaded gasoline.

Prevalence: Apparently rare.

Age of Onset: Any age.

Sex Ratio: Not known.

Familial Pattern: None known.

Pathology: Many changes can occur, depending on the specific toxin. Central-nervous-system pathology is usually only seen in the most severe cases of poisoning. Fatty degeneration of the heart, liver, and kidneys and bone-marrow depression may also occur with exposure to many organic toxins.

Complications: Complications secondary to the sleep symptoms associated with these syndromes are minor relative to the organ toxicity. Renal failure, coma, and death may result in severe cases.

Polysomnographic Features: No polysomnographic information is available; however, it is expected that all-night polysomnography would show features of insomnia, including an increased sleep latency, reduced sleep efficiency, frequent awakenings, or early morning awakening. Specific electroencephalographic changes associated with the toxin may be seen. Patients with features of excessive sleepiness are expected to have objective evidence of sleepiness on the multiple sleep latency test (MSLT).

Other Laboratory Test Features: Disturbances may be noted in renal function, liver function, and in hematologic function (hemoglobin, hematocrit, white-blood-cell count, bone marrow). Measures of cardiac function may be abnormal, and nerve-conduction changes can also occur. Testing of body fluids may reveal the toxin or its metabolite (e.g., urinary lead and porphyrin levels). Serial measurement of the excretion of the toxin in the urine is often helpful in determining the course of the syndrome. Patient susceptibility to the specific toxin can vary, and clinical features may not correlate directly with the laboratory testing values. The clinical features can also be delayed up to 1 month after exposure to the toxin.

Differential Diagnosis: Sleep disorders related to the use of or withdrawal from hypnotics or stimulants must be ruled out. In patients with symptoms of excessive sleepiness, a diagnosis of idiopathic hypersomnia should also be ruled out, as should medical disorders other than those directly related to the effects of the toxin.

Diagnostic Criteria: Toxin-Induced Sleep Disorder (780.54-6)

A. The patient has a complaint of insomnia or excessive sleepiness.
B. The complaint is temporally associated with the presence of an environmental or ingested toxic agent (e.g., heavy metal or organic toxin, etc.).
C. Polysomnographic monitoring demonstrates either of the following:
   1. An increased sleep latency, reduced sleep efficiency, frequent awakenings, or an early morning awakening
   2. An MSLT that shows excessive sleepiness
D. No mental or medical disorder, other than the one associated with the toxicity, accounts for the complaint.
E. The symptoms do not meet the diagnostic criteria for any other sleep disorder causing a complaint of insomnia or excessive sleepiness.

Minimal Criteria: A plus B plus D plus E.

Severity Criteria:

Mild: Mild insomnia or mild sleepiness, as defined on page 23.
Moderate: Moderate insomnia or moderate sleepiness, as defined on page 23.
Severe: Severe insomnia or severe sleepiness, as defined on page 23.

Duration Criteria:

Acute: 7 days or less.
Subacute: More than 7 days but less than 3 months.
Chronic: 3 months or longer.

Bibliography:

Friedman PA. Poisoning and its management. In: Braunwald E, Isselbacher KJ, Petersdorf RG, Wilson JD, Martin JB, Fauel AS, eds. Harrison's principles of internal medicine, 11th ed. New York: McGraw-Hill, 1987.

Kilburn KH, Seidman BC, Warshaw R. Neurobehavioral and respiratory symptoms of formaldehyde and xylene exposure in histology technicians. Arch Environ Health 1985; 40:229–233.

Valciukas JA, Lilis R, Eisinger J, Blumberg WE, Fischbein A, Selikoff IJ. Behavioral indicators of lead neurotoxicity: Results of a clinical field survey. Int Arch Occup Environ Health 1978; 41: 217–236.

DYSSOMNIAS

CIRCADIAN-RHYTHM SLEEP DISORDERS

1. Time Zone Change (Jet Lag) Syndrome (307.45-0) 118
2. Shift Work Sleep Disorder (307.45-1)......................... 121
3. Irregular Sleep-Wake Pattern (307.45-3)...................... 125
4. Delayed Sleep-Phase Syndrome (780.55-0) 128
5. Advanced Sleep-Phase Syndrome (780.55-1) 133
6. Non-24-Hour Sleep-Wake Disorder (780.55-2)................... 137
7. Circadian Rhythm Sleep Disorder Not Otherwise Specified (780.55-9)

Circadian Rhythm Sleep Disorders

The circadian rhythm sleep disorders comprise a third section of dyssomnias and are grouped because they share a common underlying chronophysiologic basis. The major feature of these disorders is a misalignment between the patient's sleep pattern and the sleep pattern that is desired or regarded as the societal norm. When internal factors, such as neurologic disease, or external factors, such as environmental or social circumstances, produce a circadian rhythm sleep disorder, diagnostic subtypes can be specified with the diagnosis of intrinsic type or extrinsic type, respectively. Three circadian rhythm sleep disorders have intrinsic and extrinsic subtypes: delayed sleep-phase syndrome, advanced sleep-phase syndrome, and non-24-hour sleep-wake disorder.

In most circadian rhythm sleep disorders, the underlying problem is that the patient cannot sleep when sleep is desired, needed, or expected. As a result of sleep episodes occurring at inappropriate times, the corresponding wake periods may occur at undesired times. Therefore, the patient complains of insomnia or excessive sleepiness. For several of the circadian rhythm sleep disorders, once sleep is initiated, the major sleep episode is of normal duration with normal REM and non-REM cycling. However, intermittent sleep episodes may occur in some disorders, including the irregular sleep-wake pattern.

In the 1979 *Diagnostic Classification of Sleep and Arousal Disorders,* the sleep-wake schedule disorders were divided into two groups: transient and persistent disorders. This subdivision has not been retained in the *International Classification of Sleep Disorders* because the duration of a disorder can now be specified and coded separately on axis A. Consequently, the disorder "frequently changing sleep-wake schedule" is no longer a useful diagnostic entity.

For additional information on the chronophysiologic basis of this group of disorders, the reader is referred to current texts on circadian rhythms, chronobiology, and chronophysiology.

It should be pointed out that the appropriate timing of sleep within the 24-hour day can be disturbed in many other sleep disorders, particularly those disorders associated with insomnia. If the cause of the altered sleep timing is another sleep disorder, sole diagnosis should be of the specific sleep disorder; diagnosis of the associated circadian rhythm sleep disorder should not be stated. For example, patients with narcolepsy can have a pattern of sleepiness that is identical to that described as due to an irregular sleep-wake pattern. Because the primary sleep diagnosis is narcolepsy, however, the patient should not receive a second diagnosis of a circadian rhythm sleep disorder unless the disorder is unrelated to the narcolepsy. For example, a diagnosis of time zone change (jet lag) syndrome could be stated along with a diagnosis of narcolepsy, if appropriate. Similarly, patients with mood disorders or psychoses can, at times, have a sleep pattern similar to that of delayed sleep-phase syndrome. Only the primary psychiatric diagnosis should be stated, however, unless the sleep pattern is unrelated to the mental disorder or the mental disorder is in remission and the sleep disorder is the predominant diagnosis.

Some disturbance of sleep timing is a common feature of patients who have a diagnosis of inadequate sleep hygiene. Only if the timing of sleep is the predominant cause of the sleep disturbance and is outside the societal norm would a diagnosis of a circadian rhythm sleep disorder be stated. Limit-setting sleep disorder also is associated with an altered time of sleep within the 24-hour day. However, the timing of sleep in this disorder is not within the patient's control nor is it intrinsically induced. If the setting of limits is a function of a caretaker, the sleep disorder is more appropriately diagnosed within the extrinsic subsection of the dyssomnias (i.e., as a limit-setting sleep disorder).

Most of the names of the circadian rhythm sleep disorders have remained the same as those previously presented in the *Diagnostic Classification of Sleep and Arousal Disorders*. One or two minor changes have been made. The word *rapid* has been deleted from the name *rapid time zone change (jet lag) syndrome* because a rapid transit across the time zones is now implied in the name of the disorder. The simpler term *shift work sleep disorder* is preferred to the previous longer and more cumbersome term, *work shift change in conventional sleep-wake schedule.*

Time Zone Change (Jet Lag) Syndrome (307.45-0)

Synonyms and Key Words: Jet lag, transmeridian flight desynchronosis, air travel, transmeridian dyschronism.

Essential Features:

Time zone change (jet lag) syndrome consists of varying degrees of difficulties in initiating or maintaining sleep, excessive sleepiness, decrements in subjective daytime alertness and performance, and somatic symptoms (largely related to gastrointestinal function) following rapid travel across multiple time zones.

The severity and duration of the symptoms vary considerably, depending on the number of time zones crossed, the direction (east or west) of the travel, the timing of takeoff and arrival, and individual susceptibility. The sleep-wake disturbances generally abate after two to three days in the arrival location. Symptoms are often associated with, but are not entirely dependent upon, sleep deprivation. Symptoms typically last longer following eastward flights. Adaptation of the timing of physiologic functions other than sleep and waking may take eight or more days. Individuals who routinely travel back and forth across time zones (e.g., airline flight personnel, diplomats, multinational corporation executives) may experience chronic symptoms of sleep disturbance, daytime malaise, irritability, and performance impairment similar to those experienced by shift workers.

Associated Features: Social or occupational dysfunction may occur, related to decrements in daytime alertness and performance in the new time zone. Jet lag symptoms should be distinguished from the usually short-lived symptoms of dry itching eyes, irritated nasal passages, muscle cramps, headaches, nausea, abdominal distention, dependent edema, and intermittent dizziness that can occur solely or largely as a function of airplane cabin conditions and are not truly symptoms of jet lag.

Course: For most individuals, this syndrome represents an occasional minor inconvenience, which, although sometimes severe, is self-limiting, with very few apparent symptoms by the third day after the flight. Depending on the degree of sleep deprivation during the flight, sleep may be subjectively good on the first night after arrival only to deteriorate on the second and, possibly, into the third night. An alternating pattern of good and poor sleep may also occur for up to a week.

Predisposing Factors: Reports are mainly anecdotal, but some experimental evidence suggests that individuals over age 50 are more likely to suffer from jet lag than are younger individuals. Neurotic extroverts have been found to phase adjust faster than neurotic introverts and, thus, would be expected to experience less jet lag.

Prevalence: Not known.

Age of Onset: All ages are presumably susceptible, but individuals over age 50 appear to be more likely to develop jet lag than are those under age 30.

Sex Ratio: Not known.

Familial Pattern: Not known.

Pathology: After rapid air travel across several time zones, the endogenous circadian system remains aligned to the environmental time cues of the home time zone. Because the adjustment process of the circadian system is slow, averaging 60 minutes of phase adjustment per day after a phase-advance shift (eastbound flight) and 90 minutes per day after a phase-delay shift (westbound flight), symptoms can last for several days after the flight. There appears to be no difference in the amount of jet lag experienced in homeward versus outward directions per se. Daytime symptoms are thought to be caused by (1) waking behaviors suddenly occurring in the "sleepy" phases of the unadjusted sleep-wake cycle; (2) sleep disruption due to the person's attempt to sleep during the unadjusted "awake" phases of the cycle; and (3) malaise that results from the loss of harmony (dissociation) among the various rhythms governed by the circadian system, some of which phase adjust more rapidly than others.

Complications: Subjective distress about not sleeping well and social embarrassment because of falling asleep at inappropriate times may occur. Self-treatment, especially involving the use of large amounts of alcohol, may complicate the clinical picture. Menstrual irregularities in female air crew have been attributed to repeated jet lag, but clear and convincing data on this subject are lacking. Patients with bipolar (manic-depressive) disorder may experience an exacerbation, with a higher likelihood of mania following eastward flights and depression after westbound travel.

Polysomnographic Features: In general, polysomnographic studies have shown a greater number of arousals and a greater percentage of stage 1 sleep during the first two to three sleep periods after arrival compared to home-based sleep. Sleep efficiency is consequently mildly reduced, usually no more than 10% from baseline. Prolongation of sleep latency and reduction of slow-wave sleep occur quite variably, the latter possibly more dependent on age than on the time zone change itself. Most often, the second half of the sleep period is the more severely disrupted, whether the flight was eastbound or westbound.

Other Laboratory Test Features: Actigraphy may demonstrate a disrupted sleep-wake pattern consistent with time zone (jet lag) syndrome. There may be loss of the normal pattern of circadian rhythmicity, as demonstrated by 24-hour temperature or biochemical patterns.

Differential Diagnosis: In most cases, the syndrome is self-limited and does not come to clinical attention. Persistence of symptoms beyond 2 weeks after the flight suggests the probability of some other disorder producing insomnia or excessive sleepiness, such as psychophysiologic insomnia or the obstructive sleep apnea syndrome.

Diagnostic Criteria: Time Zone Change (Jet Lag) Syndrome (307.45-0)

A. The patient has a primary complaint of insomnia or excessive sleepiness.
B. There is a disruption of the normal circadian sleep-wake cycle.
C. The symptoms began within 1 or 2 days after air travel across at least two time zones.
D. At least two of the following symptoms are present:
   1. Decreased daytime performance

2. Altered appetite or gastrointestinal function
   3. An increase in the frequency of nocturnal awakenings to urinate
   4. General malaise
E. Polysomnography and the multiple sleep latency test demonstrate loss of a normal sleep-wake pattern evidence (i.e., a disturbed chronobiologic rhythmicity).
F. No medical or mental disorder accounts for the symptoms.
G. The symptoms do not meet criteria for any other sleep disorder producing insomnia or excessive sleepiness (e.g., shift-work sleep disorder).

Minimal Criteria: A plus C.

Severity Criteria:

Mild: Mild insomnia or mild excessive sleepiness, as defined on page 23.
Moderate: Moderate insomnia or moderate excessive sleepiness, as defined on page 23.
Severe: Severe insomnia or severe excessive sleepiness, as defined on page 23.

Duration Criteria:

Acute: 7 days or less.
Subacute: More than 7 days but less than 3 months; symptoms are associated with more than one episode of time-zone change.
Chronic: 3 months or longer; symptoms are associated with multiple episodes of time-zone change.

Bibliography:

Aschoff J, Hoffman K, Pohl H, Wever R. Re-entrainment of circadian rhythms after phase shifts of the Zeitgeber. Chronobiologia 1975; 2: 23–78.
Sleep and wakefulness in international aircrews. Aviat Space Environ Med 1986; 57: whole supplement.
Klein KE, Wegmann HM, Hunt BI. Desynchronization of body temperature and performance circadian rhythm as a result of outgoing and homecoming transmeridian flights. Aerospace Med 1972; 43: 119–132.
Sasaki M, Endo S, Nakagawa S, Kitahara T, Mori A. A chronobiological study on the relation between time zone changes and sleep. Jikeiaki Med J 1985; 32: 83–100.
Winget CM, DeRoshia CW, Markley CL, Holley DC. A review of human physiological and performance changes associated with desynchronosis of biological rhythms. Aviat Space Environ Med 1984; 55: 1085–1096.

Shift Work Sleep Disorder (307.45-1)

Synonyms and Key Words: Night shift, irregular work hours, transient insomnia, transient excessive sleepiness, "work-shift" change in conventional sleep-wake schedule, acute-phase shift of sleep, frequently changing sleep-wake schedule.

Essential Features:

***Shift work sleep disorder** consists of symptoms of insomnia or excessive sleepiness that occur as transient phenomena in relation to work schedules.*

The work is usually scheduled during the habitual hours of sleep (i.e., shift work–rotating or permanent shifts), roster work, or irregular work hours. The sleep complaint typically consists of an inability to maintain a normal sleep duration when the major sleep episode is begun in the morning (6 a.m. to 8 a.m.) after a night shift. The reduction in sleep length usually amounts to one to four hours (mainly affecting REM and stage 2 sleep). Subjectively, the sleep period is perceived as unsatisfactory and unrefreshing. The insomnia appears despite the patient's attempts to optimize environmental conditions for sleep. The condition usually persists for the duration of the work-shift period. Early morning work shifts (starting between 4 a.m. and 7 a.m.) may also be associated with complaints of difficulty in sleep initiation as well as difficulty in awakening. Work on permanent evening shifts can be associated with difficulties initiating the major sleep episode. Excessive sleepiness usually occurs during shifts (mainly night) and is associated with the need to nap and impaired mental ability because of the reduced alertness.

Associated Features: Reduced alertness, which occurs not only during the work shift, may be associated with reduced performance capacity, with consequences for safety. Also, major portions of the individual's free time may have to be used for recovery of sleep, which in many cases will have negative social consequences such as marital disharmony and impaired social relationships. There have also been reports of increased irritability, presumably related to the lack of sleep or to the conflict between demands for sleep and demands for social activities.

Course: The course is closely associated with the shift schedule. There can be improvement in symptoms after the first week of a new shift, but the symptoms usually persist to some degree until a conventional daytime shift is established. After rotation to another shift from the night shift, sleep-onset disorders rather than maintenance difficulties can occur for several days. Adaptation rarely occurs despite many years of night-shift work, in part because of resumption of full daytime activities and nighttime sleep during weekends and vacations.

Predisposing Factors: It is known that a normal, full sleep episode during the daytime becomes more difficult with increasing age. Also, individuals described as morning types appear to obtain shorter daytime sleep after a night shift. Presumably, individuals with a strong need for stable hours of sleep may be at particular risk.

Prevalence: The prevalence depends on the prevalence of shift work in the population. It appears that most individuals experience sleep difficulties after a night shift. Depending on which country is considered, between 5% and 8% of the population is exposed to night work on a regular or irregular basis. Thus, a prevalence of shift work sleep disturbance of 2% to 5% may be a reasonable estimate. These figures, however, do not involve individuals with early morning work, which may comprise another group at risk.

Age of Onset: Variable, depending upon the age at which shift work is commenced.

Sex Ratio: None known.

Familial Pattern: None known.

Pathology: No known anatomic or biochemical pathology has been described. The condition is directly related to the circadian interference with sleep during the morning and evening, which conflicts with the shift worker's need to sleep at these times. The excessive sleepiness during night work appears to be partly related to the lack of sleep and partly related to the conflict between the requirement of working at night and the circadian sleepiness propensity during the night hours.

Complications: It is hypothesized that the condition may lead to chronic sleep disturbances, although very little empirical evidence is available. Gastrointestinal disorders may be exacerbated or produced by the effects of shift work. There are also indications that cardiovascular disease may result. Disruptions of social and family life are frequent. Drug and alcohol dependency may result from attempts to improve the sleep and decrease the wakefulness disturbances produced by shift work.

Polysomnographic Features: The disorder is usually able to be diagnosed by history. Polysomnographic recordings may be useful if the sleep disorder is severe or the etiology of the sleep disturbance is in question. Ideally, the sleep recording is performed during the habitual "shifted" sleep period and in the work environment of the individual. A 24-hour recording over the first and last of the series of rotating shifts should be performed. Monitoring of an episode of usual daytime wakefulness and night sleep during a daytime shift is ideal for comparative purposes. If excessive sleepiness is part of the complaint, a multiple sleep latency test should be carried out in the standard manner at least three times: at the beginning, middle, and end of the work shift.

If field (at home and at work) polysomnography is not feasible, an alternative evaluation involves polysomnography in the sleep laboratory during simulated shift work sleep and wake patterns. One night of recording is performed during the habitual sleep period, followed by an MSLT performed over a period that conforms to the work shift. Polysomnography may demonstrate impaired quality of the habitual sleep period, with either a prolonged sleep latency or shortened total sleep time, depending on the timing of the sleep period in relation to the underlying phase of the circadian timing system. The sleep period may be fragmented, with frequent arousals and awakenings. The MSLT may demonstrate excessive sleepiness during the time of the work shift.

Other Laboratory Test Features: Actigraphy may be helpful to demonstrate a disrupted sleep-wake pattern consistent with shift work sleep disorder. There may be a loss of the normal pattern of circadian rhythmicity, as demonstrated by 24-hour temperature or biochemical patterns.

Differential Diagnosis: Sleep disturbances before early morning work may be mistaken for another disorder of initiating sleep, whereas the disturbance after the night shift might be mistaken for another disorder of sleep maintenance. The excessive sleepiness should be differentiated from that due to narcolepsy or sleep apnea syndrome. Sometimes, patients with sleep disorders such as narcolepsy tend to adopt shift work as an attempt to rationalize symptoms of excessive sleepiness. Conversely, patients suffering from insomnia may adopt nighttime work patterns. Furthermore, both the insomnia and the excessive sleepiness might be mistakenly attributed to a persistent circadian rhythm sleep disorder. However, historic information on the relation between the occurrence of disturbed sleep and work-hour distribution should provide sufficient information to indicate the correct diagnosis. Drug- and alcohol-dependency sleep disorders can occur concomitantly.

Diagnostic Criteria: Shift Work Sleep Disorder (307.45-1)

A. The patient has a primary complaint of insomnia or excessive sleepiness.
B. The primary complaint is temporally associated with a work period (usually night work) that occurs during the habitual sleep phase.
C. Polysomnography and the MSLT demonstrate loss of a normal sleep-wake pattern (i.e., disturbed chronobiologic rhythmicity).
D. No medical or mental disorder accounts for the symptoms.
E. The symptoms do not meet criteria for any other sleep disorder producing insomnia or excessive sleepiness (e.g., time-zone change [jet lag] syndrome).

Minimal Criteria: A plus B.

Severity Criteria:

Mild: Mild insomnia or mild excessive sleepiness, as defined on page 23; the sleep deficit is often one to two hours.
Moderate: Moderate insomnia or moderate excessive sleepiness, as defined on page 23; the sleep deficit is often two to three hours.
Severe: Severe insomnia or severe excessive sleepiness, as defined on page 23; the sleep deficit is greater than three hours.

Duration Criteria:

Acute: 7 days or less.
Subacute: More than 7 days but less than 3 months.
Chronic: 3 months or longer.

Bibliography:

Coleman RM, Dement WC. Falling asleep at work: a problem for continuous operations. Sleep Res 1986; 15: 265.
Foret J, Benoit O. Shift work: The level of adjustment to schedule reversal assessed by a sleep study. Waking Sleeping 1978; 2: 107–112.
Tilley AJ, Wilkinson RT, Warren PS, Watson B, Drud M. The sleep and performance of shift workers. Human Factors 1982; 24: 629–641.
Torsvall L, Akerstedt T. Sleepiness on the job: Continuously measured EEG changes in train drivers. Electroencephalogr Clin Neurophysiol 1987; 66: 502–511.
Walsh JK, Tepas DI, Moss PD. The EEG sleep of night and rotating shift workers. In: Johnson LC, Tepas DI, Colquhoun WP, Colligan MJ, eds. Biological rhythms, sleep and shift work. New York: SP Medical & Specific Books, 1981; 347–356.

Irregular Sleep-Wake Pattern (307.45-3)

Synonyms and Key Words: No circadian rhythm, disregard of zeitgebers, grossly disturbed sleep-wake rhythm, low-amplitude circadian rhythms.

Essential Features:

Irregular sleep-wake pattern consists of temporally disorganized and variable episodes of sleeping and waking behavior.

Although patients with irregular sleep-wake patterns may have a total 24-hour average sleep time that is within normal limits for age, no single sleep period is of normal length, and the likelihood of being asleep at any particular time of day is unpredictable. Depending on the source of the sleep complaint, the clinical manifestation may be inability to initiate and maintain sleep at night, frequent daytime napping, or both. Ambulatory patients living in the community may emphasize the nocturnal insomnia and view the daytime napping as a necessary result of their difficulty at night. The nighttime caretakers of institutionalized patients with this disorder may resort to physical or chemical restraints to control concomitant symptoms of nocturnal wandering and agitation, while the family of the same patient complains that the patient is seldom awake when they come to visit.

Unlike in patients with the advanced sleep-phase, delayed sleep-phase, and non-24-hour syndromes, a well-kept sleep-wake log by patients with this disorder shows no recognizable ultradian or circadian patterns of sleep onset or wake time. Instead, sleep is broken up into three or more short blocks in each 24 hours, with marked day-to-day variability in the timing of sleep and wakefulness. The pattern is reminiscent of that of newborn infants, except that sleep occupies a much smaller fraction of the 24-hour day in patients with this disorder than in infants.

Associated Features: Subjective cognitive impairment and sleepiness characterize the awake intervals between the sleep episodes, particularly in ambulatory outpatients. The syndrome is probably most common in patients with severe congenital, developmental, or degenerative brain dysfunction, but rare cases have been described in cognitively intact patients who have ceased adhering to a clear rest-activity pattern, spend extremely excessive time in bed, and may not adhere even to a regular pattern of eating. Rhythms of endocrine, temperature, and other functions that normally display regular circadian periodicity may lose their expected fluctuations and show flattened amplitudes. Neither the cognitively intact nor the impaired have any understanding that the napping and insomnia may be mutually reinforcing.

Course: The condition tends to be chronic, punctuated by futile diagnostic and treatment efforts, the latter including the use of hypnotic and analeptic medication.

Predisposing Factors: Diffuse brain dysfunction, especially if the patient's environment lacks a regular and unvarying daily routine, may predispose patients to developing this condition. Cognitively intact individuals who are in a position to spend excessive time in bed and nap frequently may also be at risk. Chronically depressed patients occasionally show this pattern, and patients who have undergone prolonged enforced bed rest for medical reasons may develop it.

Prevalence: The disorder is apparently rare in the general population. The prevalence in patients with diffuse brain dysfunction is unknown, but the syndrome is probably not uncommon in severely impaired, institutionalized patients.

Age of Onset: Presumably dependent on the age of onset of diffuse brain dysfunction.

Sex Ratio: Not known.

Familial Pattern: None, although many degenerative brain diseases, including senile dementia of the Alzheimer's type, have known or suspected familial or genetic patterns of occurrence.

Pathology: In patients with diffuse brain disease, an irregular sleep-wake pattern may be the result of pathologic involvement of either the endogenous circadian timing system or the systems governing sleep and wakefulness that receive the output of the timing system, or both. In neurologically intact patients, the pattern is presumably initiated by an initial voluntary failure to attend to conventional social and environmental time cues; the pattern is then perpetuated by ongoing nocturnal insomnia and frequent daytime napping.

Complications: Significant drug dependence or toxicity may occur, the former more likely in cognitively intact outpatients, the latter in elderly patients with chronic brain dysfunction.

Polysomnographic Features: Polysomnographic confirmation of this syndrome has seldom been reported, and all reported cases have been of patients with varying but generally severe degrees of diffuse brain dysfunction. Continuous polygraphic recordings lasting 72 hours or longer and in the presence of conventional social and environmental time cues show variable and irregular periods of sleep and wakefulness. In some cases, evidence of a "skeletal" circadian pattern may be present in the form of either short (two- to three-hour) sleep or wakeful periods that reoccur at nearly the same time each day. Frequent, around-the-clock behavioral state ratings by trained observers or ambulatory wrist actigraphic monitoring for several consecutive days may yield adequate data to confirm the diagnosis in institutionalized or homebound patients. The sleep electroencephalogram may show a paucity of sleep spindles or K-complexes, as well as reduced or absent slow-wave sleep, particularly in the elderly patient with degenerative brain disease.

Other Laboratory Test Features: Brain-imaging tests may demonstrate the presence of intracerebral pathology in patients with the intrinsic form of the disorder.

Differential Diagnosis: In cognitively intact patients, this condition should be differentiated on historic grounds from shift work sleep disorder, in which similar symptoms may be present if the patient's work schedule changes frequently. For example, police and fire departments often use rapidly shifting work schedules. The inability to nap in the daytime separates many, if not most, patients with insomnia associated with other causes. Occasionally, patients with clear-cut narcolepsy display a sleep and nap pattern that resembles the irregular sleep-wake pattern.

Diagnostic Criteria: Irregular Sleep-Wake Pattern (307.45-3)

A. The patient has a complaint of either insomnia or excessive sleepiness.
B. The patient has an irregular pattern of at least three sleep episodes during a 24-hour period.
C. The sleep pattern has been present for at least three months.
D. Total average sleep time per 24-hour period is normal for age.
E. Disturbed chronobiologic rhythmicity is demonstrated by either of the following:
   1. Continuous polysomnographic monitoring for at least 24 hours shows a loss of the normal sleep-wake pattern
   2. Continuous temperature monitoring for at least 24 hours shows a loss of the normal temperature
F. No medical or mental disorder accounts for the symptom.
G. The symptoms do not meet the criteria for any other sleep disorder causing insomnia or excessive sleepiness.

Note: If the sleep disorder is believed to be socially or environmentally induced, state and code as irregular sleep-wake pattern (extrinsic type). If there is evidence that the sleep disorder is due to an abnormal circadian pacemaker, its entrainment mechanism, or brain dysfunction, state and code as irregular sleep-wake pattern (intrinsic type).

Minimal Criteria: A plus B plus C, or B plus E.

Severity Criteria:

Mild: Mild insomnia or mild excessive sleepiness, as defined on page 23.
Moderate: Moderate insomnia or moderate excessive sleepiness, as defined on page 23.
Severe: Severe insomnia or severe excessive sleepiness, as defined on page 23.

Duration Criteria:

Acute: 6 months or less.
Subacute: 6 to 12 months.
Chronic: 1 year or longer.

Bibliography:

Allen SR, Seiler WO, Stahelin HB, Spiegel R. Seventy-two hour polygraphic and behavioral recordings of wakefulness and sleep in a hospital geriatric unit: comparison between demented and nondemented patients. Sleep 1987; 10: 143–159.

Hauri P. The sleep disorders. Michigan: The Upjohn Company, 1977; 10–12.

Okawa M, Takahashi K, Sasaki H. Disturbance of circadian rhythms in severely brain-damaged patients correlated with CT findings. J Neurol 1986; 233: 274–282.

Wagner DR. Sleep (in Alzheimer's disease). Generations--J West Gerontol Soc 1984; 9(2): 31–37.

Delayed Sleep-Phase Syndrome (780.55-0)

Synonyms and Key Words: Phase lag, phase delay, sleep-onset insomnia, morning sleepiness, stable asynchrony relative to typical environmental pattern.

Essential Features:

Delayed sleep-phase syndrome is a disorder in which the major sleep episode is delayed in relation to the desired clock time, resulting in symptoms of sleep-onset insomnia or difficulty in awakening at the desired time.

Delayed sleep-phase syndrome (DSPS) is marked by: (1) sleep-onset and wake times that are intractably later than desired, (2) actual sleep-onset times at nearly the same daily clock hour, (3) little or no reported difficulty in maintaining sleep once sleep has begun, (4) extreme difficulty awakening at the desired time in the morning, and (5) a relatively severe to absolute inability to advance the sleep phase to earlier hours by enforcing conventional sleep and wake times. Typically, the patients complain primarily of chronic difficulty in falling asleep until between 2 a.m. and 6 a.m. or difficulty awakening at the desired or necessary time in the morning to fulfill social or occupational obligations. Daytime sleepiness, especially in the morning hours, occurs variably, depending largely on the degree of sleep loss that ensues due to the patient's attempts to meet his or her social obligations by getting up "on time." When not obliged to maintain a strict schedule (e.g., on weekends or during vacations), the patient sleeps normally but at a delayed phase relative to local time.

Associated Features: Patients with DSPS are usually perplexed that they cannot find a way to fall asleep more quickly. Their efforts to advance the timing of sleep onset (early bedtime, help from family or friends in getting up in the morning, relaxation techniques, or the ingestion of hypnotic medications) yield little permanent success. Hypnotics in normal doses are often described as having little or no effect at all in aiding sleep onset and may only aggravate the daytime symptoms of difficulty awakening and sleepiness. Chronic dependence on hypnotics or alcohol for sleep is unusual but, when present, complicates the clinical situation. More commonly, patients give a history of having tried multiple sedating agents, which were abandoned because of only transient efficacy.

Patients with DSPS typically score high as "night people" on the owl-lark questionnaire and state that they feel and function best and are most alert during the late evening and night hours. In pure cases of DSPS, a carefully kept sleep-wake log documents a consistent pattern of sleep onsets, usually later than 2 a.m.; few to no awakenings once sleep is achieved; curtailed sleep during the work or school week (if the patient has not given up on getting up); and lengthy (9- to 12-hour) sleeps, with late morning to midafternoon arising times on weekends. In cases where the clinical situation is complicated by chronic alcohol or hypnotic use or abuse, or in the context of major mental difficulties, sleep-wake logs may also show frequent awakenings during the delayed sleep period. Sleep-wake logs obtained during periods when morning social obligations are lessened or absent (vacations, long weekends, unemployment, school suspension) show fairly consistent, but also consistently "late," sleep and arising times.

Although some degree of psychopathology is present in about half of adult patients with DSPS, there appears to be no particular psychiatric diagnostic category into which these patients fall. Psychopathology is not particularly more common in DSPS patients compared to patients with other forms of "insomnia." In adolescents, failure to cooperate with a plan to reschedule the patient's sleep may be a sign of clinical depression.

Course: The duration of DSPS symptomatology varies from months to decades in cases reported in the literature. Adolescence appears to be a particularly vulnerable life stage for the development of the syndrome. However, the histories of some adult patients extend back to early childhood, and pediatric sleep clinicians have described prepubertal children with the syndrome.

When DSPS occurs in the context of severe psychopathology or is complicated by sedative or alcohol abuse, the course may be quite protracted and the symptoms may be refractory to behavioral intervention until these complicating factors are dealt with specifically.

Predisposing Factors: Many DSPS patients report that their difficulties began after a period of late-night studying or partying, or after employment on the evening or night shift, following which they found it impossible to resume sleeping on a conventional schedule despite the resumption of conventional work or school hours. DSPS may be induced by alterations in the photoperiod, such as is seen in individuals living at latitudes above the Arctic Circle. In such cases, the onset of the disorder is precipitated by the dark period of the seasonal light-dark cycle.

Prevalence: The exact prevalence is unknown, but the disorder is probably uncommon, representing a small proportion (5% to 10%) of patients presenting to sleep disorders centers with the complaint of insomnia. The prevalence in the general population is unknown. One survey study of adolescents found evidence suggesting a 7% prevalence in this age group. There may be individuals who adapt to the pattern by taking evening or night jobs.

Age of Onset: Adolescence appears to be the most common period of life for the onset of DSPS, but childhood cases have been reported. Onset after age 30 is rare.

Sex Ratio: Case series in the literature have varied between a 10:1 male:female ratio in adolescents to 1:1 in a mixed series of adults and adolescents.

Familial Pattern: None known.

Pathology: The current understanding of the pathophysiology of DSPS rests on the application of the principles of phase-response curves, largely derived from experiments in lower animals, to the human sle
are thought to have a relatively weak ability to
tems in response to normal environmental
sources of sleep-onset delay (late-night studyi
illnesses), which are ordinarily dealt with wit
normal phase-response capability, unmask thi
patient with DSPS. That some ability to phase
strated by the regular, albeit late-to-bed-late-
adopt during vacations.

Complications: Occupational, school, a
degrees are a typical accompaniment of DSI
that brings the patient to clinical attention. A
poorly tolerated in the school and day-shift
DSPS come to be regarded as lazy, unmotiv
peers, and superiors in the business or scho
otherwise good social and mental function
clinical depression, or vice versa, is unkno
erable despair and hopelessness over sleepi
alcohol use or abuse accompanies some ca

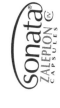

Polysomnographic Features: The
polysomnographic recordings of patients
greater than 30 minutes) sleep latency when the recordings
patients' habitual sleeping hours (e.g., 4 a.m. to noon). Sleep efficiencies tend to be somewhat low for age (75% to 85%), but most of the inefficiency is due to the prolonged sleep latency. Some patients have modest shortening of the REM latency (e.g., to 50 to 70 minutes). Sleep is largely free of arousals once the patient is asleep. Sleep architecture and amount are also within normal limits for age in

cases that are not complicated by concurrent drug or alcohol use or a major mental disorder. No pathologies of sleep (e.g., sleep apnea syndrome or periodic limb movement disorder) that could account for the complaints of insomnia and daytime sleepiness are present.

When patients are recorded at the socially acceptable or preferred time, that is earlier than their habitual sleep time (e.g., 11 p.m. to 7 a.m.), the sleep latency is prolonged and the patients experience difficulty in awakening. A multiple sleep latency test (MSLT) performed after such a sleep period can show shorter sleep latencies on the morning naps compared to the afternoon naps.

Other Laboratory Test Features: Continuous core body temperature monitoring in a small group of DSPS patients who were sleeping on their habitual schedules showed that their average absolute low temperature values occurred at or after the mid-low phase (midpoint of that portion of the rhythm below the mean) of the temperature rhythm. By contrast, in normal age- and sex-matched subjects, the absolute low temperature occurred before the mid-low phase.

Differential Diagnosis: A pattern of delayed sleep onset occurs in some previously unaffected individuals with the start of major mental disturbances, in particular in the excited phase of bipolar affective disorder and during schizophrenic decompensations. In bipolar mania, however, sleep is also typically shortened, and such patients have no difficulty arising at a conventional hour. In addition, the delayed sleep pattern is usually transient in major mental disorders and covaries with the mental symptoms in severity over time. Persistence of phase-delayed sleep after remission of the mental symptoms suggests that the patient has DSPS that was unmasked by the initial mental disturbance.

Patients with DSPS should also be differentiated from individuals who habitually go to sleep and awaken late for social reasons but then complain of sleep-onset insomnia and difficult morning awakening on the sporadic days that they must go to bed and get up early. Such individuals suffer instead from a transient sleep-wake-cycle disturbance, compounded by sleep loss, which usually accompanies an acute-phase shift. Such cases are better categorized as inadequate sleep hygiene. Reestablishment of a regular, more conventional sleep schedule achieves rapid and appreciable success in the transient case, whereas it is ineffective in DSPS.

A chronic pattern of sleep-phase delay is sometimes seen in patients with nocturnal panic attack or in phobic, avoidant, and introverted individuals. With such patients, it may be difficult to decide whether sleeping late represents avoidance of social interaction or a wholly independent process (i.e., DSPS). A history of stable entrainment at earlier, more-conventional hours (e.g., at camp, in the military, or during a hospitalization) at any time during the period of DSPS symptoms strongly suggests that the patient has a normal endogenous phase-resetting capacity and that DSPS is therefore unlikely.

Another important differentiation is from non-24-hour sleep-wake syndrome, in which incremental sequential delays of the sleep phase occur even during periods of vacation or unemployment. Although a pattern of sequential phase delays of sleep onset can also occur in patients with DSPS, the delays are smaller (0.5 to

2 hours), phase advances appear in the pattern every few days, and patients with DSPS can maintain a stable sleep-wake period at or close to 24 hours during vacations, etc. In either syndrome, occasional noncircadian days may occur (i.e., sleep is "skipped" for an entire day and night plus some portion of the following day), followed by a sleep period lasting 12 to 18 hours.

Cases of insufficient nocturnal sleep, in which most of the sleep curtailment is due to voluntarily staying up late, may be confused with DSPS. In general, insufficient sleepers do not stay up as late as do patients with DSPS, although they may sleep as late into the day on weekends. However, most insufficient sleepers complain of daytime sleepiness in the afternoon and evening rather than in the morning, as do patients with DSPS. In addition, nocturnal polysomnographic sleep latency in insufficient sleepers is normal to short, and an increase in delta sleep is also often present.

A number of sleep disorders that are nearly exclusive to childhood must be differentiated from childhood-onset DSPS in children with complaints of sleep-onset insomnia. These sleep disorders include limit-setting sleep disorder, sleep-onset association disorder, and idiopathic insomnia. Differentiation can usually be made on the basis of history and polysomnographic study.

Diagnostic Criteria: Delayed Sleep-Phase syndrome (780.55-0)

A. The patient has a complaint of an inability to fall asleep at the desired clock time, an inability to awaken spontaneously at the desired time of awakening, or excessive sleepiness.
B. There is a phase delay of the major sleep episode in relation to the desired time for sleep.
C. The symptoms are present for at least 1 month.
D. When not required to maintain a strict schedule (e.g., vacation time), patients will exhibit all of the following:
   1. Have a habitual sleep period that is sound and of normal quality and duration
   2. Awaken spontaneously
   3. Maintain stable entrainment to a 24-hour sleep-wake pattern at a delayed phase
E. Sleep-wake logs that are maintained daily for a period of at least two weeks must demonstrate evidence of a delay in the timing of the habitual sleep period.
F. One of the following laboratory methods must demonstrate a delay in the timing of the habitual sleep period:
   1. Twenty-four-hour polysomnographic monitoring (or by means of two consecutive nights of polysomnography and an intervening multiple sleep latency test)
   2. Continuous temperature monitoring showing that the time of the absolute temperature nadir is delayed into the second half of the habitual (delayed) sleep episode
G. The symptoms do not meet the criteria for any other sleep disorder causing inability to initiate sleep or excessive sleepiness.

Note: If the sleep disorder is believed to be socially or environmentally induced, state and code as delayed sleep-phase syndrome (extrinsic type). If there is evidence that the sleep disorder is due to an abnormal circadian pacemaker or its entrainment mechanism, state and code as delayed sleep-phase syndrome (intrinsic type).

Minimal Criteria: A plus B plus C plus D plus E.

Severity Criteria:

Mild: The patient has a habitual inability to fall asleep within a mean of two hours of the desired sleep time, over at least a one-month period, and the disorder is associated with little or mild impairment of social or occupational functioning.

Moderate: The patient has a habitual inability to fall asleep within a mean of three hours of the desired sleep time, over at least a one-month period, and the disorder is associated with moderate impairment of social or occupational functioning.

Severe: The patient has a habitual inability to fall asleep within a mean of four hours of the desired sleep time, over at least a one-month period, and the disorder is associated with severe impairment of social or occupational functioning.

Duration Criteria:

Acute: 3 months or less.
Subacute: More than 3 months but less than 1 year.
Chronic: 1 year or longer.

Bibliography:

Czeisler CA, Richardson GS, Coleman RM, et al. Chronotherapy: resetting the circadian clock of patients with delayed sleep phase insomnia. Sleep 1981; 4: 1–21.

Lingjaerde O, Bratlid T, Hansen T. Insomnia during the "dark period" in northern Norway. An explorative, controlled trial with light treatment. Acta Psychiatr Scand 1985; 71: 506–512.

Thorpy MJ, Korman E, Spielman AJ, Glovinsky PB. Delayed sleep-phase syndrome in adolescents. J Adolesc Health Care 1988; 9: 22–27.

Weitzman ED, Czeisler CA, Coleman RM, et al. Delayed sleep-phase syndrome. A chronobiological disorder with sleep-onset insomnia. Arch Gen Psychiatry 1981; 38: 737–746.

Advanced Sleep-Phase Syndrome (780.55-1)

Synonyms and Key Words: Phase advance, stable asynchrony relative to typical environmental patterns, evening somnolence and early morning wakefulness, extreme larkishness.

Essential Features:

Advanced sleep-phase syndrome is a disorder in which the major sleep episode is advanced in relation to the desired clock time, resulting in symptoms of compelling evening sleepiness, an early sleep onset, and an awakening that is earlier than desired.

Advanced sleep-phase syndrome is marked by a patient's intractable and chronic inability to delay the onset of evening sleep or extend sleep later into the morning hours by enforcing more conventional social sleep and wake times. The major presenting complaint may concern either the inability to stay awake in the evening, or early morning awakening insomnia, or both. Unlike other sleep maintenance disorders, the early morning awakening occurs after a normal amount of otherwise undisturbed sleep. In pure cases, there is no major mood disturbance during the waking hours. Unlike in other causes of excessive sleepiness, daytime school or work activities are not affected by somnolence. However, evening activities are routinely curtailed by the need to retire much earlier than the social norm. Typical sleep-onset times are between 6 p.m. and 8 p.m., and no later than 9 p.m., and wake times are between 1 a.m. and 3 a.m., and no later than 5 a.m. These sleep-onset and wake times occur despite the patient's best efforts to delay sleep to later hours.

Associated Features: Negative personal or social consequences may occur due to leaving activities in the early to midevening hours in order to go to sleep. Attempts to delay sleep onset to a time later than usual may result in falling asleep during social gatherings, or may have more serious consequences, such as drowsiness or falling asleep while driving in the evening. Afflicted individuals who attempt to work evening or night shifts would presumably have marked difficulty staying awake during the evening and early morning hours. If patients are chronically forced to stay up later for social or vocational reasons, the early-wakening aspect of the syndrome could lead to chronic sleep deprivation and daytime sleepiness or napping.

Course: Not known.

Predisposing Factors: None known.

Prevalence: Apparently rare.

Age of Onset: Given the apparent shortening of the endogenous period of the circadian timing system that accompanies aging, advance sleep-phase syndrome is theoretically more likely to occur in elderly individuals.

Sex Ratio: Not known.

Familial Pattern: None known.

Pathology: Patients with advanced sleep-phase syndrome have only rarely come to clinical attention, and no particular anatomic or biochemical pathology has been described. The disorder is presumed to be the converse of the delayed sleep-phase syndrome in terms of circadian-system pathophysiology (i.e., a partially deficient phase-delay capability resulting in the symptoms of evening sleepiness and early morning awakening). However, almost all normal humans studied in time-isolation facilities have shown endogenous timing systems with periods of longer than 24 hours, implying that the normal task of synchronizing to the 24-hour day may require only a phase-advance capability. Thus, alternative explanations of advanced sleep-phase syndrome might include an inherently "fast" endogenous circadian timing system or a too-powerful or oversensitive phase-advance capability.

Complications: See Associated Features.

Polysomnographic Features: In order to determine the sleep-wake cycle, polysomnography is best performed over two consecutive nights, with an intervening multiple sleep latency test (MSLT). The first night is performed over the patient's habitual sleep period (e.g., 7 p.m.-2 a.m.), as ascertained from a sleep-wake log. The MSLT should begin two hours after the patient's time of habitual awakening. (Alternatively, the MSLT can be performed over a period terminating two hours before bedtime of the second night of recording.) The second night of polysomnography should commence at the patient's desired bedtime and extend to the desired time of awakening (e.g., 11 p.m.-7 a.m).

During the first night of recording, the patient's sleeping hours, sleep onset, sleep latency (less than 20 minutes), sleep staging, and sleep duration are normal for age. The MSLT demonstrates normal daytime alertness (mean sleep latency greater than 10 minutes), with normal sleep latency on the first nap two hours after spontaneous awakening. (If the MSLT is performed in the alternative manner as described above, the sleep latency on the last nap will be normal or short in duration.) The second night of recording will demonstrate an initial sleep latency that is normal or short in duration and a prolonged period of wakefulness at the end of the recording, with normal sleep before the terminal awakening.

Other Laboratory Test Features: None helpful.

Differential Diagnosis: A mild degree of phase-advanced sleep may be a normal accompaniment of the aging process and may account for the early awakening pattern of many elderly individuals. The early morning awakening of patients with major affective disorder, which actually occurs in only about one third of such patients, is usually accompanied by other sleep and somatic symptoms and altered mood. Polysomnography in depressed patients is typically abnormal, with diminished to absent slow-wave sleep, shortened latency to the first REM period, and numerous awakenings. The inability to sleep late differentiates patients with advanced sleep-phase syndrome from those with insufficient nocturnal sleep, in which evening sleepiness and napping are common.

Diagnostic Criteria: Advanced Sleep-Phase Syndrome (780.55-1)

A. The patient complains of an inability to stay awake until the desired bedtime or an inability to remain asleep until the desired time of awakening.
B. There is a phase advance of the major sleep episode in relation to the desired time for sleep.
C. The symptoms are present for at least three months.
D. When not required to remain awake until the desired (later) bedtime, patients will exhibit the following findings:
  1. Have a habitual sleep period that is of normal quality and duration, with a sleep onset earlier than desired
  2. Awaken spontaneously earlier than desired
  3. Maintain stable entrainment to a 24-hour sleep-wake pattern
D. Polysomnographic monitoring during a 24- to 36-hour period demonstrates an advance in the timing of the habitual sleep period.
E. The symptoms do not meet the criteria for any other disorder causing inability to maintain sleep or excessive sleepiness.

Note: If the sleep disorder is believed to be socially or environmentally induced, state and code as advanced sleep-phase syndrome (extrinsic type). If there is evidence that the sleep disorder is due to an abnormal circadian pacemaker or its entrainment mechanism, state and code as advanced sleep-phase syndrome (intrinsic type).

Minimal Criteria: A plus C plus E.

Severity Criteria:

Mild: The patient is habitually unable, over a two-week period, to stay awake until within two hours of the desired sleep time; the disorder is usually associated with mild insomnia or mild excessive sleepiness.
Moderate: The patient is habitually unable, over a two-week period, to stay awake until within three hours of the desired sleep time; the disorder is usually associated with moderate insomnia or moderate excessive sleepiness.
Severe: The patient is habitually unable, over a two-week period, to stay awake until within four hours of the desired sleep time; the disorder is usually associated with severe insomnia or severe excessive sleepiness

Duration Criteria:

Acute: 6 months or less.
Subacute: More than 6 months but less than 1 year.
Chronic: 1 year or longer.

Bibliography:

Kamei R, Hughes L, Miles L, Dement W. Advanced-sleep-phase syndrome studied in a time isolation facility. Chronobiologia 1979; 6: 115.
Moldofsky H, Musisi S, Phillipson EA. Treatment of a case of advanced sleep-phase syndrome by phase advance chronotherapy. Sleep 1986;9:61–65.

Non-24-Hour Sleep-Wake Syndrome (780.55-2)

Synonyms and Key Words: Free-running pattern, incremental asynchrony relative to typical environmental pattern, periodic insomnia, periodic excessive sleepiness, blindness, hypernycthemeral syndrome.

Essential Features:

Non-24-hour sleep-wake syndrome consists of a chronic steady pattern comprising one- to two-hour daily delays in sleep onset and wake times in an individual living in society.

Patients with non-24-hour sleep-wake syndrome exhibit a sleep-wake pattern that is reminiscent of that found in normal individuals living without environmental time cues (i.e., sleep-onset and wake times occur at a period of about every 25 hours). At times, one or more noncircadian (longer than 27 hours) sleep-wake cycles may occur in the patient with the non-24-hour syndrome, similar to the phenomenon of internal desynchrony observed in some time-isolation experiments. Such individuals are literally sleeping "around the (24-hour) clock," despite the presence of 24-hour social and environmental time cues. In the long run, their sleep phase periodically travels in and out of phase with the conventional social hours for sleep. When "in phase," the patient may have no sleep complaint, and daytime alertness is normal. As incremental phase delays in sleep occur, the complaint will consist of difficulty initiating sleep at night coupled with oversleeping into the daytime hours or inability to remain awake in the daytime. Therefore, over long periods of time, patients alternate between being symptomatic and asymptomatic, depending on the degree of synchrony between their internal biologic rhythm and the 24-hour world.

Some individuals with this condition intermittently or permanently give up attempting to synchronize their sleep with conventional hours. In these patients, a sleep-wake diary or log will appear similar to that of the free-running pattern of time-isolated normals. Most patients, however, attempt to sleep and wake at conventional social times. These attempts produce progressively less sleep, with secondary daytime sleepiness interfering with functioning at work or school. In addition, sleep may be skipped for 24 to 40 hours, followed by sleeping for 14 to 24 hours without awakening. Unlike patients with the delayed sleep-phase syndrome, who share some of the above symptoms, the patient with a non-24-hour disorder does not achieve a stable pattern of normal sleep at a delayed phase during vacations from work or school.

Associated Features: Typically, individuals with this condition are partially or totally unable to function in scheduled social activities on a daily basis, and most are unable to work at conventional jobs. Most of the patients described in the medical literature have been blind, either congenitally or on an acquired basis, and some have been mentally retarded as well. Less commonly, a severely schizoid or avoidant personality disorder may accompany the condition. One patient who was initially described as having this disorder was later discovered to have a large pituitary adenoma that involved the optic chiasma.

Efforts to induce sleep at conventional times in these patients often include the use of, and dependency on, hypnotic and analeptic medication, at times in very large doses. A history that such medications alternate between apparent efficacy and progressive loss of efficacy with no change in dose suggests that the non-24-hour syndrome may be the underlying cause of the patient's sleep-wake symptoms.

Course: Depending mostly on associated conditions, the non-24-hour syndrome may be chronic and intractable or may respond well to the institution of strict and regular 24-hour time cues. Some blind individuals, mostly in institutionalized settings, have responded to strict 24-hour scheduling, consisting of strong social time cues.

Predisposing Factors: See Associated Features.

Prevalence: This disorder is apparently rare in the general population. Although the prevalence in the blind is unknown, one survey of blind individuals revealed a high incidence of sleep-wake complaints, with 40% of the respondents having recognized that their symptoms occurred in a cyclic pattern.

Age of Onset: The syndrome has been described in congenitally blind infants as well as in blind middle-aged and elderly individuals. Onset in normal-sighted individuals appears variable.

Sex Ratio: Not known.

Familial Pattern: None known.

Pathology: Various causes of blindness involving the optic chiasma or prechiasmatic visual structures have been present in blind patients with the non-24-hour syndrome, suggesting that the blindness itself underlies the syndrome, rather than being the cause of the syndrome. This theory is in keeping with the likelihood that the environmental light-dark cycle, acting through the retino-hypothalamic tract on the suprachiasmatic nucleus of the hypothalamus, is a major source of 24-hour time information for humans as well as lower animals. Blindness deprives the endogenous circadian timing system of this crucial information, and, particularly when other brain abnormalities are present, social zeitgebers may be ineffective. In sighted individuals, a suprachiasmatic tumor may have been the cause of the syndrome in one case, but personality factors appear to be paramount. In such cases, the conscious or unconscious disregard of entraining cues may serve an adaptive, albeit a pathologic, function for the patient.

Complications: The complications relate to impaired psychosocial functioning.

Polysomnographic Features: Little specific information is available. Recordings done at fixed times over several successive days would be expected to show progressively longer sleep latencies and progressively less total sleep, but normal age-related sleep-stage architecture across the period of study. Electroencephalographic abnormalities, such as reduced sleep spindles and K-complexes, may be present in brain-damaged or retarded patients.

Other Laboratory Test Features: Sighted individuals, as well as those with blindness of unknown etiology, should undergo a neurologic evaluation that includes imaging of the suprasellar region (computed tomography scan or magnetic resonance imaging scan).

Differential Diagnosis: A carefully kept sleep-wake log that is recorded for a lengthy period of time is essential to making this diagnosis. Non-24-hour sleep-wake syndrome should be differentiated from delayed sleep-phase syndrome and irregular sleep-wake pattern. In the delayed sleep-phase syndrome, stable entrainment to a 24-hour schedule with sleep at a delayed phase from conventional hours is present during vacations. Patients with the non-24-hour sleep-wake syndrome continue in a pattern of progressive delays of sleep. The diagnosis should be suspected in any blind individual with sleep or somnolence complaints.

Diagnostic Criteria: Non-24-Hour Sleep-Wake Syndrome (780.55-2)

A. The patient has a primary complaint of either difficulty initiating sleep or difficulty in awakening.
B. Sleep onset and offset are progressively delayed, with the patient unable to maintain stable entrainment to a 24-hour sleep-wake pattern.
C. The sleep pattern has been present for at least six weeks.
D. Progressive sequential delay of the sleep period is demonstrated by one of the following methods:
   1. Polysomnography performed over several consecutive days on a fixed 24-hour bedtime and waketime schedule
   2. Continuous 24-hour temperature monitoring over at least five days that shows a progressive delay of the temperature nadir
E. The symptoms do not meet the criteria for any other sleep disorder causing inability to initiate sleep or excessive sleepiness.

Note: If the sleep disorder is believed to be socially or environmentally induced, state and code as non-24-hour sleep-wake syndrome (extrinsic type). If there is evidence that the sleep disorder is due to an abnormal circadian pacemaker or its entrainment mechanism, state and code as non-24-hour sleep-wake syndrome (intrinsic type).

Minimal Criteria: A plus B plus C.

Severity Criteria:

Mild: Mild insomnia or mild excessive sleepiness, as defined on page 23; usually associated with a mild impairment of social or occupational functioning.

Moderate: Moderate insomnia or moderate excessive sleepiness, as defined on page 23; usually associated with a moderate impairment of social or occupational functioning.

Severe: Severe insomnia or severe excessive sleepiness, as defined on page 23; usually associated with a severe impairment of social or occupational functioning.

Duration Criteria:

Acute: 6 months or less.
Subacute: More than 6 months but less than 1 year.
Chronic: 1 year or longer.

Bibliography:

Kokkoris CP, Weitzman ED, Pollak CP, et al. Long-term ambulatory monitoring in a subject with a hypernychthemeral sleep-wake cycle disturbance. Sleep 1977;1:177–190.

Miles LE, Raynal DM, Wilson MA. Blind man living in normal society has circadian rhythms of 24.9 hours. Science 1973; 198: 421–423.

Miles LE, Wilson MA. High incidence of cyclic sleep-wake disorders in the blind. Sleep Res 1977; 6: 192.

Okawa M. Sleep-waking rhythm and its central mechanism in humans: Studies of biological rhythm, computed tomography and autopsy of severely brain-damaged children. Adv Neurol 1985; 29: 346–365.

Okawa M, Nanami T, Wada S, et al. Four congenitally blind children with circadian sleep-wake rhythm disorder. Sleep 1987; 10: 101–110.

Weber AL, Cary MS, Conner N, Keyes P. Human non-24-hour sleep-wake cycles in an everyday environment. Sleep 1980; 2: 347–354.

PARASOMNIAS

The parasomnias consist of clinical disorders that are not abnormalities of the processes responsible for sleep and awake states per se but, rather, are undesirable physical phenomena that occur predominantly during sleep. The parasomnias are disorders of arousal, partial arousal, and sleep-stage transition. Many of the parasomnias are manifestations of central nervous system activation. Autonomic nervous system changes and skeletal muscle activity are the predominant features of this group of disorders.

In the *Diagnostic Classification of Sleep and Arousal Disorders,* the parasomnias were not subdivided into groups. With the recognition of additional parasomnias, however, some subgrouping is now necessary. The parasomnias are subdivided into arousal disorders, sleep-wake transition disorders, parasomnias usually associated with REM sleep, and other parasomnias.

The arousal disorders consist of the classic disorders of arousal, sleepwalking and sleep terrors, and an additional newly described disorder: confusional arousals. The sleep-wake transition disorders include those disorders that occur in the transition from wakefulness to sleep or from sleep to wakefulness. This group does not include those disorders that are clearly associated with REM sleep, such as sleep paralysis. Although some of the sleep-wake transition disorders can occur during sleep or even in wakefulness (e.g., rhythmic movement disorder–jactatio capitis nocturna), the most typical occurrence of these disorders is in the transition from wakefulness to sleep. Restless legs syndrome could be considered a sleep-wake transition disorder; however, this disorder is not a parasomnia, as it is associated primarily with a complaint of insomnia and, therefore, is listed within the dyssomnias.

The parasomnias usually associated with REM sleep include six disorders that have a close association with the REM sleep stage. Although sleep paralysis generally occurs in the transition from wakefulness to sleep or from sleep to wakefulness, sleep paralysis is listed in this subsection. The association of the other disorders with REM sleep is clear.

The fourth subsection contains parasomnias that are not classified in the previous three sections (i.e., the other parasomnias).

PARASOMNIAS

AROUSAL DISORDERS

1. Confusional Arousals (307.46-2) 142
2. Sleepwalking (307.46-0). 145
3. Sleep Terrors (307.46-1). 147

Arousal Disorders

The disorders of arousal are grouped together because impaired arousal from sleep has been postulated as a cause for these disorders. The onset of these disorders in slow-wave sleep is a typical feature. Although originally included as a disorder of arousal, sleep enuresis can occur during any sleep stage and is not associated solely with an arousal from slow-wave sleep. Confusional arousals are newly described, although their presence was first alluded to in the original description of the disorders of arousal. Confusional arousals most commonly occur in children and have features in common with both sleepwalking and sleep terrors. They are probably partial manifestations of sleepwalking and sleep-terror episodes. They can occur in people who have either or both disorders. Or confusional arousals may occur as an isolated sleep disorder. The diagnosis of confusional arousal is only stated if the arousal occurs as an isolated sleep disorder.

Confusional Arousals (307.46-2)

Synonyms and Key Words: Sleep drunkenness, excessive sleep inertia, Schlaftrunkenheit, l'ivresse du sommeil.

Essential Features:

Confusional arousals consist of confusion during and following arousals from sleep, usually from deep sleep in the first part of the night.

The individual is disoriented in time and space, is slow of speech and mentation, and responds poorly and slowly to command or questioning. There is major memory impairment, both retrograde and anterograde in type. Behavior may be very inappropriate, such as picking up a lamp to talk when the sleeper believed the telephone had rung. The confusional behavior may last from several minutes to several hours. Confusional arousals can be precipitated by forced awakenings, mainly in the first third of the night.

Associated Features: Persons who are in occupations demanding high levels of performance and who have marked confusional arousals when called at night may react inappropriately.

Course: The course of the childhood form is usually benign. Marked confusional arousals become progressively less frequent and then disappear with age. In adults, the condition is usually fairly stable, varying only with the main predisposing factors.

Predisposing Factors: Any factor that deepens sleep and impairs ease of awakening can be a predisposing factor. Major factors include young age; recovery from sleep deprivation; circadian rhythm sleep disorders (shift work, jet lag, etc.); the use of medications, particularly central nervous system depressants, such as hypnotics, sedatives, tranquilizers, alcohol, and antihistamines; and metabolic, hepatic, renal, toxic, and other encephalopathies. Confusional arousals are often seen in hypersomnias characterized by deep sleep, such as idiopathic hypersomnia (in which the parasomnias may occur whenever the patient is awakened, more or less throughout the night and even in the morning). They may also occur in the many forms of symptomatic hypersomnia, as well as in some patients with narcolepsy or sleep apnea syndrome. Episodes of confusional arousals are particularly frequent in sufferers of sleep terrors and sleepwalking. Excessive exercise is a less convincing factor but sometimes appears to play a role.

Prevalence: Repeated confusional arousals are almost universal in young children before the age of about five years; they become much less common in older childhood. Confusional arousals are fairly rare in adulthood, during which their precise prevalence is undocumented.

Sex Ratio: No difference.

Familial Pattern: There appears to be a strong familial pattern in the cases of the idiopathic confusional arousals seen in families of deep sleepers. Formal genetic studies have not been performed.

Pathology: Rare organic cases generally show lesions in areas impairing arousal, such as the periventricular gray, the midbrain reticular area, and the posterior hypothalamus.

Complications: Personal injury has occasionally resulted. Confused subjects who are restrained may resist and become aggressive.

Polysomnographic Features: Polysomnographic recordings during confusional arousals have typically shown their onset in arousals from slow-wave sleep. Confusional arousals most commonly occur in the first third of the night but also occur in afternoon naps and, occasionally, in awakenings from lighter stages of NREM sleep. They appear to be very rare in REM awakenings, during which return to clear mentation is usually rapid. Electroencephalographic monitoring during the confusion period may show brief episodes of delta activity, stage 1 theta patterns, repeated microsleeps, or a diffuse and poorly reactive alpha rhythm.

Other Laboratory Test Features: Cerebral evoked potentials may be altered during the confusional period.

Differential Diagnosis: Confusional arousals must be differentiated from a number of other parasomnias in which mental confusion during the sleep period is prominent. For example, sleep terrors have acute signs of fear and often are associated with a blood-curdling cry. Sleepwalking has the appearance of complex motor automatisms such as leaving the bed and walking about. Subjects with REM sleep behavior disorder often show explosive movements such as fighting or diving out of bed, but a full awakening does not occur. Rare sleep-related epileptic seizures of the partial complex type with confusional automatisms are associated with an epileptic electroencephalographic discharge, and similar attacks usually occur in the daytime.

Diagnostic Criteria: Confusional Arousals (307.46-2)

A. The patient has or an observer notes that the patient has recurrent mental confusion upon arousal or awakening.
B. Spontaneous confusional episodes can be induced by forced arousal.
C. The patient has an absence of fear, walking behavior, or intense hallucinations in association with the episodes.
D. Polysomnography demonstrates arousals from slow-wave sleep.
E. The symptoms are not associated with other medical disorders such as partial complex seizures.
F. The symptoms do not meet the diagnostic criteria for other sleep disorders causing the complaint (e.g., sleep terrors, sleepwalking).

Minimal Criteria: A plus B plus E plus F.

Severity Criteria:

Mild: Fewer than one episode per month.
Moderate: Episodes that occur more than once per month but less than weekly.
Severe: Episodes that occur more than once per week.

Duration Criteria:

Acute: 1 month or less.
Subacute: More than 1 month but less than 6 months.
Chronic: 6 months or longer.

Bibliography:

Broughton RJ. Sleep disorders: disorders of arousal? Enuresis, somnambulism, and night mares occur in confusional states of arousal, not in "dreaming sleep." Science 1968; 159: 1070–1078.

Ferber R. Sleep disorders in infants and children. In: Riley TL, ed. Clinical aspects of sleep and sleep disturbance. Boston: Butterworth, 1985; 113–158.

Gastaut H, Broughton R. A clinical and polygraphic study of episodic phenomena during sleep. In: Wortis J, ed. Recent advances in biological psychiatry, Volume 7. New York: Plenum Press, 1965; 197–223.

Roth B, Nevsimalova S, Sagova V, Paroubkova D, Horakova A. Neurological, psychological and polygraphic findings in sleep drunkenness. Arch Suisse Neurol Neurochirurg Psychiatr 1981; 129: 209–222.

Sleepwalking (307.46-0)

Synonyms and Key Words: Somnambulism, semipurposeful automatisms, amnesia, nonepileptic.

Essential Features:

Sleepwalking consists of a series of complex behaviors that are initiated during slow-wave sleep and result in walking during sleep.

Episodes can range from simple sitting up in bed to walking and even to apparent frantic attempts to "escape." The patient may be difficult to awaken but, when awakened, often is mentally confused. The patient is usually amnestic for the episode's events. Sleepwalking originates from slow-wave sleep and, therefore, is most often evident during the first third of the night or during other times of increased slow-wave sleep, such as after sleep deprivation. The motor activity may terminate spontaneously, or the sleepwalker may return to bed, lie down, and continue to sleep without reaching alertness at any point. Sleep talking can also be observed during these events.

Associated Features: Sleepwalking can include inappropriate behavior, such as urinating in a closet, and these behaviors are especially common in children. Sleepwalking can result in falls and injuries. Physical harm can result from the attempt to "escape" or simply from walking into dangerous situations. Walking out of a door into the street or through a window is not uncommon. Rarely, homicide or suicide during an apparent sleepwalking episode has been reported. The person attempting to awaken the patient can be violently attacked. Other parasomnia activity, such as sleep terrors, can also occur in patients who are sleepwalkers.

Course: Sleepwalking episodes can occur as soon as a child is able to walk, but reach a peak prevalence between ages four and eight years, and usually disappear spontaneously after adolescence. They can occur several times a week or only when precipitating factors are present.

Predisposing Factors: The use of several medications, such as thioridazine hydrochloride, chloral hydrate, lithium carbonate, prolixin, perphenazine, and desipramine hydrochloride, can exacerbate or induce sleepwalking. Fever and sleep deprivation, which can be self-induced or can occur as a result of a medical disorder, can produce an increased frequency of sleepwalking episodes. Obstructive sleep apnea syndrome and other disorders that produce severe disruption of slow-wave sleep can be associated with sleepwalking episodes. Internal stimuli, such as a distended bladder, or external stimuli, such as noises, can also precipitate episodes.

Prevalence: The incidence of sleepwalking is between 1% and 15% of the general population. This disorder is more common in children than in adolescents and adults.

Age of Onset: Sleepwalking can occur at any time after the child is able to walk, but episodes most commonly occur for the first time between ages four and eight years. Rarely, episodes occur for the first time in adults.

Sex Ratio: In children, sleepwalking occurs equally in both sexes; in adults, the sex ratio is not known.

Familial Pattern: Several studies have demonstrated the presence of this disorder in families. The incidence of sleepwalking increases in relation to the number of affected parents; the incidence is 22% when neither parent has the disorder, 45% if one is affected, and 60% when both are affected. Several relatives may be affected.

Pathology: None known.

Complications: The child who avoids visiting friends or summer camp because of sleepwalking episodes may suffer embarrassment or social isolation. Physical harm can occur, and even homicide and suicide have been reported.

Polysomnographic Features: Sleepwalking begins in stage 3 or stage 4 sleep, most commonly at the end of the first or second episode of slow-wave sleep.

Other Laboratory Test Features: Electroencephalography does not demonstrate epileptic features.

Differential Diagnosis: It can be difficult to clinically distinguish sleepwalking from sleep terrors with an attempt to "escape" from the terrifying stimulus. Intense fear and panic coupled with an initial scream are characteristics of sleep terrors. REM sleep behavior disorder is characterized by polysomnographic and clinical features of episodes occurring in REM sleep, as opposed to sleepwalking, which occurs in slow-wave sleep. Sleep-related epilepsy can be distinguished by the absence of clinical and electroencephalographic features of epilepsy. Patients with obstructive sleep apnea syndrome can be confused during the night and can have episodes of sleepwalking. The nocturnal eating syndrome is often associated with eating and ambulatory behavior that resembles sleepwalking.

Diagnostic Criteria: Sleepwalking (307.46-0)

A. The patient exhibits ambulation that occurs in sleep.
B. The onset typically occurs in prepubertal children.
C. Associated features include:
   1. Difficulty in arousing the patient during an episode
   2. Amnesia following an episode
D. Episodes typically occur in the first third of the sleep episode.
E. Polysomnographic monitoring demonstrates the onset of an episode during stage 3 or stage 4 sleep.
F. Other medical and mental disorders can be present but do not account for the symptom.
G. The ambulation is not due to other sleep disorders, such as REM sleep behavior disorder or sleep terrors.

Note: If episodes are associated with obstructive sleep apnea syndrome or nocturnal eating syndrome, state one diagnosis only on axis A along with the symptom (e.g., obstructive sleep apnea syndrome, with sleepwalking, 780.53-0).

Minimal Criteria: A plus B plus C.

Severity Criteria:

Mild: The episodes of sleepwalking occur less than once per month and do not result in harm to the patient or others.
Moderate: The episodes of sleepwalking occur more than once per month, but not nightly, and do not result in harm to the patient or others.
Severe: The episodes of sleepwalking occur almost nightly or are associated with physical injury to the patients or others.

Duration Criteria:

Acute: 1 month or less.
Subacute: More than 1 month but less than 3 months.
Chronic: 3 months or longer.

Bibliography:

Broughton RJ. Sleep disorders: disorders of arousal? Enuresis, somnambulism, and night mares occur in confusional states of arousal, not in "dreaming sleep." Science 1968; 159: 1070–1078.

Gastaut H, Broughton R. A clinical and polygraphic study of episodic phenomena during sleep. In: Wortis J, ed. Recent advances in biological psychiatry, Volume 7. New York: Plenum Press, 1965; 197–223.

Kales A, Soldatos CR, Bixler EO, et al. Hereditary factors in sleepwalking and night terrors. Br J Psychiatry 1980; 137: 111–118.

Sleep Terrors (307.46-1)

Synonyms and Key Words: Pavor nocturnus, incubus, severe autonomic discharge, night terrors.

Essential Features:

Sleep terrors *are characterized by a sudden arousal from slow-wave sleep with a piercing scream or cry, accompanied by autonomic and behavioral manifestations of intense fear.*

Sleep terrors manifest as a severe autonomic discharge, with tachycardia, tachypnea, flushing of the skin, diaphoresis, mydriasis, decreased skin resistance, and increased muscle tone. The patient usually sits up in bed, is unresponsive to external stimuli, and, if awakened, is confused and disoriented. Amnesia for the episode occurs, although sometimes there are reports of fragments or very brief vivid dream images or hallucinations. The episode may be accompanied by incoherent vocalizations or micturition.

Associated Features: Attempts to escape from bed or to fight can result in harm to the patient or others. Mental evaluations of adults indicate that psychopathology may be associated with sleep terrors. Children with sleep terrors do not have a higher incidence of psychopathology than do children in the general population.

Course: Sleep terrors typically are observed in children between the ages of 4 and 12 and, as in sleepwalking, tend to resolve spontaneously during adolescence.

Predisposing Factors: Sleep terror episodes can be precipitated by fever, sleep deprivation, or the use of central nervous system depressant medications.

Prevalence: The prevalence is approximately 3% of children and less than 1% of adults.

Age of Onset: Sleep terrors commonly occur in prepubertal children but can occur at any age. In adults, they are most prevalent in individuals between 20 and 30 years of age.

Sex Ratio: Sleep terrors are more frequent in males than in females.

Familial Pattern: Sleep terrors can occur in several members of a family.

Pathology: None known.

Complications: Social embarrassment about the episodes can impair social relationships in both children and adults. Attempts to escape or fight can result in harm to the patient or others.

Polysomnographic Features: Sleep terrors begin in stage 3 or stage 4 sleep, usually in the first third of the major sleep episode. However, episodes can occur in slow-wave sleep at any time. Partial arousals from slow-wave sleep without full terror are more common than are full sleep terrors. Tachycardia usually occurs during both clinical episodes of sleep terrors and partial arousals.

Other Laboratory Test Features: When differentiating between sleep terrors and sleep-related epilepsy, such as temporal-lobe epilepsy, an electroencephalogram with nasopharyngeal leads could be indicated.

Differential Diagnosis: Sleep terrors should be differentiated from nightmares. The nightmare sufferer usually remembers the dream content in vivid detail. Nightmares occur during the last third of the night, as opposed to sleep terrors, which occur at the beginning. Nightmares usually do not involve major motor activity. There is considerably less anxiety, vocalization, and autonomic discharge during a nightmare than during a sleep terror. When awakened during a nightmare, the patient exhibits good intellectual function, whereas the patient with sleep terror is usually confused. Nightmares occur out of REM sleep, as opposed to out of slow-wave sleep for sleep terrors.

Confusional arousals are awakenings from slow-wave sleep without terror or ambulation.

The differential diagnosis includes sleep-related epilepsy; confusional states; and other sleep disorders that produce anxiety during the night, including obstructive sleep apnea syndrome and nocturnal cardiac ischemia.

Diagnostic Criteria: Sleep Terrors (307.46-1)

A. The patient complains of a sudden episode of intense terror during sleep.
B. The episodes usually occur within the first third of the night.
C. Partial or total amnesia occurs for the events during the episode.
D. Polysomnographic monitoring demonstrates the onset of episodes during stage 3 or stage 4 sleep. Tachycardia usually occurs in association with the episodes.
E. Other medical disorders (e.g., epilepsy, are not the cause of the episode).
F. Other sleep disorders (e.g., nightmares, can be present).

Minimal Criteria: A plus B plus C.

Severity Criteria:

Mild: The episodes of sleep terrors occur less than once per month and do not result in harm to the patient or others.
Moderate: The episodes occur less than once per week and do not result in harm to the patient or others.
Severe: The episodes occur almost nightly or are associated with physical injury to the patient or others.

Duration Criteria:

Acute: 1 month or less.
Subacute: More than 1 month but less than 3 months.
Chronic: 3 months or longer.

Bibliography:

Broughton RJ. Sleep disorders: disorders of arousal? Enuresis, somnambulism, and night mares occur in confusional states of arousal, not in "dreaming sleep." Science 1968; 159: 1070–1078.

Fisher C, Kahn E, Edwards A, Davis DM. A psychophysiological study of nightmares and night terrors. I. Physiological aspects of the stage 4 night terror. J Nerv Ment Dis 1973; 157: 75–98.

Gastaut H, Broughton R. A clinical and polygraphic study of episodic phenomena during sleep. In: Wortis J, ed. Recent advances in biological psychiatry, Volume 7. New York: Plenum Press, 1965; 197–223.

Kales A, Soldatos CR, Bixler EO, et al. Hereditary factors in sleepwalking and night terrors. Br J Psychiatry 1980; 137: 111–118.

PARASOMNIAS

SLEEP-WAKE TRANSITION DISORDERS

1. Rhythmic Movement Disorder (307.3) 151
2. Sleep Starts (307.47-2) 155
3. Sleep Talking (307.47-3) 157
4. Nocturnal Leg Cramps (729.82) 159

Sleep-Wake Transition Disorders

The sleep-wake transition disorders occur in the transition from wakefulness to sleep; in the transition from sleep to wakefulness; or, more rarely, in sleep-stage transitions. All of these disorders can occur commonly in otherwise healthy persons and, therefore, are regarded as altered physiology rather than pathophysiology. Each can occur with an exceptionally high frequency or severity, however, which can lead to discomfort, pain, embarrassment, anxiety, or disturbance of a bedpartner's sleep.

The term *rhythmic movement disorder* is a preferred term for headbanging or jactatio capitis nocturna. The term *headbanging* applies to only one form of rhythmic stereotype, and several other forms can exist without headbanging. Although this disorder commonly occurs out of sleep stages, it is more commonly associated with drowsiness during sleep onset or in the transition from wakefulness to sleep. Rhythmic movement disorder also can occur during full wakefulness and alertness, particularly in individuals who are mentally retarded. Sleep starts (hypnic jerks) are included as a disorder because they can rarely cause sleep-onset insomnia. Sleep talking does not usually have any direct consequences to the patient but is a source of embarrassment and can be disturbing to the sleep of the bedpartner. The term *sleep* in such terms as *sleep starts* and *sleep talking*, is preferred over previously used terms such as *hypnic* or *hypnogenic* and refers to phenomena that occur in sleep. In contrast, the term *nocturnal* applies to phenomena that more commonly occur at night but not necessarily in sleep. Hence, the term *nocturnal leg cramps* is preferred because these muscle contractions can occur in wakefulness or during sleep but most commonly occur at night, usually when the person is in bed.

Rhythmic Movement Disorder (307.3)

Synonyms and Key Words: Jactatio capitis nocturna, headbanging, headrolling, bodyrocking, bodyrolling, rhythmie du sommeil. The term *rhythmic movement disorder* is preferred because different body areas may be involved in the movement activity. The term *headbanging* is less acceptable because it refers to only one form of behavior.

Essential Features:

> ***Rhythmic movement disorder*** *comprises a group of stereotyped, repetitive movements involving large muscles, usually of the head and neck; the movements typically occur immediately prior to sleep onset and are sustained into light sleep.*

The most commonly recognized variant is headbanging, which itself has several forms. The child may lie prone, repeatedly lifting the head or entire upper torso, forcibly banging the head back down into the pillow or mattress. The child may rock on hands and knees, banging the vertex or frontal region of the head into the headboard or wall. Or, the child may sit with the back of the head against the headboard or wall, repeatedly banging the occiput. Headrolling consists of side-to-side head movements, usually with the child in the supine position. Bodyrocking occurs when the child rocks forward and backward without headbanging. Bodyrocking may involve the entire body, with the child on hands and knees, or it may be limited to the torso, with the child sitting. Less common rhythmic movement forms include bodyrolling, legbanging, or legrolling. Rhythmic humming or chanting may accompany any of the rhythmic movements and may be quite loud.

Episodes typically occur at sleep onset, although they may also occur during quiet wakeful activities, such as listening to music or traveling in vehicles. The movement frequency varies greatly, but the rate is usually between 0.5 and 2 per second. Duration of the individual cluster of movements also varies greatly but generally is less than 15 minutes. Cessation of movements following disturbance or being spoken to suggests the occurrence of the disorder in wakefulness or lighter stages of sleep.

Associated Features: The vast majority of affected individuals are otherwise normal infants and children. However, when it persists into older childhood or beyond, rhythmic-movement disorder of sleep may be associated with mental retardation, autism, or other significant psychopathology.

Course: This condition commonly occurs in infants and toddlers and usually resolves in the second or third year of life. Persistence beyond four years of age is unusual. The symptoms may decrease in both intensity and duration and may not disappear but may persist into adulthood.

Prevalence: Some form of rhythmic activity is found in two thirds of all infants at nine months of age. By 18 months, the prevalence has declined to less than half, and by four years, it is only 8%. Bodyrocking is more common in the first year, but headbanging and headrolling are more frequent in older children.

Predisposing Factors: The soothing effect of vestibular stimulation has been proposed as the initiating factor in infants and toddlers. Environmental stress and lack of environmental stimulation have also been proposed as factors. Self-stimulation and auto-erotic behavior have been suggested as factors, particularly in retarded, autistic, and emotionally disturbed children. The activity may be an attention-getting behavior or a form of passive-aggressive behavior.

Age of Onset: Bodyrocking has a mean age of onset of six months, headbanging of nine months, and headrolling of 10 months. The vast majority of patients have the onset prior to one year of age. The condition rarely may present at an older age following central nervous system trauma. Spontaneous onset in adolescence or adulthood is very rare.

Sex Ratio: The disorder is more common in males, with a 4:1 male-to-female ratio.

Familial Pattern: A familial pattern has been occasionally reported, as has occurrence in identical twins.

Pathology: None known.

Complications: Headbanging is the most disturbing form of the disorder. Traumatic injury is uncommon but may result in subdural hematoma and retinal petechiae. Chronic skull irritation can produce callus formation. Carotid dissection related to headbanging has been reported. Violent rhythmic body movements can produce loud noises when the patient hits the bed frame or when the bed vibrates against the wall or floor. The noises can be very disturbing to other family members. Parental concern is common, and psychosocial consequences in the older individual can be most distressing.

Polysomnographic Features: The few reported polysomnographic studies have shown the activity to occur during presleep drowsiness and mainly in light NREM sleep, although the activity has also been detected in deep slow-wave sleep. Rarely, the behavior may occur solely during REM sleep. An epileptic etiology has been reported in one individual.

Other Laboratory Test Features: An electroencephalogram may be necessary to differentiate the behavior from that due to epilepsy. Electroencephalographic studies have shown normal activity between episodes of rhythmic behavior.

Differential Diagnosis: Rhythmic movement disorder of sleep must be distinguished from other repetitive movements involving restricted small muscle groups, such as bruxism, thumbsucking, and rhythmic sucking of the pacifier, as well as less stereotyped activity, including periodic limb movement disorder. There are usually few diagnostic problems, but, rarely, the disorder needs to be differentiated from epilepsy.

Diagnostic Criteria: Rhythmic Movement Disorder (307.3)

A. The patient exhibits rhythmic body movements during drowsiness or sleep.
B. At least one of the following types of disorder is present:
   1. The head is forcibly moved in an anterior-posterior direction (head-banging type)
   2. The head is moved laterally while in a supine position (headrolling type)
   3. The whole body is rocked while on the hands and knees (bodyrocking type)
   4. The whole body is moved laterally while in a supine position (body-rolling type)
C. Onset typically occurs within the first two years of life.
D. Polysomnographic monitoring during an episode demonstrates both of the following findings:
   1. Rhythmic movements during any stage of sleep or in wakefulness
   2. No other seizure activity occurs in association with the disorder
E. No other medical or mental disorder (e.g., epilepsy, causes the symptom).
F. The symptoms do not meet the diagnostic criteria for other sleep disorders producing abnormal movements during sleep (e.g., sleep bruxism).

Note: Specify the predominant type of activity (e.g., rhythmic-movement disorder–headbanging type).

Minimal Criteria: A plus B.

Severity Criteria:

Mild: Episodes occur less than once per week, without evidence of personal injury or impairment of psychosocial functioning.
Moderate: Episodes occur more than once per week but less than nightly, with evidence of mild impairment of psychosocial functioning.
Severe: Episodes occur nightly or almost nightly, with evidence of physical injury or significant psychosocial consequences.

Duration Criteria:

Acute: 1 month or less.
Subacute: More than 1 month but less than 6 months.
Chronic: 6 months or longer.

Bibliography:

De Lissovoy V. Head banging in early childhood. Child Dev 1962; 33: 43–56.
Klackenburg G. Rhythmic movements in infancy and early childhood. Acta Paediatr Scand [1] 1971; 224: 74–83.
Sallustro F, Atwell CW. Body rocking, head banging, and head rolling in normal children. J Pediatr 1978; 93: 704–708.
Thorpy MJ, Glovinsky PB. Headbanging (jactatio capitis nocturna). In: Kryger MH, Roth T, Dement WC, eds. Principles and practice of sleep medicine. Philadelphia: WB Saunders, 1989; 648–654.

Sleep Starts (307.47-2)

Synonyms and Key Words: Hypnagogic jerks, predormital myoclonus, hypnic jerks.

Essential Features:

Sleep starts are sudden, brief contractions of the legs, sometimes also involving the arms and head, that occur at sleep onset.

Sleep starts usually consist of a single contraction that often affects the body asymmetrically. The jerks may be either spontaneous or induced by stimuli. Sleep starts are sometimes associated with the subjective impression of falling, a sensory flash, or a visual hypnagogic dream or hallucination. A sharp cry may occur. The patient may not recall a jerk that was noted by a bedpartner if the sleep start does not cause awakening. Multiple jerks occasionally occur in succession.

Associated Features: When particularly intense, and especially if multiple, sleep starts may lead to a sleep-onset insomnia.

Course: Usually benign.

Predisposing Factors: Excessive caffeine or other stimulant intake, prior intense physical work or exercise, and emotional stress can increase the frequency and severity of sleep starts.

Prevalence: Sleep starts are an essentially universal component of the sleep-onset process, although they often are not recalled. A prevalence of 60% to 70% has been reported. Sleep starts are rare in the extreme form and can cause sleep-onset difficulties.

Age of Onset: Sleep starts may occur at any age. As a subjective complaint, however, they are usually encountered in adulthood.

Sex Ratio: No difference.

Familial Pattern: Not known.

Pathology: None described.

Complications: Chronic severe sleep starts may lead to fear of falling asleep and chronic anxiety. Sleep deprivation may also occur. Sleep-onset insomnia may result either from repeated awakenings induced by the starts or from anxiety about falling asleep. Injury, such as bruising a foot against a bedstead or kicking a sleeping companion, may occasionally occur.

Polysomnographic Features: Sleep starts occur during transitions from wakefulness to sleep, mainly at the beginning of the sleep episode. Superficial electromyographic recordings of the muscles involved show brief (generally 75- to 250-millisecond) high-amplitude potentials, either singly or in succession. The electroencephalogram typically shows drowsiness or stage 1 sleep patterns, sometimes with a negative-vertex sharp wave occurring at the time of the jerk. Tachycardia may follow an intense jerk. After the jerk, return to sustained wakefulness or a brief transient arousal may occur.

Polysomnographic monitoring may be useful to differentiate episodes of sleep starts from other causes of movement activity during the sleep period. Two nights of recording may be necessary if the disorder is suspected of causing insomnia.

Other Laboratory Test Features: None.

Differential Diagnosis: Sleep starts must be differentiated from a number of movement disorders that occur at sleep onset or during sleep. Excessive startling may occur as part of the hyperexplexia syndrome, in which generalized myoclonus is easily elicitable by stimuli during either wakefulness or sleep. Brief epileptic myoclonus can be differentiated by coexistent electroencephalographic discharge, the presence of other features of epileptic seizures, and the occurrence of the myoclonus in both wakefulness and during sleep rather than at sleep onset. The muscle contractions of periodic limb movement disorder are much longer in duration, involve mainly the feet and lower legs, show periodicity, and occur within sleep. Restless legs syndrome consists of slower and repetitive semivoluntary movements at sleep onset that are associated with deep, unpleasant, and sometimes unbearable sensations, which are temporarily relieved by getting up and exercising. Fragmentary myoclonus consists of brief, small-amplitude jerks or twitches that occur in an asynchronous, symmetrical, and bilateral manner. Fragmentary myoclonus occurs at sleep onset as well as within all sleep stages; in the pathologic form, the twitches are mainly present throughout NREM sleep. Finally, benign neonatal sleep myoclonus consists of marked twitching of the fingers, toes, and face during sleep in infants.

Diagnostic Criteria: Sleep Starts (307.47-2)

A. The patient has a complaint of either difficulty initiating sleep or an intense body movement at sleep onset.
B. The patient complains of sudden brief jerks at sleep onset, mainly affecting the legs or arms.
C. The jerks are associated with at least one of the following:
   1. A subjective feeling of falling
   2. A sensory flash
   3. A hypnagogic dream
D. Polysomnographic monitoring during an episode demonstrates one or more of the following:
   1. Brief, high-amplitude muscle potentials during transition from wakefulness to sleep
   2. Arousals from light sleep
   3. Tachycardia following an intense episode

E. No other medical or mental disorder (e.g., hyperexplexia, accounts for the symptoms).
F. Sleep starts can occur in the presence of other sleep disorders that produce insomnia.

Minimal Criteria: A plus B.

Severity Criteria:

Mild: Episodes occur less than once per week, without evidence of impairment of psychosocial functioning. The sleep starts cause subjective complaint or interfere with sleep onset but can be considered normal.
Moderate: Episodes occur more than once per week but less than nightly, with some personal complaint and degree of interference with sleep onset. Mild insomnia may be present, as defined on page 23.
Severe: Episodes involve nightly, regular jerks at sleep onset, leading to moderate or severe insomnia, as defined on page 23.

Duration Criteria:

Acute: 1 month or less.
Subacute: More than 1 month but less than 6 months.
Chronic: 6 months or longer.

Bibliography:

Broughton R. Pathological fragmentary myoclonus, intensified sleep starts and hypnagogic foot tremor: Three unusual sleep-related disorders. In: Koella WP, ed. Sleep 1986. New York, Stuttgart: Fischer-Verlag, 1988; 240–243.
Kennard MA, Schartzman AE, Millar TP. Sleep consciousness and the alpha electroencephalographic rhythm. Arch Neurol Psychiatry 1958; 79: 328–342.
Oswald I. Sudden bodily jerks on falling asleep. Brain 1959; 82: 92–93.

Sleep Talking (307.47-3)

Synonyms and Key Words: Somniloquy, utterances, moans, verbalization.

Essential Features:

Sleep talking is the utterance of speech or sounds during sleep without simultaneous subjective detailed awareness of the event.

The utterances may be annoying to bedpartners or other household members, even to neighbors. The sleep talking usually is brief, infrequent, and devoid of signs of emotional stress. However, it can consist of frequent, nightly, longer speeches and can include a content infused with anger and hostility. Sleep talking may be spontaneous or induced by conversation with the sleeper.

Associated Features: None.

Course: The course is usually self-limited and benign. The disorder may be present for a few days only or may last for several months or many years. Sleep talking associated with psychopathology or medical illness occurs more commonly in persons over 25 years of age.

Predisposing Factors: Sleep talking may be precipitated by emotional stress; febrile illness; or sleep disorders such as sleep terror, confusional arousals, obstructive sleep apnea syndrome, and REM sleep behavior disorder.

Prevalence: Not known, but apparently very common. Sleep talking that significantly disturbs others is rare.

Age of Onset: Not known.

Sex Ratio: May be more common in males than in females.

Familial Pattern: A familial tendency has been reported.

Pathology: None known.

Complications: None known.

Polysomnographic Features: Polysomnographic studies have demonstrated sleep talking during all stages of sleep. Dream mentation is associated with episodes occurring out of REM sleep in 79% of patients with sleep talking, stage 2 sleep in 46%, and slow-wave sleep in 21%. In sleepwalkers, episodes of sleep talking are likely to occur during arousals out of slow-wave sleep, and in patients with REM sleep behavior disorder, episodes are more likely to occur out of REM sleep. Sleep talking can occur during arousals from sleep in individuals with obstructive sleep apnea syndrome.

Other Laboratory Test Features: None.

Differential Diagnosis: Sleep talking, when severe, should be differentiated from talking during periods of wakefulness that interrupt sleep, which may be normal phenomena or reflect psychopathology. Sleep talking also frequently occurs in association with other sleep disorders, such as obstructive sleep apnea syndrome, REM sleep behavior disorder, or sleep terrors.

Diagnostic Criteria: Sleep Talking (307.47-3)

A. The patient exhibits speech or utterances during sleep.
B. Episodes are not associated with subjective awareness of talking.
C. Polysomnography demonstrates episodes of sleep talking that can occur during any stage of sleep.
D. Sleep talking can be associated with medical or mental disorders (e.g., anxiety disorders or febrile illness).

E. Sleep talking can be associated with other sleep disorders (e.g., sleepwalking, obstructive sleep apnea syndrome, or REM sleep behavior disorder).

Note: Sleep talking is only stated and coded as a sole diagnosis when it is the patient's predominant complaint. If sleep talking is a major complaint associated with another sleep disorder, state and code both disorders on axis A.

Minimal Criteria: A plus B.

Severity Criteria:

Mild: Episodes occur less than weekly.
Moderate: Episodes occur more than once per week but less than nightly and cause mild disturbance to a bedpartner.
Severe: Episodes occur nightly and may cause pronounced interruption of a bedpartner's sleep.

Duration Criteria:

Acute: 1 month or less.
Subacute: More than 1 month but less than 1 year.
Chronic: 1 year or longer.

Bibliography:

Aarons L. Evoked sleep-talking. Percept Mot Skills 1970; 31: 27–40.
Arkin AM. Sleep talking: a review. J Nerv Ment Dis 1966; 143: 101–122.
Arkin AM, Toth MF, Baker J, Hastey JM. The frequency of sleep talking in the laboratory among chronic sleep talkers and good dream recallers. J Nerv Ment Dis 1970; 151: 369–374.
Arkin AM, Toth MF, Baker J, Hastey JM. The degree of concordance between the content of sleep talking and mentation recalled in wakefulness. J Nerv Ment Dis 1970; 151: 375–393.

Nocturnal Leg Cramps (729.82)

Synonyms and Key Words: Leg cramps, muscle tightness of the leg, muscle hardness, nocturnal leg pain, "charley horse."

Essential Features:

***Nocturnal leg cramps** are painful sensations of muscular tightness or tension, usually in the calf but occasionally in the foot, that occur during the sleep episode.*

The symptom may last for a few seconds and remit spontaneously but, in some cases, may remain persistent for up to 30 minutes. The cramp often results in arousal or awakening from sleep. Patients with nocturnal leg cramps will often experience one or two episodes nightly, several times a week. The cramp can usually be relieved by local massage, application of heat, or movement of the affected limb.

Leg cramps can occur in some patients primarily during the daytime, and sleep disturbance is usually not a feature in these patients.

Associated Features: None.

Course: The natural history of leg cramps is not well understood. Many patients describe a waxing and waning course of many years' duration. Leg cramps are often seen in the elderly.

Predisposing Factors: Predisposing factors include pregnancy, diabetes mellitus, and metabolic disorders. The disorder can be associated with: prior vigorous exercise; pregnancy; use of oral contraceptives; fluid and electrolyte disturbances; endocrine disorders; neuromuscular disorders; and disorders of reduced mobility, such as arthritis and Parkinson's disease.

Prevalence: Definitive data are not available. Symptoms of nocturnal leg cramps have been identified in up to 16% of healthy individuals, particularly following vigorous exercise, with an increased incidence among the elderly.

Age of Onset: Nocturnal leg cramps have not been reported in infancy. The peak onset is usually in adulthood but may be seen for the first time in old age.

Sex Ratio: No definitive information exists. Nocturnal leg cramps may be more prevalent in females, due to the frequent occurrence of leg cramps in pregnant women.

Familial Pattern: Leg cramps are usually seen as an isolated case. Some familial characteristics are described, but no definitive pattern has been established.

Pathology: Suggestions of abnormal calcium metabolism have not been firmly established.

Complications: Complications include insomnia and occasional daytime fatigue due to interruptions in sleep. No marked mental or social dysfunction has been described due to leg cramps alone.

Polysomnographic Features: Polysomnographic studies of patients with chronic nocturnal leg cramps reveal nonperiodic bursts of gastrocnemius electromyographic activity. Episodes occur out of sleep without any specific preceding physiologic changes during sleep.

Differential Diagnosis: Chronic myelopathy, peripheral neuropathy, akathisia, restless legs syndrome, muscular pain-fasciculation syndromes, and disorders of calcium metabolism should be differentiated by clinical history and physical examination. Nocturnal leg cramps may coexist with other sleep disorders, such as periodic limb movement disorder or sleep apnea syndromes, without necessarily influencing the pathophysiology of those disorders.

Diagnostic Criteria: Nocturnal Leg Cramps (729.82)

A. The patient has a complaint of a painful sensation in the leg that is associated with muscle hardness or tightness.
B. Recurrent awakenings from sleep are associated with painful leg sensations.
C. The discomfort is relieved by local massage, movement, or application of heat.
D. Polysomnographic monitoring demonstrates increased electromyographic activity in the affected leg and an associated awakening.
E. No underlying medical disorder accounts for the sensation.
F. Other sleep disorders may be present but do not account for the symptom.

Minimal Criteria: A plus B.

Severity Criteria:

Mild: The leg cramps occur episodically, usually not more often than once or twice weekly, with minimal disruption to sleep and without causing the patient significant distress.
Moderate: The leg cramps occur on three to five nights of the week, with awakenings from sleep and moderate disruption of sleep continuity.
Severe: The leg cramps occur on a nightly basis, with repetitive wakenings from sleep and ensuing daytime symptoms.

Duration Criteria:

Acute: 1 month or less.
Subacute: More than 1 month but less than 6 months.
Severe: 6 months or longer.

Bibliography:

Jacobsen JH, Rosenberg RS, Huttenlocher PR, Spire JP. Familial nocturnal cramping. Sleep 1986; 9: 54–60.
Layzer RB, Rowland LP. Cramps. N Engl J Med 1971; 285: 31–40.
Norris FH, Gasteiger EL, Chatfield PO. An electromyographic study of induced and spontaneous muscle cramps. Electroencephalogr Clin Neurophysiol 1957; 9: 139–147.
Saskin P, Whelton C, Moldofsky H, Akin F. Sleep and nocturnal leg cramps. Sleep 1988; 11: 307–308.
Weiner IH, Weiner HL. Nocturnal leg muscle cramps. JAMA 1980; 244: 2332–2333.

PARASOMNIAS

PARASOMNIAS USUALLY ASSOCIATED WITH REM SLEEP

1. Nightmares (307.47-0) 162
2. Sleep Paralysis (780.56-2) 166
3. Impaired Sleep-Related Penile Erections (780.56-3) 169
4. Sleep-Related Painful Erections (780.56-4). 173
5. REM-Sleep-Related Sinus Arrest (780.56-8). 175
6. REM-Sleep Behavior Disorder (780.59-0) 177

Parasomnias Usually Associated with REM Sleep

These parasomnias typically are associated with the REM sleep stage. They are grouped together because some common underlying pathophysiologic mechanism related to REM sleep possibly underlies these disorders.

The term nightmares has been retained and is preferred over the term dream anxiety attacks, which had been recommended in the *Diagnostic Classification of Sleep and Arousal Disorders*. The term nightmares as used here applies to the REM sleep phenomena evident by the group heading, and therefore, there is little chance of confusing this disorder with that associated with slow-wave sleep, sleep terrors. Two newly described sleep disorders are included in this section: REM sleep-related sinus arrest and REM sleep behavior disorder. The first of these disorders appears to be relatively rare. However, the second is being recognized more often, sometimes in association with other sleep disorders such as narcolepsy.

Nightmares (307.47-0)

Synonyms and Key Words: Nightmare, dream anxiety attack, terrifying dream, REM nightmare. *Nightmare* is the preferred term and has been widely used to describe this condition for many years in pediatric and adult literature. The reason that other terms, such as *dream anxiety attack* and *REM nightmare,* have at times been suggested is to differentiate this phenomenon from sleep terrors (sometimes called *stage 4 nightmares*), assuming that *nightmare* was an overall lay term covering stage 4 as well as REM sleep. However, it is preferable to use the term *nightmares* for the REM phenomena, as they differ radically from sleep terrors.

Essential Features:

Nightmares are frightening dreams that usually awaken the sleeper from REM sleep.

The nightmare is almost always a long, complicated dream that becomes increasingly frightening toward the end. The long, dreamlike feature is essential in making the clinical differentiation from sleep terrors. The awakening occurs out of REM sleep. Sometimes there will not be an immediate awakening, but, instead recall of a very frightening dream will occur at a later time. This latter situation is not common with nightmares.

The element of fright or anxiety is an essential part of the nightmares. The frightening quality is left to the patient to judge, as some patients are frightened by content that does not appear disturbing to others.

Associated Features: Talking, screaming, striking out, or walking during the nightmare rarely occurs and differentiates nightmare from sleep terrors and REM sleep behavior disorder.

Course: A large number of children (10% to 50% of the population) will suffer from nightmares between ages three and six years. There is usually a gradual onset; parents often note nightmares even earlier, at age two to three years, but the child only starts to describe them as frightening dreams or nightmares at three to four years of age. The nightmares usually subside or decrease greatly in frequency after a period of weeks, months, or, occasionally years.

A subgroup of children continues to have nightmares into adolescence and even into adulthood. These individuals often become lifelong, frequent nightmare sufferers. The outcome of the untreated disorder is not clear. Usually no specific treatment is used for nightmares, though many of these patients do have psychotherapy at some time. Nightmares generally seem to diminish in frequency and intensity over the course of decades, but some patients at the age of 60 or 70 years still describe frequent episodes.

Predisposing Factors: Certain personality characteristics appear to be associated with the presence of frequent nightmares. A sizable proportion (20%-40%) of these patients have a diagnosis of schizotypal personality (most frequent), borderline personality disorder, schizoid personality disorder, or schizophrenia. Over 50% can be given no psychiatric diagnosis but frequently have some features of the above disorders. Those with frequent nightmares can be vulnerable to mental illness. They consider their childhood to have been difficult and complicated, though there is usually no overt trauma. Adolescence and young adulthood are characterized by severe difficulties in relationships with others. These patients are also unusually open and trusting and often have artistic or other creative inclinations.

Stressful periods of various kinds, and especially traumatic events, increase the frequency and severity of nightmares. Certain medications, including L-dopa (and related drugs) and beta-adrenergic blockers, and withdrawal of REM-suppressant medications can induce or increase the incidence of nightmares.

Prevalence: There is no definite agreement between studies. Apparently, 10% to 50% of children at the age of three to five have enough nightmares to disturb the parents. A larger percentage, probably 75%, can remember at least one or a few nightmares in the course of their childhood.

Approximately 50% of adults admit to having at least an occasional nightmare. The condition of frequent nightmares (one or more a week) occurs in perhaps 1% of the adult population.

Age of Onset: Nightmares usually start at ages three to six years but can occur at any age.

Sex Ratio: In children, there is an equal sex ratio. In adults, both in patient populations and in populations of volunteer research subjects, there is a ratio of 2:1 to 4:1 favoring women. However, the actual ratio is not certain; some evidence indicates that women are more willing to admit to having nightmares and more readily discuss them but do not actually experience more nightmares.

Familial Pattern: Not certain. One study indicates a familial pattern for the condition of frequent, lifelong nightmares.

Pathology: None known.

Complications: None known.

Polysomnographic Features: Polysomnography shows an abrupt awakening from REM sleep. The REM sleep episode is usually at least 10 minutes in duration and is associated with an increased REM density. There is increased variability in heart and respiratory rates but not the sudden doubling of pulse and respiratory rates that is found in sleep terrors. A nightmare can sometimes occur in REM sleep during a long nap.

Nightmares that follow trauma can sometimes occur in non-REM sleep, especially stage 2.

Other Laboratory Test Features: None.

Differential Diagnosis: Nightmares must be differentiated from sleep terrors and REM sleep behavior disorder. Nightmares are described as dreams, whereas sleep terrors have either no content or only a single image. Nightmares occur late during the sleep period, in the second half of the night, whereas sleep terrors occur predominantly in the first third of the night. Polysomnography can confirm the diagnosis, as nightmares involve an awakening from REM sleep, whereas sleep terrors occur on awakening from stage 3 and stage 4 sleep. The incidence of nightmares (and sleep terrors) appears to be lower in the laboratory than at home, so unless the event is described as occurring every night or several times per night, it will often not occur in the laboratory setting. Sleep terrors, but not nightmares, are associated with marked increase in heart and respiratory rate and, at times, sleepwalking.

REM sleep behavior disorder more commonly occurs in the elderly and is distinguished by violent, often explosive movement activity during REM sleep. Persons with REM sleep behavior disorder do not have the abrupt awakening to full alertness, and less fear and panic are expressed. Characteristic polysomnographic features can be seen.

Diagnostic Criteria: Nightmares (307.47-0)

A. The patient has at least one episode of sudden awakening from sleep with intense fear, anxiety, and feeling of impending harm.
B. The patient has immediate recall of frightening dream context.
C. Full alertness occurs immediately upon awakening, with little confusion or disorientation.
D. Associated features include at least one of the following:
   1. Return to sleep after the episode is delayed and not rapid
   2. The episode occurs during the latter half of the habitual sleep period
E. Polysomnographic monitoring demonstrates the following:
   1. An abrupt awakening from at least 10 minutes of REM sleep
   2. Mild tachycardia and tachypnea during the episode
   3. Absence of epileptic activity in association with the disorder
F. Other sleep disorders, such as sleep terrors and sleepwalking, can occur.

Minimal Criteria: A plus B plus C plus D.

Severity Criteria:

Mild: Episodes occur less than once per week, without evidence of impairment of psychosocial functioning.
Moderate: Episodes occur more than once per week but less than nightly, with evidence of mild impairment of psychosocial functioning.
Severe: Episodes occur nightly, with evidence of moderate or severe impairment of psychosocial functioning.

Duration Criteria:

Acute: 1 month or less.
Subacute: More than 1 month but less than 6 months.
Chronic: 6 months or longer.

Bibliography:

Fisher CJ, Byrne J, Edwards T, Kahn E. A psychophysiological study of nightmares. J Am Psychoanal Assoc 1970; 18: 747–782.
Hartman E. The nightmare. New York: Basic Books, 1984.
Hersen M. Personality characteristics of nightmare sufferers. J Nerv Ment Dis 1952; 153: 27–31.
Mack JE. Nightmares and human conflict. Boston: Little & Brown, 1970.

Sleep Paralysis (780.56-2)

Synonyms and Key Words: Isolated sleep paralysis, familial sleep paralysis, hypnagogic and hypnopompic paralysis, predormital and postdormital paralysis.

Essential Features:

Sleep paralysis consists of a period of inability to perform voluntary movements at sleep onset (hypnagogic or predormital form) or upon awakening, either during the night or in the morning (hypnopompic or postdormital form).

During sleep paralysis limb, trunk, and head movements typically are not possible, although ocular and respiratory movements are intact. The experience is usually frightening, particularly if the patient senses difficulty in being able to breathe. The sensorium is normally clear. Sleep paralysis usually lasts one to several minutes and disappears either spontaneously or upon external stimulation, especially by touch or movement induced by another person. Some patients have noted that repeated efforts to move or vigorous eye movements may help to abort the paralytic state.

Sleep paralysis may occur in an isolated form in otherwise healthy individuals, in a familial form that is transmitted genetically, and as one of the classic tetrad of symptoms of narcolepsy. The isolated cases most frequently occur on awakening, whereas in the familial form and in narcolepsy, paralysis is most common at sleep onset.

Associated Features: Acute anxiety is common since the individual is fully conscious but unable to move and feels vulnerable. Hypnagogic imagery may be present and is often threatening, adding further to the individual's discomfort. At times, dreamlike mentation is also experienced, especially if the paralyzed person becomes drowsy or light sleep occurs during an attack.

Course: The course of the condition varies with its form. Isolated cases may have sleep paralysis only under the provocation of predisposing factors. The familial form and that associated with narcolepsy tend to be more chronic, although the frequency of episodes also depends upon predisposing factors.

Predisposing Factors: Irregular sleep habits, sleep deprivation, and other disturbances of the sleep-wake rhythm predispose to the patient to developing sleep paralysis, apparently for all three forms. Isolated episodes occur during periods of shift work or rapid time zone change (jet lag). Mental stress, overtiredness, and sleeping in the supine position have also been reported as predisposing factors in some individuals.

Prevalence: Isolated sleep paralysis occurs at least once in a lifetime in 40% to 50% of normal subjects. As a chronic complaint, however, it is much less common. Surveys of normal subjects have indicated sleep paralysis in 3% to 6% of respondents, many of whom had rare episodes. Familial sleep paralysis in individuals lacking sleep attacks or cataplexy is exceptionally rare, with only a few families described in the literature. Seventeen percent to 40% of narcoleptics have been reported to have sleep paralysis.

Age of Onset: Sleep paralysis most frequently begins in adolescence or young adulthood, although onset in childhood and middle age or, sometimes later has also been reported.

Sex Ratio: Isolated cases show no sexual predominance. In the familial form. women are affected more often than are men.

Familial Pattern: Most cases are isolated, with no familial pattern. In familial sleep paralysis, the disorder is transmitted as an X-linked dominant trait.

Pathology: There have been no autopsy reports of isolated or familial cases, but the fact that neurologic examination between attacks is normal, along with the absence of documented significant pathology in narcolepsy, argues against the existence of a significant central nervous system lesion. It appears more likely that a microstructual change or a neurochemical or neuroimmunologic dysfunction exists in the mechanism controlling the normal motor paralysis of the REM state.

Complications: Episodes of sleep paralysis are generally without complications; the normal state returns between attacks. Occasionally, attacks will induce chronic anxiety or depression.

Polysomnographic Features: Recordings during sleep paralysis have shown suppression of muscle tone recorded by submental, axial, or more peripheral electromyography, which is associated with an electroencephalographic (EEG) pattern of wakefulness and the presence of waking eye movement and blink patterns in the electrooculogram. Electrically induced H-reflex studies have shown suppression of anterior motorneuron excitability similar to that present in cataplexy and in REM sleep. Subjects who become drowsy during sleep paralysis may show coexistent EEG slowing or pendular eye movements. Direct transitions into or from REM sleep have been documented.

All-night polysomnography and multiple sleep latency testing can be useful to exclude a diagnosis of narcolepsy and to document the REM association of the episodes.

Other Laboratory Test Features: None. Histocompatability testing for the antigens DR2 or DQw1 (or DR15 and DQ6 using a newer nomenclature) may be helpful in excluding a diagnosis of narcolepsy.

Differential Diagnosis: Generally, the features of sleep paralysis are sufficiently clear that diagnosis is not difficult. Isolated and familial cases should be readily distinguishable from narcolepsy, in which sleepiness, cataplexy, and often vivid hypnagogic hallucinations also usually occur. Cataplexy is differentiated by its occurrence in the awake state rather than in sleep-wake transitions, as well as by its precipitation by emotional stimuli.

Hysteric and psychotic states with immobility must be distinguished but are usually evident by their associated clinical features.

Atonic generalized epileptic seizures can be differentiated by their usual occurrence in the daytime waking state. The atonic drop attacks in patients with vertebrobasilar vascular insufficiency usually occur in older patients in wakefulness without precipitating causes (other than orthostatic hypotension) and are unrelated to sleep-wake transitions.

Localized paresis present in the morning due to peripheral-nerve compression from an unusual sleeping posture ("Saturday-night palsy") rarely may be confused with sleep paralysis.

Hypokalemic paralysis is perhaps the only condition that closely resembles sleep paralysis. The attacks usually occur during rest; paralysis occurs on awakening, as in true sleep paralysis. The condition most often occurs in adolescent males, has a familial transmission, shows low serum-potassium levels during attacks, may be provoked by the ingestion of high-carbohydrate meals or alcohol, and is readily reversed by correcting the hypokalemia.

Diagnostic Criteria: Sleep Paralysis (780.56-2)

A. The patient has a complaint of inability to move the trunk or limbs at sleep onset or upon awakening.
B. Brief episodes of partial or complete skeletal muscle paralysis are present.
C. Episodes can be associated with hypnagogic hallucinations or dreamlike mentation.
D. Polysomnographic monitoring demonstrates at least one of the following:
   1. Suppression of skeletal muscle tone
   2. A sleep-onset REM period
   3. Dissociated REM sleep
E. The symptoms are not associated with other medical or mental disorders (e.g., hysteria or hypokalemic paralysis).

Note: If the symptom is associated with a familial history, the diagnosis should be stated as sleep paralysis–familial type. If the symptom is not associated with a familial history, the diagnosis should be stated as sleep paralysis–isolated type. If the sleep paralysis is associated with narcolepsy, state only one diagnosis on axis A, if necessary, along with the symptom of sleep paralysis (e.g., narcolepsy with sleep paralysis, 347).

Minimal Criteria: A plus B plus E.

Severity Criteria:

Mild: Episodes occur less than once per month.
Moderate: Episodes occur more than once per month but less than weekly.
Severe: Episodes occur at least once per week.

Duration Criteria:

Acute: 1 month or less.
Subacute: More than 1 month but less than 6 months.
Chronic: 6 months or longer.

Bibliography:

Goode GB. Sleep paralysis. Arch Neurol 1962; 6: 228–234.
Hishikawa Y. Sleep paralysis. In: Guilleminault C, Dement WC, Passouant P, eds. Narcolepsy. New York: Spectrum, 1976; 97–124.
Nan'no H, Hishikawa Y, Koida H, Takahashi H, Kaneko Z. A neurophysiological study of sleep paralysis in narcoleptic patients. Electroencephogr Clin Neurophysiol 1970; 28: 382–390.

Impaired Sleep-Related Penile Erections (780.56-3)

Synonyms and Key Words: Impaired nocturnal penile tumescence (NPT), impotence, organic impotence, erectile dysfunction, erectile failure, and sexual dysfunction.

Essential Features:

Impaired sleep-related penile erections refers to the inability to sustain a penile erection during sleep that would be sufficiently large or rigid enough to engage in sexual intercourse.

Significant reduction or absence of sleep-related penile erections, in the presence of reasonably intact sleep architecture, usually occurs as a result of organic impotence. In some patients, sleep-related penile circumference increases without commensurate increase in penile rigidity. This dissociation between size and rigidity is an essential feature of organic impotence in patients with apparently normal sleep tumescence.

Associated Features: The patient's age must be considered when interpreting observed decrements in sleep-related tumescence. There is a natural decline in the frequency, magnitude, and duration of sleep-related erections with advancing age.

Course: Organic impotence seldom improves spontaneously without treatment. However, it is a common misconception that all forms of organic impotence are permanent and irreversible. Impotence with organic components often produces psychologic complications because of intermittent erectile failure in sexual situations. Selection of treatment and prognosis for organic impotence depend on the specifics of history, etiology, and severity.

Predisposing Factors: Virtually all diseases that compromise vascular, neural, neurotransmitter, and endocrine function are potential contributors to erectile dysfunction. The diseases most often implicated in organic impotence include diabetes mellitus, hypertension, cancer, heart disease, renal failure, spinal cord injury, alcoholism, epilepsy, pelvic injury, and multiple sclerosis. It has recently been suggested that mental illnesses, such as depression, can be associated with impaired sleep-related tumescence.

Urogenital problems are frequently associated with impaired sleep-related erections (e.g., Peyronie's disease, priapism, venous leakage, prostatectomy). New nerve-sparing procedures, however, have reduced the incidence of impotence resulting from prostate surgery. Other surgical procedures, including pelvic and spinal surgery, have been implicated as the cause of impaired tumescence.

Many prescribed and recreational drugs have been implicated as either causes or aggravators of impotence. Most notably, these include antihypertensives, antipsychotics, antidepressants, disulfiram, digoxin, amphetamine, heroin, and methadone. Additionally, alcohol abuse and cigarette smoking may contribute to impotence. The relationship between drugs and impotence, however, is largely based on clinical and anecdotal reports.

Prevalence: It is estimated that more than 10% of adult males in the United States have chronic erectile dysfunction. The majority (60%-70%) are thought to have organic impotence. Differentiation of organic and nonorganic impotence requires sophisticated testing and clinical skill. Moreover, the sample of patients at particular clinics may be biased because of selection forces created by the institutions' reputations. For these two reasons, it may be difficult to obtain precise prevalence data.

Age of Onset: Impaired sleep-related penile erections can occur at any age. Among men with erectile complaints, the percentage with an organic basis for impotence increases dramatically after 45 years of age. By age 60 years, 60% to 70% and by age 70 years, 70% to 85% of impotent men evaluated polysomnographically are likely to have diminished sleep-related erections, impaired penile rigidity during sleep-related tumescence, or both.

Sex Ratio: This disorder occurs only in male patients.

Familial Pattern: To the extent that diabetes mellitus, hypertension, heart disease, alcoholism, and other diseases implicated as the cause of organic impotence demonstrate familial patterns, sleep-related erectile impairment follows those patterns. Regardless of whether the familial pattern is genetically determined or behaviorally acquired, such an association exists. It is not known if organic impotence is a specific heritable trait.

Pathology: A number of pathologies are characteristic of patients with impaired sleep-related penile erections. Vascular insufficiency often accompanies organic impotence. Likewise, autonomic nervous system dysfunction, peripheral neuropathy, and venous leakage may be present. Decreased testosterone, elevated prolactin, and other endocrine abnormalities are also known to correlate with impaired sleep-related penile erections in some men.

Complications: A variety of mental, social, and marital problems can result from organic impotence or organically based intermittent erectile failure. These problems can have devastating effects on family stability, gender identity, and general mental status. Impotence can be associated with anxiety and depression; however, the relationship between cause and effect has not been fully elucidated.

Polysomnographic Features: Impaired sleep-related penile erections as determined by sleep-recording technology are a biologic marker for organic impotence. Polysomnographic procedures to evaluate sleep-related penile erections are regarded as the most accurate diagnostic means for differentiating organic from nonorganic impotence. Typically, two or three nights of recording are necessary.

Sleep-related penile erections are regarded as abnormal if the following minimal criteria are met:

1. The longest full tumescence episode has a duration of less than five minutes.
2. The largest increase in penile circumference recorded at the coronal sulcus never exceeds four millimeters.
3. Erectile capacity is functionally impaired if penile rigidity (buckling force) is less than 500 grams during a representative erection. Five hundred grams is the average minimal rigidity necessary for penetration. A representative erection is one during which the circumference increase is minimally 80% of the largest erection recorded for that patient. Buckling force is the amount of force applied to the tip of the penis sufficient to produce at least a 30° bend in the shaft. An organic component to an erectile problem can exist, notwithstanding the observation of an erection with a rigidity of 500 grams or more. In normal healthy men, however, the rigidity of a full erection will exceed 1,000 grams. Finally, a patient can sometimes be functionally impaired with rigidities greater than 500 grams due to an interaction of individual differences in morphology between the patient and his partner.

The manifestation of the naturally occurring penile erectile cycle depends upon the quality and quantity of sleep, especially REM sleep. The following minimal sleep criteria can be used as guidelines for valid interpretation of diminished or absent sleep-related erections:

1. At least one REM period with a duration of 15 minutes or more occurs.
2. A nightly total of sleep includes at least 30 minutes of REM sleep in one or more REM periods and 180 minutes of NREM (non-REM)sleep.
3. The recording period (total time in bed) is at least six hours. This is especially important in elderly patients because some have a prolonged erection-episode latency.
4. No severe sleep fragmentation is produced by sleep apnea syndromes, periodic limb movement disorder, or other sleep disorders disrupting REM sleep and, therefore, obscuring the erectile episodes. Additional polysomnographic features may be useful for understanding the etiologic basis of impaired sleep-related penile erections. These include reduced perineal muscle activity, reduced penileb pulsation density, and diminished penile segmental pulsatile blood flow. Reduced REM latency and REM density, with or without depression, are frequently observed in men with impaired sleep-related erections.

Other Laboratory Test Features: A number of laboratory tests are important for proper differential diagnosis of impotence. These include psychologic and psychiatric evaluations, with special attention to depression. It is useful to assess hemodynamics, bulbocavernosus reflex latency, penile sensory responses, and one or more indexes of autonomic nervous system function (e.g., Valsalva maneuver).

Although these tests may be helpful in understanding the etiologic basis of organic impotence, evidence of impaired sleep-related tumescence is the best composite measure. In 15% to 20% of cases where sleep-related erections are abnormally diminished, no daytime abnormality can be found to account for the complaint of erectile dysfunction.

In contrast, several findings can indicate organic impotence even in men who have apparently normal sleep-related erections. These include vascular "steal syndrome," endocrine abnormalities, and neural lesions in the penile sensory pathway. Although these disorders rarely occur without significantly impaired sleep-related penile erections, they are noteworthy.

Differential Diagnosis: Impaired sleep-related penile erections associated with organic impotence must be differentiated from diminished erections that result from other sleep disorders. In many older men, the latency to sleep-related erections is prolonged; therefore, a sufficient recording period must be provided.

Episodes of sleep apnea and periodic limb movements during sleep can interfere with sleep erections because these interferences reduce or disrupt sleep quality or quantity. Consequently, because sleep-related erections usually occur during REM sleep, an adequate amount of REM sleep must be present to make a valid interpretation of polysomnographic tracings. Impaired sleep-related penile erections associated with organic impotence must also be distinguished from diminished erections that are secondary to profoundly disrupted sleep by recording conditions, poor health, and pharmacologic agents.

Diagnostic Criteria: Impaired Sleep-Related Penile Erections (780.56-3)

A. The patient has a complaint of inability to achieve or maintain a penile erection adequate for sexual intercourse.
B. Erectile capability is impaired during sleep.
C. Polysomnographic monitoring demonstrates significant reduction or absence of sleep-related erections in the presence of a normal major sleep episode.
D. The symptoms can be associated with other medical or mental disorders (e.g., diabetes mellitus and depression).
E. Impaired sleep-related penile tumescence can be associated with disorders affecting sleep (e.g., obstructive sleep apnea syndrome).

Minimal Criteria: A plus B plus C.

Severity Criteria:

Mild: Episodes of sleep-related penile erections occur with expansion at both the tip and base; however, maximum rigidity ranges from 400 to 549 grams.

Moderate: Episodes of sleep-related penile erections occur, but maximum rigidity is less than 400 grams.
Severe: Sleep-related penile erections are absent, and there is no penile rigidity.

Duration Criteria:

Acute: Less than 1 month.
Subacute: More than 1 month but less than 6 months.
Chronic: 6 months or longer.

Bibliography:

Fisher C, Schiavi RC, Edwards A, Davis DM, Reitman M, Fine J. Evaluation of nocturnal penile tumescence in the differential diagnosis of sexual impotence. A quantitative study. Arch Gen Psychiatry 1979; 36: 431–437.

Karacan I. Evaluation of nocturnal penile tumescence and impotence. In: Guilleminault C, ed. Sleeping and waking disorders: Indications and techniques. Menlo Park, California: Addison-Wesley, 1982; 343–371.

Karacan I, Moore C, Sahmay S. Measurement of pressure necessary for vaginal penetration. Sleep Res 1985; 14: 269.

Karacan I, Williams RL, Thornby JI, Salis PJ. Sleep-related penile tumescence as a function of age. Am J Psychiatry 1975; 132: 932–937.

Pressman MR, DiPhillipo MA, Kendrick JI, Conroy K, Fry JM. Problems in the interpretation of nocturnal penile tumescence studies: disruption of sleep by occult sleep disorders. J Urol 1986; 136: 595–598.

Schmidt HS, Nofzinger EA. Short REM latency in impotence without depression. Biol Psychiatry 1988; 24: 25–32.

Schmidt HS, Wise HA 2d. Significance of impaired penile tumescence and associated polysomnographic abnormalities in the impotent patient. J Urol 1981; 126: 348–352.

Ware JC. Evaluation of impotence. Monitoring periodic penile erections during sleep. Psychiatr Clin North Am 1987; 10: 675–686.

Sleep-Related Painful Erections (780.56-4)

Synonyms and Key Words: Painful erections.

Essential Features:

Sleep-related painful erections *are characterized by penile pain that occurs during erections, typically during REM sleep.*

Patients with sleep-related painful erections report repeated awakenings with a partial or full erection and the experience of pain. Patients may also note that the awakenings interrupt dreaming. Repeated awakenings and sleep loss, if persistent, can produce a complaint of insomnia, anxiety, irritability, and excessive sleepiness.

Associated Features: Patients may experience anxiety, tension, and irritability during the day, presumably resulting from sleep loss, REM deprivation, and preoccupation with the disorder. Surprisingly, sexual erections in the awake state are not accompanied by pain. Peyronie's disease and phimosis may be present but rarely account for the sleep-related painful erections.

Course: It appears that this disorder gradually becomes more severe with age; however, little objective evidence is available.

Predisposing Factors: None known.

Prevalence: This disorder is rare, occurring in less than 1% of patients presenting with sexual and erectile problems.

Age of Onset: Sleep-related painful erections can begin at any age; however, patients with this condition are typically over 40 years of age.

Sex Ratio: This disorder occurs only in male patients. An analogous disorder in females with painful clitoral erections has not been described.

Familial Pattern: None known.

Pathology: Painful erections occur without apparent penile pathology. It has been noted, however, that anatomic abnormalities of the penis, such as Peyronie's disease, may be present.

Complications: Because sleep-related penile tumescence normally occurs in conjunction with REM sleep, repeated awakenings produced by painful erections can produce REM fragmentation and deprivation. Complaints of excessive sleepiness or insomnia can become severe.

Polysomnographic Features: Polysomnographic monitoring demonstrates an awakening during an episode of sleep-related penile tumescence. The patient attributes the awakening to the painful sensation.

Other Laboratory Test Features: None.

Differential Diagnosis: This disorder must be differentiated from other disorders producing penile pain, such as Peyronie's disease, infections, or phimosis. In sleep-related painful erections, the pain occurs only with erections during sleep and not with sexually induced erections in the awake state. There is usually no difficulty in differentiating this condition from other disorders of insomnia or excessive sleepiness. Patients are quite aware that their awakenings result from painful erections.

Diagnostic Criteria: Sleep-Related Painful Erections (780.56-4)

    A. The patient has a complaint of painful penile erections during sleep.
    B. Erections during wakefulness are not painful.

C. Polysomnographic monitoring demonstrates penile tumescence associated with awakenings from REM sleep.
D. The symptoms are not associated with other medical or mental disorders (e.g., Peyronie's disease or phimosis).
E. Other sleep disorders (e.g., nightmares, may be present but do not account for the symptom).

Note: If associated with Peyronie's disease or phimosis, the diagnosis is not sleep-related painful erections but that of the underlying disease (e.g., Peyronie's disease).

Minimal Criteria: A plus B plus D plus E.

Severity Criteria:

Mild: Episodes occur less than once per week.
Moderate: Episodes occur several times per week.
Severe: Episodes occur every night or more than once per night.

Duration Criteria:

Acute: 7 days or less.
Subacute: More than 7 days but less than 1 month.
Chronic: 1 month or longer.

Bibliography:

Hinman F Jr. Etiologic factors in Peyronie's disease. Urol Int 1980; 35: 407–413.
Karacan I. Painful nocturnal penile erections. JAMA 1971; 215: 1831.
Matthews BJ, Crutchfield MB. Painful nocturnal penile erections associated with rapid eye movement sleep. Sleep 1987; 10: 184–187.

REM Sleep-Related Sinus Arrest (780.56-8)

Synonyms and Key Words: Nocturnal asystole, sinus arrest.

Essential Features:

REM sleep-related sinus arrest is a cardiac rhythm disorder that is characterized by sinus arrest during REM sleep in otherwise healthy individuals.

Electrocardiographic monitoring demonstrates periods of asystole during sleep that may last up to nine seconds and that occur repeatedly during REM sleep. These periods of asystole are associated with neither sleep apnea nor sleep disruption.

Associated Features: Some patients may complain of vague diurnal chest pain, tightness, or intermittent palpitations. Upon abrupt awakening, lightheadedness, faintness, and blurred vision may occur. Some patients report infrequent syncope while ambulatory at night. Electrocardiographic and angiographic findings during wakefulness are usually completely normal.

Course: Not known.

Predisposing Factors: None known.

Prevalence: Not known. Because the disorder in most cases is asymptomatic and presumably undiagnosed, this information will be difficult to obtain.

Age of Onset: REM sleep-related sinus arrest has been observed only in young adults. It may occur, however, in other age-groups.

Sex Ratio: Too few cases have been reported to calculate a meaningful sex ratio. This disorder occurs in both sexes.

Familial Pattern: None known.

Pathology: None known.

Complications: A potential exists for loss of consciousness or even cardiac arrest in association with the asystole. Insidious impairment of mental function may also result. As a preventive measure, a patient may be given a ventricular-inhibited pacemaker with a low rate limit.

Polysomnographic Features: The periods of asystole occur repeatedly during REM sleep, usually in clusters. They are not associated with apnea or oxygen desaturation. Neither arousals, awakenings, nor sleep-stage changes occur in conjunction with these cardiac events.

Other Laboratory Test Features: Twenty-four-hour Holter electrocardiographic monitoring will demonstrate sinus arrest exclusively during REM sleep.

Differential Diagnosis: This disorder must be differentiated from the cardiac irregularities commonly associated with sleep-related breathing disorders such as the obstructive sleep apnea syndrome. Asystoles of up to 2.5 seconds may occur in normal healthy adults.

Diagnostic Criteria: REM Sleep-Related Sinus Arrest (780.56-8)

A. The patient has no related sleep complaint.
B. The patient may have a complaint of vague chest discomfort during the day.
C. An associated feature is infrequent syncope at night while ambulatory.
D. Polysomnographic monitoring demonstrates asystole, lasting greater than 2.5 seconds, occurring solely during REM sleep.
E. Other electrophysiologic and hemodynamic studies of the heart are normal.
F. There is no evidence of any medical disorder that produces cardiac irregularity.
G. There is no evidence of any other sleep disorder that could account for the finding (e.g., obstructive sleep apnea syndrome).

Minimal Criteria: A plus D plus F plus G.

Severity Criteria:

Mild: Episodes of sinus arrest up to three seconds in duration, occurring more than twice per night.
Moderate: Episodes of sinus arrest of between three and five seconds in duration, occurring several times per night.
Severe: Episodes of sinus arrest greater than five seconds in duration, occurring five or more times per night.

Duration Criteria:

Acute: 7 days or less.
Subacute: More than 7 days and less than 1 month.
Chronic: 1 month or longer.

Bibliography:

Guilleminault C, Connolly SJ, Winkle RA. Cardiac arrhythmia and conduction disturbances during sleep in 400 patients with sleep apnea syndrome. Am J Cardiol 1983; 52: 490–494.
Guilleminault C, Pool P, Motta J, Gillis AM. Sinus arrest during REM sleep in young adults. N Engl J Med 1984; 311: 1006–1010.
Motta J, Guilleminault C. Cardiac dysfunction during sleep. Ann Clin Res 1985; 17: 190–198.

REM Sleep Behavior Disorder (780.59.0)

Synonyms and Key Words: REM sleep behavior disorder (RBD), oneirism, acting out of dreams, REM motor parasomnia.

Essential Features:

REM sleep behavior disorder is characterized by the intermittent loss of REM sleep electromyographic (EMG) atonia and by the appearance of elaborate motor activity associated with dream mentation.

Punching, kicking, leaping, and running from the bed during attempted dream enactment are frequent manifestations and usually correlate with the reported imagery.

Medical attention is often sought after injury has occurred to either the person or a bedpartner. Occasionally, a patient may present because of sleep disruption. Because RBD occurs during REM sleep, it typically appears at least 90 minutes after sleep onset. Violent episodes typically occur about once per week but may appear as frequently as four times per night over several consecutive nights.

An acute, transient form may accompany REM rebound during withdrawal from alcohol and sedative-hypnotic agents. Drug-induced cases have been reported during treatment with tricyclic antidepressants and biperiden.

Associated Features: There may be a prodromal history of sleep talking, yelling, or limb jerking. Dream content may become more vivid, unpleasant, violent, or action-filled coincident with the onset of this disorder. Symptoms of excessive daytime sleepiness may appear if sufficient sleep fragmentation exists.

Course: The idiopathic form usually begins in late adulthood, progresses over a variable period of time (months to years), and then may stabilize.

Predisposing Factors: Approximately 60% of cases are idiopathic; advanced age is an apparent predisposing factor. The remaining cases are associated with neurologic disorders such as dementia, subarachnoid hemorrhage, ischemic cerebrovascular disease, olivopontocerebellar degeneration, multiple sclerosis, and brain-stem neoplasm. There is no associated psychopathology.

Prevalence: RBD is apparently rare; however, many cases are probably masquerading as other parasomnias (see differential diagnosis).

Age of Onset: RBD usually presents in the sixth or seventh decade; however, it may begin at any age (particularly the symptomatic variety).

Sex Ratio: The reported cases indicate that RBD is much more predominant in males than in females.

Familial Pattern: A familial pattern occasionally is suggested by history, but insufficient information is available.

Pathology: Autopsy studies have not been reported. An identical syndrome is seen in cats with experimentally induced bilateral peri-locus coeruleus lesions. Extensive neurologic evaluations in humans suffering from both the idiopathic and symptomatic forms have not identified specific lesions; however, findings in some patients suggest that diffuse lesions of the hemispheres, bilateral thalamic abnormalities, or primary brain-stem lesions may result in the RBD.

Complications: Injury (lacerations, ecchymoses, fractures) to self or bedpartner and damage to surroundings are the major complications. Social consequences, especially those involving the relationship with the bedpartner, may be significant.

Polysomnographic Features: During REM sleep, affected individuals display persistent and possibly augmented muscle tone. Prominent and often prolonged periods of extremity activity (usually far in excess of normal REM sleep-related twitches) are present. These motor phenomena may be highly integrated (repeated punching and kicking or more complex limb and trunk movements) and often are associated with emotionally charged utterances. If awakened during an episode, the subject may report dream mentation appropriate to the observed behavior. In NREM (non-REM) sleep, periodic movements involving the legs, and occasionally the arms, and periodic movements of all extremities have been reported. There is frequently a pronounced increase in both the REM density and percentage of slow-wave sleep.

Other Laboratory Test Features: The results of the neurologic history and examination may indicate the need for other neurologic testing, including a computed tomographic scan or magnetic resonance imaging of the brain.

Differential Diagnosis: The differential diagnosis includes sleep-related seizures, confusional arousals, sleepwalking, sleep terrors, posttraumatic stress syndrome, and nightmares. Precipitous arousals can be seen with obstructive sleep apnea syndrome, cardiopulmonary and gastrointestinal disorders, and panic attacks.

Diagnostic Criteria: REM Sleep Behavior Disorder (780.59-0)

A. The patient has a complaint of violent or injurious behavior during sleep.
B. Limb or body movement is associated with dream mentation.
C. At least one of the following occurs:
   1. Harmful or potentially harmful sleep behaviors
   2. Dreams appear to be "acted out"
   3. Sleep behaviors disrupt sleep continuity
D. Polysomnographic monitoring demonstrates at least one of the following electrophysiologic measures during REM sleep:
   1. Excessive augmentation of chin electromyography (EMG) tone
   2. Excessive chin or limb phasic EMG twitching, irrespective of chin EMG activity and one or more of the following clinical features during REM sleep
   a. Excessive limb or body jerking
   b. Complex, vigorous, or violent behaviors
   c. Absence of epileptic activity in association with the disorder
E. The symptoms are not associated with mental disorders but may be associated with neurologic disorders.
F. Other sleep disorders (e.g., sleep terrors or sleepwalking) can be present but are not the cause of the behavior.

Minimal Criteria: B plus C.

Severity Criteria:

Mild: REM sleep behavior occurs less than once per month and causes only mild discomfort for the patient or bedpartner.
Moderate: REM sleep behavior occurs more than once per month but less than once per week and is usually associated with physical discomfort to the patient or bedpartner.
Severe: REM sleep behavior occurs more than once per week and is associated with physical injury to the patient or bedpartner.

Duration Criteria:

Acute: 1 month or less.
Subacute: More than 1 month but less than 6 months.
Chronic: 6 months or longer.

Bibliography:

Hishikawa Y, Sugita Y, Iijima S, Teshima Y, Shimizu T. Mechanisms producing "stage 1-REM" and similar dissociations of REM sleep and their relation to delirium. Adv Neurol Sci (Tokyo) 1981; 25: 1129–1147.

Jouvet M, Sastre J-P, Sakai K. Toward an etho-ethnology of dreaming. In: Karacan I, ed. Psychophysiological aspects of sleep. Park Ridge: Noyes Medical, 1981; 204–214.

Schenck CH, Bundlie SR, Ettinger MG, Mahowald MW. Chronic behavioral disorders of human REM sleep: A new category of parasomnia. Sleep 1986; 9: 293–306.

Schenck CH, Bundlie SR, Patterson AL, Mahowald MW. Rapid eye movement sleep behavior disorder: A treatable parasomnia affecting older males. JAMA 1987; 257: 1786–1789.

PARASOMNIAS

OTHER PARASOMNIAS

1. Sleep Bruxism (306.8) 182
2. Sleep Enuresis (788.36) 185
3. Sleep-Related Abnormal Swallowing Syndrome (780.56-6) 188
4. Nocturnal Paroxysmal Dystonia (780.59-1) 190
5. Sudden Unexplained Nocturnal Death Syndrome (780.59-3) 193
6. Primary Snoring (786.09)................................... 195
7. Infant Sleep Apnea (770.80)................................. 198
8. Congenital Central Hypoventilation Syndrome (770.81)............. 205
9. Sudden Infant Death Syndrome (798.0) 209
10. Benign Neonatal Sleep Myoclonus (780.59-5) 212
11. Other Parasomnia Not Otherwise Specified (780.59-9)

Other Parasomnias

This group of parasomnias comprises those parasomnias that cannot be classified in other sections of this text. In future editions of the *International Classification of Sleep Disorders,* some common attributes may be focused on to subdivide what is likely to be a growing list.

The terms *sleep bruxism* and *sleep enuresis* are preferred over the previously used terms *nocturnal bruxism* and *nocturnal enuresis* in order to denote the association with sleep rather than the time of day. A new entry, primary snoring, is included because snoring may be associated with the presence of altered cardiovascular status and can be a forerunner to the development of obstructive sleep apnea syndrome. Primary snoring can not only lead to impaired health but also cause social embarrassment and disturb the sleep of a bedpartner. Snoring that is associated with obstructive sleep apnea syndrome is not diagnosed as primary snoring. The disorder of sleep-related abnormal swallowing syndrome is retained in this classification, although it is noted that there are few additional reports since the original description. Nocturnal paroxysmal dystonia is a newly described disorder that primarily is associated with non-REM sleep, although it can occur in wakefulness during the major sleep episode. Because this disorder is solely a sleep phenomenon, it is classified here rather than as a sleep disorder associated with neurologic disease.

Sudden unexplained nocturnal death syndrome is also a relatively newly described syndrome that has a specific association with sleep and, therefore, is classified here. Similarly, benign neonatal sleep myoclonus is a disorder of muscle activity that occurs solely during sleep in infants.

Included in this group are sudden infant death syndrome and the infant sleep-related breathing disorders: infant sleep apnea and congenital central hypoventilation syndrome. The infant sleep-related breathing disorders can produce dyssomnia features of insomnia or excessive sleepiness. These symptoms are not predominant complaints, however, and the disorders usually are associated with a sudden event noticed to occur during sleep; therefore, they are listed in the parasomnia section. The inclusion of these infant breathing disorders as sleep disorders requires further explanation.

The newborn and young infant sleep a great portion of the day, and the majority of apnea and related respiratory disorders are observed during sleep. Apnea, hypoventilation, and periodic breathing are intrinsic features of infancy, reflecting immaturity of the respiratory system rather than pathology. Although there is general agreement that apnea associated with prematurity requires diagnosis, surveillance, and treatment, there is far less agreement about the boundaries between pathologic and normal manifestations of sleep-related respiratory instabilities in term infants or premature infants who have reached 37 weeks postconceptional age. Whereas the clinical significance of congenital central hypoventilation and obstructive apnea due to a narrow airway is beyond doubt, controversy about the significance of other infant sleep apnea and breathing patterns is of such magnitude that some clinicians will be concerned while others will view the same infant as healthy and the observed phenomena as a variation of normal. The fear that respiratory instability during sleep may predispose some infants to developing sudden infant death syndrome (SIDS) confers urgency to clinical management. The majority of SIDS cases happen during a time when the infant is presumed to be asleep. However, even though infant sleep apnea has been implicated as a precursor to SIDS, there is no definitive evidence establishing a direct link; therefore, SIDS is discussed separately.

Sleep Bruxism (306.8)

Synonyms and Key Words: Nocturnal bruxism, nocturnal tooth grinding, tooth clenching.

Essential Features:

Sleep bruxism is a stereotyped movement disorder characterized by grinding or clenching of the teeth during sleep.

The sounds made by friction of the teeth are usually perceived by a bedpartner as being unpleasant. The disorder is typically brought to medical attention to eliminate the disturbing sounds, although the first signs of the disorder may be recognized by a dentist. Bruxism can lead to abnormal wear of the teeth, periodontal tissue damage, or jaw pain.

Bruxism can also occur during wakefulness. Sleep-related and waking bruxism appear to be etiologically different phenomena, although the effects on dentition may be similar.

Associated Features: Additional symptoms include a variety of muscle and tooth sensations, atypical facial pain, or headache. There is great variability in the intensity and duration of bruxism, but typically hundreds of events can occur during the night. These events are not usually associated with an awakening but can produce brief arousals from sleep.

Although most often reported in healthy children and adults, the disorder is also commonly reported in children with cerebral palsy and mental retardation. Psychologic assessment of otherwise healthy adults suggests a close correlation with stress from situational or psychologic sources.

Course: Little is known about the natural history of sleep bruxism. There is a close relationship of the disorder to stress, and it varies with the degree of perceived emotional tension; however, the disorder may be chronic, without any apparent association with stress.

Predisposing Factors: Minor anatomic defects, including rough cusp ends and malocclusion, may be predisposing factors. There is no evidence that correction of such abnormalities leads to resolution of the bruxism. A correlation has frequently been reported between anxiety and bruxism.

Prevalence: Eight-five percent to 90% of the population grind their teeth to some degree during their lifetime. In approximately 5% of these patients, bruxism will present as a clinical condition. Children appear to be affected as frequently as adults, but longitudinal studies are not available.

Age of Onset: Bruxism in adults usually begins at age 10 to 20 years. Bruxism is seen in over 50% of normal infants, with a median age of onset at 10.5 months, soon after the eruption of the deciduous incisors.

Sex Ratio: No difference.

Familial Pattern: Bruxism has occasionally been reported to occur in families. Children of sleep bruxists are more likely to be affected than are the children of individuals who never had the problem or who suffer from daytime bruxism only.

Pathology: None known.

Complications: Dental damage with abnormal wear to the teeth is the most frequent sign of the disorder. Damage to the structures surrounding the teeth can include recession and inflammation of the gums and resorption of the alveolar bone. Hypertrophy of the muscles of mastication can occur, and bruxism can lead to temporomandibular joint (TMJ) disorders, often associated with facial pain.

Polysomnographic Features: Polysomnographic monitoring demonstrates increased masseter and temporalis muscle activity during sleep. Sleep bruxism can occur during all stages of sleep, but it is most common in stage 2 sleep. In some individuals, it takes place predominantly in REM sleep. The sound of bruxism can be very loud and unpleasant.

If polysomnography is indicated to demonstrate the disorder or to rule out associated epilepsy, two nights of recording may be necessary. Even a two-night sleep evaluation will produce a number of false-negative studies because bruxism, even in patients with significant clinical conditions, may not occur for several nights.

Other Laboratory Test Features: Dental examination may be indicated in severely afflicted patients. No other laboratory studies have proven useful. An electroencephalogram may be indicated if a seizure disorder is suspected.

Differential Diagnosis: The disorder seldom poses diagnostic problems, but evaluation for TMJ disorders or primary dental or periodontal disease is indicated. The rhythmic jaw movements associated with partial complex or generalized seizure disorders need to be considered in the differential diagnosis.

Diagnostic Criteria: Sleep Bruxism (306.8)

A. The patient has a complaint of tooth-grinding or tooth-clenching during sleep.
B. One or more of the following occurs:
   1. Abnormal wear of the teeth
   2. Sounds associated with the bruxism
   3. Jaw muscle discomfort
C. Polysomnographic monitoring demonstrates both of the following:
   1. Jaw muscle activity during the sleep period
   2. Absence of associated epileptic activity
D. No other medical or mental disorders (e.g., sleep-related epilepsy, accounts for the abnormal movements during sleep).
E. Other sleep disorders (e.g., obstructive sleep apnea syndrome, can be present concurrently).

Minimal Criteria: A plus B.

Severity Criteria:

Mild: Episodes occur less than nightly, without evidence of dental injury or impairment of psychosocial functioning.
Moderate: Episodes occur nightly, with evidence of mild impairment of psychosocial functioning.
Severe: Episodes occur nightly, with evidence of dental injury, TMJ disorders, other physical injury, or moderate or severe impairment of psychosocial functioning.

Duration Criteria:

Acute: 7 days or less.
Subacute: More than 7 days and less than 1 month.
Chronic: 1 month or longer.

Bibliography:

Funch DP, Gale EN. Factors associated with nocturnal bruxism and its treatment. J Behav Med 1980; 3: 385–397.
Gastaut H, Broughton R. A clinical and polygraphic study of episodic phenomena during sleep. Rec In: Wortis J, ed. Recent advances in biological psychiatry, Volume 7. New York: Plenum Press, 1965; 197–223.
Glaros AG, Rao SM. Bruxism: a critical review. Psychol Bull 1977; 84: 767–781.
Kravitz H, Boehm JJ. Rhythmic habit patterns in infancy: Their sequence, age of onset, and frequency. Child Dev 1971; 42: 399–413.
Reding GR, Zepelin H, Robinson JE Jr, Zimmerman SO, Smith VH. Nocturnal teeth-grinding: All-night psychophysiologic studies. J Dent Res 1968; 47: 786–797.
Rugh JD, Harlan J. Nocturnal bruxism and temporomandibular disorders. Adv Neurol 1988; 49: 329–341.
Ware JC, Rugh JD. Destructive bruxism: Sleep stage relationship. Sleep 1988; 11: 172–181.

Sleep Enuresis (788.36)

Synonyms and Key Words: Enuresis nocturna; nocturnal bed-wetting; primary, familial, functional, idiopathic, symptomatic, or essential enuresis; night wetting. *Sleep enuresis* is the preferred term because it refers to the inability to maintain urinary control during sleep. *Primary enuresis* refers to the inability to attain urinary control from infancy, whereas secondary enuresis denotes an enuretic relapse after control has been achieved.

Essential Features:

Sleep enuresis is characterized by recurrent involuntary micturition that occurs during sleep.

Persistent bed-wetting after age five in the absence of urologic, medical, or mental pathology is considered a primary enuretic disorder. Typically, the child has never achieved continuous dry nights. In secondary enuresis, the child has had at least three to six months of dryness. Enuretic episodes occur throughout all sleep stages, as well as during nocturnal awakenings. Most episodes occur in the first third of the night. Bladder control during the daytime can be normal.

Associated Features: Primary enuresis is continuous from infancy, with children wetting from once or twice a week to nightly and often several times a night. The customary bed-wetting during sleep in infancy and early childhood persists to an age when it can no longer be regarded as normal (i.e., after the age of five years). Small functional bladder capacity and an irritable bladder are associated with multiple wettings at night and also with increased frequency of voiding and urgency during the day.

In some enuretics, toilet training is not encouraged or achieved early in childhood. This finding may account for the increased prevalence of enuresis in lower-socioeconomic groups, where parenting skills or expectations may be less developed.

Dreaming is vaguely and infrequently reported in conjunction with bed-wetting, particularly when it occurs in the first hours of the night. Typically, the sleeper dreams of being in the bathroom; this occurs more commonly with older enuretics. Such dreams are initiated after the onset of micturition and are not precipitating events.

Obstructive breathing and sleep apnea may be precipitating factors, particularly in children who have loud snoring. When obstructive sleep apnea syndrome is diagnosed, both the apnea and the enuresis often resolve after treatment of the apnea.

Allergies may play a role in the perseverance of enuresis. Some children with the disorder have been shown to be allergic to milk products and to suffer bladder irritability.

Course: Sleep enuresis is normal in infancy and usually resolves spontaneously before age six years. The prevalence decreases by 14% to 16% per year in children aged 5 to 19.

Predisposing Factors: The incidence of sleep enuresis is higher in institutionalized children and in children with a lower-socioeconomic background. Acquired metabolic or endocrine disorders may predispose a person to developing enuresis. Obstructive sleep apnea syndrome also can be associated with enuresis in children and adults.

Prevalence: Enuresis is estimated to occur in 30% of 4-year-olds, 10% of 6 year olds, 5% of 10 year olds, and 3% of 12 year olds. One percent to 3% of 18 year olds continue to have enuretic episodes. Primary enuresis comprises 70% to 90% of all cases of the disorder, with secondary enuresis representing the remaining 10% to 30%. In adults, primary enuresis is rare.

Age of Onset: Primary enuresis is continuous from infancy. Secondary enuresis can occur at any age.

Sex Ratio: Males are affected more often than females. At age five, the male to female ratio is 3:2.

Familial Pattern: A hereditary factor involving a single recessive gene is suspected in children with primary enuresis. There is often a high prevalence of enuresis among the parents, siblings, and other relatives of the child with primary enuresis. Studies suggest an incidence of 77% when both parents were enuretic as children and a rate of 44% in children when one parent has a positive history for enuresis.

Pathology: The pathologic basis of primary enuresis is largely unknown. Evidence suggests a neurophysiologic maturational delay. Small bladder size or increased bladder contractility may be present. Genitourinary malformations and disorders and metabolic, neurogenic, mental, or endocrine disorders account for most cases of secondary enuresis. Sleep apnea can be a cause.

Complications: Sleep enuresis is often kept secret when it persists beyond childhood because it causes embarrassment and inconvenience to both the sufferer and the caretaker. Daily changing of sheets and concerns about odor are typical. Primary enuresis tends to restrict the child's range of activities, such as spending the night with a friend or going on school trips, on vacations, and to sleep-away camp. The psychologic trauma is often the most serious complication.

Polysomnographic Features: Enuretic episodes can occur in all sleep stages and during nocturnal wakefulness. Episodes may correlate with the presence of obstructive sleep apnea. Sleep cystometrography in enuretic children reveals elevated intravesical pressure and spikelike detrusor contractions during bladder filling, similar to those occurring in infantile bladders.

Other Laboratory Test Features: Micturating cystometry and metabolic and endocrine tests may be helpful.

Differential Diagnosis: Primary sleep enuresis is diagnosed by exclusion when secondary enuresis has been ruled out. Primary enuretics should have a physical examination that includes a urinalysis, complete enuresis history, and a sleep history. Causes of secondary enuresis can be organic, medical, or psychologic.

Organic pathology of the urinary tract is more likely if the child has daytime enuresis, abnormalities in the initiation of micturition, or abnormal urinary flow. Urinary-tract infection, diabetes mellitus, diabetes insipidus, epilepsy, sickle cell anemia, and neurologic disorders can all cause enuresis.

Enuresis may be associated with obstructive sleep apnea syndrome.

Diagnostic Criteria: Sleep Enuresis (788.36)

A. The patient exhibits episodic involuntary voiding of urine during sleep.
B. The enuresis occurs at least twice per month in children between the ages of three and six years and at least once per month in older individuals.
C. Polysomnographic monitoring during an episode demonstrates both of the following:
   1. Voiding of urine during the sleep period
   2. Absence of epileptic activity in association with the voiding
D. The enuresis can be associated with medical or mental disorders, such as diabetes, urinary-tract infection, or epilepsy.
E. Other sleep disorders (e.g., obstructive sleep apnea syndrome, can be the cause of the symptom).

Note: Specify the type of sleep enuresis (e.g., sleep enuresis–primary type or sleep enuresis–secondary type). If the enuresis is associated with obstructive sleep apnea syndrome or other sleep disorders, specify both diagnoses on axis A. If the enuresis is associated with another medical diagnosis, specify on axis C.

Minimal Criteria: A plus B.

Severity Criteria:

Mild: Episodes occur less than once per week, without evidence of impairment of psychosocial functioning.

Moderate: Episodes occur more than once per week but less than nightly, with mild impairment of psychosocial functioning.

Severe: Episodes occur nightly, with moderate or severe impairment of psychosocial functioning.

Duration Criteria:

Acute: 1 month or less.
Subacute: More than 1 month but less than 6 months.
Chronic: 6 months or longer.

Bibliography:

Agarwal A. Enuresis. Am Fam Physician 1982; 25: 203–207.
Forsythe WI, Redmond A. Enuresis and spontaneous cure rate. Study of 1129 enuretics. Arch Dis Childhood 1974; 49: 259–263.
Mikkelsen EJ, Rapoport JL. Enuresis: Psychopathology, sleep stage, and drug response. Urol Clin North Am 1980; 7 : 361–377.
Scharf MB. Waking up dry: How to end bedwetting forever. Ohio: Writer's Digest Books, 1986.
Schmitt BD. Nocturnal enuresis: an update on treatment. Pediatr Clin North Am 1982; 29: 21–36.
Weider DJ, Hauri PJ. Nocturnal enuresis in children with upper airway obstruction. Int J Pediatr Otolaryngol 1985; 9: 173–182.

Sleep-Related Abnormal Swallowing Syndrome (780.56-6)

Synonyms and Key Words: Deficient swallowing, choking, coughing, aspiration.

Essential Features:

Sleep-related abnormal swallowing syndrome is a disorder in which inadequate swallowing of saliva results in aspiration, with coughing, choking, and brief arousals or awakenings from sleep.

Patients report the perceived sense of choking and blocked breathing at night. Polysomnographic recording does not demonstrate significant sleep apnea, only short-lived episodes of coughing and gagging following periods of "gurgling" sounds that are probably due to pooling of saliva in the hypopharynx. Sleep is restless and can be greatly disrupted. The symptoms usually do not occur at sleep onset; therefore, return to sleep is unimpeded. The episodes cease momentarily with awakening.

Associated Features: Elderly patients with sleep-related abnormal swallowing syndrome may be prone to developing respiratory infections due to aspiration.

Course: Not known.

Predisposing Factors: Administration of hypnotic agents and other central-nervous-system-depressant medications.

Prevalence: Apparently rare.

Age of Onset: Typically occurs in middle age.

Sex Ratio: Not known.

Familial Pattern: Not known.

Pathology: Not known. Presumed to be due to an inability to swallow saliva during sleep.

Complications: Not known.

Polysomnographic Features: Polysomnography demonstrates frequent awakenings from sleep of short duration (5-10 minutes). Slow-wave sleep has been reported to be absent. Studies of swallowing during sleep have shown abnormal swallowing, with accumulation of saliva in the hypopharynx and aspiration into the trachea. These episodes are associated with an electroencephalographic arousal or complete awakening.

Polysomnographic monitoring will help rule out obstructive sleep apnea syndrome and central sleep apnea syndrome, both of which have similar manifestations.

Other Laboratory Test Features: Endoscopy of the upper airway is necessary to examine vocal cord function and to exclude upper-airway pathology.

Differential Diagnosis: The complaint of arrested respiration during sleep may suggest a diagnosis of obstructive sleep apnea syndrome. However, in obstructive sleep apnea syndrome, patients are usually unaware of breathing difficulty. The presenting symptom with sleep apnea syndrome is almost invariably excessive sleepiness, whereas with abnormal swallowing syndrome, it is restlessness or insomnia.

Episodes of gastroesophageal reflux may also lead to coughing and choking during sleep, but the awakenings typically are associated with heartburn and chest pain as well. A complaint of acid reflux is sufficient to distinguish gastroesophageal reflux from the sleep-related abnormal swallowing syndrome.

Sleep terrors are characteristically associated with sensations of impaired breathing or choking during sleep, as well as with panting, agitation, and rapid pulse on awakening. However, they occur out of slow-wave sleep and rarely recur during the night. The initial scream, panic, and fear of sleep terrors separates this condition from the sleep-related abnormal swallowing syndrome.

The sleep choking syndrome is a disorder of presumed psychogenic etiology, characterized by recurrent reports of choking during sleep but no objective evidence of choking.

The sleep-related laryngospasm rarely is able to be documented in the sleep laboratory; "gurgling" sounds are not a feature of sleep-related laryngospasm.

Diagnostic Criteria: Sleep-Related Abnormal Swallowing Syndrome (780.56-6)

A. The patient has a complaint of sudden awakenings associated with choking or of insomnia.
B. Choking, associated with "gurgling" sounds from the upper airway, occurs during sleep.
C. Polysomnography demonstrates frequent arousals from sleep that are associated with "gurgling" sounds.
D. No other medical or mental disorders (e.g., panic attacks, are present that could account for the symptoms).
E. The symptoms do not meet the diagnostic criteria for any other sleep disorder that could account for the symptom (e.g., obstructive sleep apnea syndrome or sleep-related gastroesophageal reflux).

Minimal Criteria: A plus B plus D plus E.

Severity Criteria:

Mild: Mild insomnia, as described on page 23; choking episodes occur less than nightly.
Moderate: Moderate insomnia, as described on page 23; choking episodes occur on average once per night.
Severe: Severe insomnia, as described on page 23; choking episodes occur many times per night.

Duration Criteria:

Acute: 7 days or less.
Subacute: More than 7 days but less than 3 months.
Chronic: 3 months or longer.

Bibliography:

Guilleminault C, Eldridge FL, Phillips JR, Dement WC. Two occult causes of insomnia and their therapeutic problems. Arch Gen Psychiatry 1976; 33: 1241–1245.

Nocturnal Paroxysmal Dystonia (780.59-1)

Synonyms and Key Words: Hypnogenic paroxysmal dystonia; non-REM sleep-related dystonic-dyskinetic episodes; extrapyramidal seizures, choreoathetotic seizures; paroxysmal choreoathetosis (PCA); ballistic or paroxysmal kinesigenic dystonia; paroxysmal dystonic episodes; short-episode, prolonged-episode dystonic-dyskinetic episodes.

Essential Features:

Nocturnal paroxysmal dystonia (NPD) is characterized by repeated dystonia or dyskinetic (ballistic, choreoathetoid) episodes that are stereotypical and occur during NREM sleep.

Two clinical varieties of NPD exist: one with short episodes, 15 to 60 seconds in duration, and another with prolonged episodes, up to 60 minutes in duration.

The short episode type of NPD is characterized by movements not more than one minute in duration. Episodes can recur up to 15 times per night, usually preceded by a clinical and electroencephalographic arousal. They occur every or nearly every night. The eyes open, and almost immediately dystonic posturings occur that are associated with ballistic or choreoathetoid movements. The episodes are stereotypic and often associated with vocalizations. At the end of the episode, the patient is coherent and, when left undisturbed, usually resumes sleep. The prolonged episode type shows similar clinical features, but episodes can last up to one hour.

Associated Features: Episodes of NPD can cause severe sleep disruption and produce a complaint of insomnia. The sleep of a bedpartner may also be disturbed. The movements may be so severe that injuries due to striking a hard object can occur. The prolonged episode type has been known to antedate the onset of Huntington's disease by as much as 20 years.

Short-lasting dystonic-dyskinetic episodes, similar to those that occur during sleep, rarely can also occur during wakefulness. Generalized tonic-clonic epilepsy has been reported in patients with the short episode type of NPD. There also may be sporadic, unclassifiable episodes, such as a sudden urge to start walking or, on the contrary, a feeling of being unable to start moving. These particular episodes are suggestive of frontal-lobe epileptic seizures, although evidence of NPD being a manifestation of a seizure disorder has not been established.

Carbamazepine, sometimes at low doses, usually produces therapeutic benefit.

Course: The dystonic episodes usually do not subside spontaneously. Patients have been known to have had episodes for over 20 years.

Predisposing Factors: Not known.

Prevalence: Not known.

Age of Onset: Onset typically occurs from infancy to the fifth decade of life.

Sex Ratio: No difference.

Familial Pattern: Has been reported to occur with a familial pattern.

Pathology: Not known.

Polysomnographic Features: Episodes of NPD mainly appear out of sleep in stage two but also can occur out of stage 3 and stage 4 NREM sleep. Electroencephalographic desynchronization, indicating arousal, usually precedes the motor events by a few seconds. The motor phenomena may also be preceded by a central respiratory pause, slowed heart rate, and electrodermal changes.

During the event, the electroencephalogram (EEG) is often obscured by movement artifact, but epileptiform features are not seen either preceding, during, or immediately following the dystonic episodes.

Other Laboratory Test Features: A computed tomographic scan of the brain is typically normal. Routine EEG may demonstrate epileptiform features that are not associated with paroxysmal dystonia episodes.

Differential Diagnosis: Nocturnal paroxysmal dystonia must be differentiated from parasomnias such as sleep terrors and REM sleep behavior disorder. The duration of episodes, the dystonic-dyskinetic features, and the recurrence rate are distinguishing features.

Nocturnal paroxysmal dystonia should also be differentiated from the epilepsies. Epileptic seizures originating in the frontal lobe most closely resemble NPD. The lack of paroxysmal EEG discharges both during and in between episodes precludes a firm diagnosis of frontal-lobe epilepsy. Only one patient has been reported to have associated epilepsy. If NPD with brief episodes should eventually be shown to be an epileptic syndrome, it could represent the extrapyramidal, choreoathetoid, epilepsy described by Marchand and Ajuriaguerra. However, this old epileptic category probably represents patients now defined as having paroxysmal choreoathetosis.

Diagnostic Criteria: Nocturnal Paroxysmal Dystonia (780.59-1)

A. The patient has a complaint of abnormal motor activity during sleep.
B. Dystonic or dyskinetic episodes occur mainly during sleep.
C. Short-duration episodes typically last 15 to 60 seconds, and prolonged-duration episodes typically last 60 minutes.
D. Polysomnography demonstrates dystonic or dyskinetic movements occurring out of NREM sleep.
E. No medical or mental disorder (e.g., frontal-lobe epilepsy, can account for the symptoms).
F. The symptoms do not meet the diagnostic criteria for other sleep disorders, such as REM-sleep behavior disorder or sleep terrors.

Note: Specify and code the type of NPD according to duration of episodes (e.g., nocturnal paroxysmal dystonia–short-episode type).

Minimal Criteria: A plus B plus E plus F.

Severity Criteria:

Mild: Episodes occur less than nightly.
Moderate: Episodes occur nightly.
Severe: Episodes occur nightly and cause severe sleep disruption.

Duration Criteria:

Acute: 1 month or less.
Subacute: More than 1 month and less than 6 months.
Chronic: More than 6 months.

Bibliography:

Lee BI, Lesser RP, Pippenger CE, et al. Familial paroxysmal hypnogenic dystonia. Neurology 1985; 35: 1357–1360.

Lugaresi E, Cirignotta F. Hypnogenic paroxysmal dystonia: Epileptic seizures or a new syndrome? Sleep 1981; 4: 129–138.

Lugaresi E, Cirignotta F, Montagna P. Nocturnal paroxysmal dystonia. J Neurol Neurosurg Psychiatry 1986; 49: 375–380.

Sudden Unexplained Nocturnal Death Syndrome (780.59-3)

Synonyms and Key Words: Sudden unexplained death syndrome. Synonyms (translations) include "non-laita" (sleep death) in Laotian, "gangungut" (to arise and moan) in Tagalog, and "pokkuri" (sudden death) in Japanese.

Essential Features:

Sudden unexplained nocturnal death syndrome (SUND) is characterized by sudden death during sleep in healthy young adults, particularly of Southeast Asian descent.

Neither clinical history nor autopsy results provide an explanation for the cause of death. According to witnesses of SUND, the first signs are choking, gasping, and labored respiration (without wheezing or stridor). Attempts to awaken the person are unsuccessful. In several successfully resuscitated patients, ventricular fibrillation was subsequently detected.

Associated Features: Laotian, Kampuchean, and Vietnamese male refugees between the ages of 25 and 44 years are most often the victims. There are descriptive terms in the Asian language that suggest that SUND has long been recognized.

Studies have failed to identify any social, religious, or work-related activity, rituals, or specific daytime events that could be associated with SUND. Acutely stressful events were found in 4 of 51 cases. Neither exposure to chemical and biologic toxins nor use of drugs or alcohol has been implicated in the deaths. Sleep terrors have been reported to occur frequently in patients who subsequently have been victims of SUND.

Course: Fatal.

Predisposing Factors: A high incidence of SUND has occurred among Southeast Asian refugees in the United States. Of those who have died in the United States, the median length of time in the United States was 17 months. Laotians, Kampucheans, and Vietnamese are particularly afflicted. More than 50% of cases have been reported to occur in the Hmong, an ethnic subgroup from the highlands of northern Laos.

Structural abnormalities of the cardiovascular system and stress have been suggested as predisposing factors.

Prevalence: Over 100 cases have been reported. The rates for different Southeast Asian groups with SUND among male refugees settled in the United States are as follows:

  A. Hmong Laotians: 92 per 100,000
  B. Other Laotians: 82 per 100,000
  C. Kampucheans: 59 per 100,000

Age of Onset: The SUND syndrome occurs mostly in men between the ages of 24 and 44 years (median 33 years). When the disorder occurs in older men, cardiovascular pathology that could explain the sudden death is more likely to be found. The fatal event most often occurs within two years after arrival in the United States.

Sex Ratio: This syndrome is seen predominantly in males. There have been very few cases reported in females.

Familial Pattern: None known.

Pathology: No postmortem pathology has been found with this disorder.

Complications: Death.

Polysomnographic Features: No reports of polysomnography exist in the current literature.

Other Laboratory Test Features: All patients who were successfully resuscitated after sudden cardiac arrest during sleep were in ventricular fibrillation when examined by paramedics.

Differential Diagnosis: The SUND syndrome is differentiated from other forms of sudden sleep-related death by negative findings of cardiac disease or other known precipitants of cardiac arrhythmias.

Diagnostic Criteria: Sudden Unexplained Nocturnal Death Syndrome (780.59-3)

A. Sudden cardiorespiratory arrest occurs during sleep.
B. The disorder occurs in persons of Southeast Asian descent.
C. Associated features include one or more of the following:
   1. Male sex
   2. Choking, gurgling, gasping, or labored breathing occur during the episode
   3. The episode occurs during the habitual sleep period
   4. The patient has a history of prior sleep terrors
D. Polysomnographic monitoring of survivors has not been reported.
E. Cardiac studies of survivors have demonstrated spontaneous ventricular fibrillation after initial resuscitation.
F. No other medical or mental disorder (e.g., ischemic heart disease, accounts for the features).
G. The disorder may be associated with sleep terrors, but the symptoms do not meet the criteria for other sleep disorders producing a risk of cardiopulmonary arrest (e.g., obstructive sleep apnea syndrome or REM-sleep-related sinus arrest).

Minimal Criteria: A plus B plus C.

Severity Criteria: Always severe.

Duration Criteria: Always acute.

Bibliography:

Aponte G. The enigma of "gangungut." Ann Intern Med 1960; 52: 1259–1263.
Baron RC, Thacker SB, Gorelkin L, Vernon AA, Taylor WR, Choi K. Sudden death among Southeast Asian refugees. An unexplained nocturnal phenomenon. JAMA 1983; 250: 2947–2951.
Cobb LA. Cardiac arrest during sleep. N Engl J Med 1984; 311: 1044–1045.
Lown B. Sudden cardiac death: Biobehavioral perspective. Circulation 1987; 76: I186–I197.
Otto CM, Tauxe RV, Cobb LA, et al. Ventricular fibrillation causes sudden death in Southeast Asian immigrants. Ann Intern Med 1984; 101: 45–47.

Primary Snoring (786.09)

Synonyms and Key Words: Simple snoring, snoring without sleep apnea, noisy breathing during sleep, benign snoring, rhythmic snoring, continuous snoring.

Essential Features:

Primary snoring is characterized by loud upper-airway breathing sounds in sleep, without episodes of apnea or hypoventilation.

Snoring usually produces sufficiently loud inspiratory or expiratory sounds to disturb the bedpartner or others nearby. The patient occasionally is aware of the snoring. The snoring typically occurs while the patient is in the supine position and is usually continuous, present with each breath, and not accompanied by arousals or other evidence of sleep disturbance. The patient has no complaint of insomnia or excessive sleepiness.

Associated Features: The patient may experience a dry mouth, which can lead to awakenings with a desire to drink water.

Course: It is suspected that some patients with primary snoring may be predisposed to developing obstructive sleep apnea syndrome, especially following weight gain or administration of central-nervous-system depressants such as alcohol, anxiolytics, or hypnotics.

Predisposing Factors: Enlarged tonsils; retrognathia; the use of central-nervous-system depressants, such as anxiolytics, hypnotics, or alcohol; the supine body position during sleep; nasal congestion or obstruction; and obesity can all predispose an individual to primary snoring.

Prevalence: With age, the prevalence of snoring increases in both men and women, occurring in 40% to 50% of men and women over age 65 years.

Age of Onset: Primary snoring can occur at any age but is most prevalent during middle age, especially in overweight men.

Sex Ratio: Primary snoring is more prevalent in men than women at all ages.

Familial Pattern: This disorder has been described in families, often in siblings with a similar body habitus.

Pathology: The sound usually is produced by vibration of pharyngeal tissues (posterior base of the tongue, soft palate, uvula, posterior pharyngeal wall) on inspiration due to turbulent air flow through a narrow oropharyngeal or nasopharyngeal space.

Complications: Snorers are more likely to have hypertension, ischemic heart disease, and cerebrovascular disease, but it is uncertain whether these disorders are due to upper-airway obstruction, obesity, or other causes.

Polysomnographic Features: Polysomnography demonstrates noncyclic periods of snoring, usually associated with the inspiratory and, less often, the expiratory phase of breathing. The partial upper-airway obstruction may be associated with increased respiratory effort. Although some distortion of rib cage or abdominal-wall movements may be observed, the snoring is not accompanied by arousals, oxygen desaturation, or cardiac arrhythmias. The snoring may be louder and more frequent during REM sleep or while the patient is in the supine position.

Other Laboratory Test Features: None.

Differential Diagnosis: Differentiation from obstructive sleep apnea syndrome may require polysomnography. The coarser and lower-pitched character of pharyngeal snoring can usually be differentiated from the higher-pitched inspiratory sound associated with sleep-related laryngospasm. Vocalization during sleep occasionally may be confused with snoring.

Diagnostic Criteria: Primary Snoring (786.09)

A. A complaint of snoring is made by an observer.
B. There is no evidence of insomnia or excessive sleepiness resulting from the snoring.
C. The patient complains of dryness of the mouth upon awakening.
D. Polysomnographic monitoring demonstrates all of the following
   1. Inspiratory or expiratory sounds often occurring for prolonged episodes during the total sleep time
   2. No associated abrupt arousals, arterial oxygen desaturation, or cardiac disturbances
   3. Normal sleep pattern
   4. Normal respiratory pattern during sleep
E. The symptoms do not meet the diagnostic criteria of other sleep disorders (i.e., central sleep apnea syndrome, obstructive sleep apnea syndrome, central alveolar hypoventilation syndrome, or sleep-related laryngospasm).

Minimal Criteria: A plus B.

Severity Criteria:

Mild: Snoring occurs less than nightly and only when the patient is in the supine position.
Moderate: Snoring occurs nightly, occasionally disturbs others, and is usually abolished by change in body position.
Severe: Snoring occurs nightly, disturbs others, and is not altered by change in body position. Bedpartners may have to sleep in another room due to the loudness of the snoring.

Duration Criteria:

Acute: 3 months or less.
Subacute: More than 3 months but less than 1 year.
Chronic: 1 year or longer.

Bibliography:

Lugaresi E, Cirignotta F, Montagna P. Snoring: Pathogenic, clinical, and therapeutic aspects. In: Kryger MH, Roth T, Dement WC, eds. Principles and practice of sleep medicine. Philadelphia: WB Saunders, 1989; 494–500.

Waller PC, Bhopal RS. Is snoring a cause of vascular disease? An epidemiological review. Lancet 1989; 1: 143–146.

Infant Sleep Apnea (770.80)

Synonyms and Key Words: Unexplained apnea, idiopathic apnea, sleep apnea, breathing pause, stop breathing episode, periodic breathing, periodic apnea. Four terms relating to infant sleep apnea are recommended: apnea of prematurity (AOP), apparent life-threatening event (ALTE), apnea of infancy (AOI), and obstructive sleep apnea syndrome (OSAS). Undesirable terms include near-miss sudden infant death syndrome (SIDS), near-SIDS, aborted SIDS, and aborted crib death. The term AOP is restricted to apnea that occurs in infants below 37 weeks of gestation and apnea that is not due to an explainable cause except respiratory immaturity. An ALTE is a clinical syndrome and may be associated with an unexplained apnea or an apnea of known cause. The diagnosis of AOI is reserved for infants who are older than 37 weeks of gestation at the onset of the apnea and for whom no specific cause of ALTE or apnea can be identified.

Essential Features:

Infant sleep apnea is characterized by central or obstructive apneas that occur during sleep.

Apnea of prematurity refers to recurrent pauses in breathing of more than 20 seconds duration or shorter pauses associated with cyanosis, abrupt pallor, or hypotonia. Two thirds of the apneic events occur during sleep, and the remainder occur during episodes of increased motor activity when infants appear awake. It is estimated that 10% of the events are purely obstructive, with the site of the obstruction in the pharynx. Cyanosis usually occurs after 20 seconds of apnea. With few exceptions, mixed and obstructive apnea terminate with spontaneous opening of the airway, and central apnea terminates with resumption of respiratory movements. Sensory stimulation can help the infant resume ventilation. Cardiopulmonary resuscitation occasionally is necessary.

The diagnosis of ALTE associated with an apnea is based on a careful clinical history. The initial apnea may be central, mixed, or obstructive and is typically accompanied by color change (usually cyanotic or pallid but occasionally erythematous or plethoric) and by marked change in muscle tone (usually marked limpness). These apneas require vigorous stimulation or mouth-to-mouth resuscitation for termination, are frightening to the observer, and suggest to some observers that the infant has died. Approximately 90% of the apneas occur during sleep; the remainder occur during wakefulness. Infants presenting with ALTE undergo a diagnostic evaluation to rule out identifiable and treatable causes for the ALTE. If an identifiable or treatable cause for the ALTE cannot be found and the presence of an apnea has been established, the diagnosis of AOI is made.

Because the respiratory system of infants is immature, many systemic conditions include apnea as a presenting sign. In some cases, treatment of the specific disorder will result in resolution of the apnea, whereas in other cases the apnea may only decrease in frequency or severity, suggesting that the other disorder only exacerbated what turns out to be AOI.

The OSAS is characterized by repetitive episodes of complete inspiratory upper-airway (extrathoracic) obstruction during sleep, defined as cessation of airflow at the nose and mouth with continued respiratory effort. In addition, repetitive or persistent partial upper-airway obstruction without apnea may result in hypoventilation or hypoxia during sleep.

Associated Features: Apnea of prematurity may be associated with clinically significant bradycardia. However, cardiorespiratory monitoring of the preterm infant reveals that almost all apneas associated with transient episodes of mild bradycardia are of little clinical significance.

It is uncertain whether some associated features of ALTE or AOI are symptoms of a prior central nervous system disorder or a result of the hypoxic event. Moreover, there is no consistency in the presenting signs. In some infants, lethargy and impeded rate of growth or decreased upper-extremity tone have been observed. A finding of blood in the nasopharynx is rare.

The signs and symptoms of OSAS are more subtle in the infant than in the adult, thus the diagnosis is more difficult to make and should be confirmed by polysomnography. During infancy, snoring, which is characteristic of adult OSAS, may not be present. Infants more commonly present with noisy breathing, stridor, or inspiratory retractions on physical examination. These signs may be absent, however, if the infant is examined during wakefulness. Infants do not manifest excessive sleepiness, but if the resulting hypoxia is severe, infants may be lethargic or hypotonic while awake. Excessive sweating may occur. Failure to thrive is commonly seen and may be the only presenting sign.

Course: Apnea of prematurity may occur infrequently, such as only once a week, or may occur several times per hour. An inverse relationship exists between gestational age and AOP. For instance, infants who are born after 26 weeks of gestation may exhibit apnea up to 80 days after birth, whereas infants who are born after 31 weeks of gestation tend to exhibit apnea for less than 28 days. Apnea persists for longer than seven days in only about 5% of asymptomatic preterm infants who are born after 34 weeks of gestation. Because hospitalized infants are monitored and treated, death from AOP in the hospital is rare. Although prematurity is associated with an increased risk for SIDS, there is no conclusive evidence that AOP confers a significant additional SIDS risk above that due to prematurity alone.

The course of apnea associated with ALTE will depend on the underlying etiology. In approximately 30% of infants with AOI, the episodes will occur as isolated events and will not be followed by a subsequent episode. Fifty percent of the infants will exhibit one or more recurrent clinically defined episodes within the same week. It is estimated that of all episodes of reported apnea recognized after an ALTE or AOI, 7% were perceived to be severe enough to require cardiopulmonary resuscitation. One out of five infants may continue to exhibit these episodes during their first year of life, with most episodes probably subsiding before the infant is six months old. Infants who experienced their AOI while awake or during the first week of life are at a lesser risk for recurrence than are those infants who experienced the AOI during sleep or at an older age.

When reports of subsequent recurrent apnea are based on home apnea monitoring, incidence rates are elevated. The measured variable is the monitor alarm, which is not the best estimate of the recurrence of clinically significant apnea for two reasons. First, the bradycardia criteria include heart-rate levels that are seen in healthy infants. Second, when simultaneous telemetric recordings are made, monitoring alarms that lead to parental intervention are not accompanied by bradycardia.

Progression of OSAS may be slow or rapid, but once complications develop (especially pulmonary hypertension), progression is accelerated. Many infants and children never reach that point, however. The development of pulmonary hypertension and cor pulmonale can cause death.

Predisposing Factors: While any infant's respiratory system is predisposed to apnea, that of the preterm infant is even more susceptible. AOP can be triggered by spontaneous or intervention-related neck flexion, squirming induced by a painful stimulus, hiccup, regurgitation, and feeding. Susceptibility to AOP is also enhanced by general anesthesia and the use of other medications that depress the central nervous system.

Preterm infants with significant clinically defined prolonged AOP that occurs after the first week of life but before 37 weeks postconceptional age probably have an enhanced risk for the occurrence of ALTE or AOI.

There is no systematic relationship between ALTE, AOI, and bouts of upper-respiratory infection or immunizations, but it can be argued that the latter are stresses (like sleep deprivation, travel, or fever) and can induce recurrences of apnea in some vulnerable infants.

Infants with OSAS usually have a congenital anomaly of the upper airway that is associated with increased upper-airway resistance, such as choanal atresia or stenosis, mid-face hypoplasia, micrognathia, Pierre Robin syndrome, Down syndrome, or cleft palate. A severe upper-respiratory infection or chronic allergic rhinitis may cause transient obstructive sleep apnea.

Prevalence: Estimates of AOP before 31 weeks of gestation range between 50% and 80%, with a sharp reduction in infants older than 31 weeks. Only 12% to 15% of infants born after 32 weeks of gestation tend to exhibit apnea, and this value is further reduced to about 7% in infants born between 34 and 35 weeks of gestation.

There are no definitive data about the prevalence of clinically defined apnea recognized after an ALTE or AOI. The lowest estimate reported is 1.6 per thousand live births. In one study, parents of 3 out of 100 healthy infants reported having seen an ALTE or unexplained apnea; this number was doubled in infants who subsequently died of SIDS. This estimate is almost certainly too high because the recognition of the event relied on parental memory and these recollections are unlikely to duplicate the clinical definition outlined here.

The prevalence of OSAS in infants is unknown but appears to be uncommon.

Age of Onset:

AOP: The onset of AOP can occur after the first or second day of life, and the onset of AOP may appear after discontinuation of ventilatory support in neonates with respiratory distress syndrome.

Apnea with an ALTE and AOI: The peak time of the first ALTE with an apnea or of AOI is four to eight weeks of age, with a large spread up to eight months of age. The apneas have their onset sporadically beyond this age.

OSAS: OSAS may begin at any age.

Sex Ratio:

AOP: No difference.

ALTE with Apnea and AOI: Five percent to 10% higher incidence in males.

OSAS: No difference.

Familial Patterns:

AOP: None.

ALTE with Apnea, and AOI: Not known, but probably no inherited or familial pattern.

OSAS: Insufficient evidence exists to implicate an inherited or familial pattern, but there are isolated reports of a familial component.

Pathology: Apnea of prematurity is due to immaturity of the respiratory system. Preterm infants with AOP exhibit a decreased carbon-dioxide sensitivity, coupled with a decreased minute ventilation. Sensitivity normalizes after resolution of the apnea.

There are no consistent abnormalities in chemoreceptor control of sleeping ventilatory patterns in AOI. There is a suggestion of a decreased arousal response to hypoxia.

OSAS is most commonly seen in infants with increased upper-airway resistance due to anatomically narrow airways. In addition, neurologic lesions that affect control of upper-airway skeletal muscle tone or coordination may cause OSAS. Hypoxia and hypercapnia have also been shown to produce OSAS in some infants.

Complications: In AOP, a reduction in cerebral blood flow accompanies some of the longer apneas. Preterm infants have many other causes of hypoxia; therefore, long-term outcome studies have failed to distinguish the sequelae of hypoxia due to other causes from those due to apnea alone. The sequelae may turn out to be more severe if apnea is accompanied by decreased cerebral blood flow.

Periodic breathing occurs in 85% of healthy preterm infants between 32 and 36 weeks postconceptional age. Although these pauses cause slight reductions in transcutaneous oxygen levels, there is no convincing evidence that any but the most-severe episodes are of clinical significance.

There does not appear to be a relationship between the periodic breathing and the incidence of AOP in this age range.

Infants with AOI are at increased risk of dying from SIDS. The best estimate is between 2% and 6%, with a significant but not exclusive increased risk if the infant needed positive-pressure resuscitation. Although a few infants have severe sequelae, such as regression to a vegetative state, after ALTE or AOI, thus far few studies have documented a systematic increase in morbidity. It has been estimated that 1% of infants with AOI have significant cardiac arrhythmias, including sinus arrest. One percent of infant sleep apnea results from OSAS.

Pulmonary hypertension and cor pulmonale are life-threatening complications of OSAS. Systemic hypertension can be seen, but in contrast to the occurrence in adults with OSAS, cardiac arrhythmias in infant OSAS are probably rare. Polycythemia occurs in infants as a result of chronic intermittent hypoxia.

Polysomnographic Features: Limited evidence suggests that in AOP, the apneic events are less frequent during quiet sleep than during active sleep, with the longest apneas (>40 seconds) restricted to active sleep; the latter are more often associated with bradycardia appearing both early and late after cessation of breathing. Apnea of infancy can be defined as a single pause or repetitive respiratory pauses of unknown etiology in excess of 20 seconds or pauses shorter than 20 seconds if associated with cyanosis. However, most long-term polysomnographic tracings from infants with ALTE or AOI, compared with tracings from healthy infants, do not reveal abnormalities. A few reveal abnormal findings, such as a fixed heart rate, excessive periodic breathing, excessive numbers of apneas, or short obstructive pauses. The significance of isolated episodes of hypoxia, measured by transcutaneous oxygen ($PtcO_2$) or arterial oxygen saturation (SaO_2), awaits comparison with normative values.

The most reliable technique for making the diagnosis of OSAS is a tight-fitting face mask with a pneumotachograph to measure airflow and an intraesophageal balloon to measure intrathoracic pressure swings. However, these devices are not well tolerated by infants, who often will not sleep with the devices in place. While there is a lack of normative data for $PtcO_2$ and $PtcCO_2$ or SaO_2 in infants, some infants with OSAS demonstrate chronic hypercapnia or hypoxia during sleep ($PtcCO_2 >50$ or $SaO_2 <85\%$). Polysomnographic tracings, under most circumstances, will confirm the diagnosis of OSAS, although a daytime nap may be too brief to reveal obstructive apneas.

Other Laboratory Test Features: The pneumogram, a 12-hour overnight two-channel recording of chest-wall impedance, respirations, and electrocardiogram (ECG), can be employed in the hospital or at home. The pneumogram often fails to confirm the diagnosis of ALTE with apnea or AOI and cannot be considered a conclusive diagnostic test or a reliable predictor of either subsequent apnea or death. It cannot detect obstructive sleep apnea.

In children with severe OSAS, arterial blood gases obtained during wakefulness may be normal but can show hypercapnia and hypoxia. Lateral neck radiographs, which visualize the upper airway, may show tonsillar or adenoidal hypertrophy or other causes of upper-airway narrowing. The chest radiograph may show cardiomegaly or pulmonary edema in severe cases. Pulmonary hypertension may be evidenced by findings of ECG and echocardiogram (right-ventricular dimensions, pulmonic-valve systolic time intervals, septal morphology, pulmonic-valve "a" dip, pulmonic-valve early systolic closure, and acceleration time of pulmonary-artery flow [Doppler]). Elevated hemoglobin and hematocrit levels may indicate polycythemia from chronic intermittent hypoxia.

Differential Diagnosis: In preterm infants, any systemic disorder or abnormality can cause apnea. The following disorders are especially prone to causing apnea: respiratory infections such as respiratory syncytial virus or chlamydia; hypothermia and hyperthermia; hypoglycemia and hyperglycemia; hypocalcemia; other electrolyte imbalances; anemia; sepsis; intraventricular hemorrhage; hypoxia; acidosis; lung disease; pneumothorax; seizures; and necrotizing enterocolitis.

Apnea of infancy must be distinguished from ALTE with apnea due to a known cause. Treatable causes are found in 15% to 25% of infants presenting to referral centers with ALTE with apnea. The proportion of infants with treatable causes of ALTE presenting to primary-care physicians may be higher. Diagnostic evaluation should include serum electrolytes, glucose, calcium, and thyroid studies; chest radiograph; ECG; arterial blood gases; clinical electroencephalogram (EEG); and a barium esophagram or gastric scintiscan. Some infants may require lumbar puncture or laryngoscopy and bronchoscopy, as indicated by history and physical examination. If functional obstructions are suspected, a polysomnogram can aid in the diagnosis.

Seizures are a common cause of ALTE with apnea in infants. Pneumonia with resultant increased work of breathing and hypoxia commonly causes apnea, especially in young infants (first two-three months of life). Similarly, chronic lung disease can cause apnea. Gastroesophageal reflux (GER) is seen in 30% to 50% of normal infants, and the association with apnea is rare. A history of spitting up following feedings is usually present. The diagnosis of GER is made by barium esophagram, gastric scintiscan, or esophageal pH-probe monitoring. Polysomnography with esophageal pH monitoring shows that documented episodes of reflux are usually not temporally associated with apneas. This finding sheds doubt on the theory that GER is an important cause of infant apnea. Sepsis can cause infant sleep apnea.

Malformations resulting in narrowing of the larynx and trachea (such as tracheal stenosis, laryngeal web, or unilateral or bilateral abductor vocal cord paralysis) can cause sleep apnea in infants. The location of the airway obstruction may be difficult to determine based upon clinical symptoms, and laryngoscopy and bronchoscopy are usually necessary.

Diagnostic Criteria: Infant Sleep Apnea (770.80)

A. The clinical presentation of infant sleep apnea includes one or more of the following:
   1. An episode of cessation of breathing during sleep
   2. An episode characterized by
      a. Color change (pallor or cyanosis)
      b. Tone change (limpness, rarely stiffness)
   3. Noisy breathing during sleep
B. Central or obstructive apneas occur during sleep.
C. The age of infant at presentation can be either:

1. Less than 37 weeks postconceptional age (for AOP)
2. Greater than 37 weeks postconceptional age (for AOI)
D. Polysomnographic monitoring demonstrates one or more of the following:
   1. Prolonged central apnea, longer than 20 seconds
   2. Obstructive apnea, longer than 10 seconds
   3. An apnea accompanied by cyanosis
   4. An apnea accompanied by transient bradycardia (defined as a drop in heart rate to levels below 50 bpm, a heart rate below 60 bpm lasting more than 10 seconds, or a drop below 60 bpm with a duration exceeding 30 seconds below baseline heart rate)
   5. Arterial oxygen saturation less than 85% during sleep
   6. Sustained hypoventilation (e.g., $PETCO_2$ >45 mm Hg) during sleep
E. An identifiable cause for the apnea was either
   1. Found following a thorough diagnostic evaluation and is believed to be the cause of the apnea (ALTE with apnea, OSAS)
   2. Not found following a thorough diagnostic evaluation (AOP, AOI)

Note: State and code the diagnosis as infant sleep apnea (770.80). If desired, specify the type according to the appropriate diagnostic features (e.g., infant sleep apnea–AOP type [770.80], infant sleep apnea–AOI-type, ALTE-with-apnea-type–OSAS-type).

Minimal Criteria:

AOP Type: A plus B plus C.1 plus D.
ALTE with Apnea: A.2 plus B plus C.2.
AOI: A.2 plus B plus C.2 plus E.2.
OSAS: A or B plus D.2.

Severity Criteria:

Mild: Intermittent apneas that resolve spontaneously. Significant complications, associated features, and significant hypoxia or hypercapnia are absent.
Moderate: Several prolonged apneas that are resolved only after vigorous stimulation; polysomnographic testing shows moderate hypoxia without hypercapnia; and symptoms interfere with normal activities or lifestyle.
Severe: One or more of the following conditions is present:

a. Apneas resolve only after full cardiopulmonary resuscitation
b. Recurrent prolonged (>20 seconds) apneas
c. Severe complications, including right-heart failure, chronic hypercapnia, and severe hypoxia

Duration Criteria:

Acute: 14 days or less.
Subacute: More than 14 days but less than 30 days.
Chronic: 30 days or longer.

Bibliography:

Brazy JE, Kinney HC, Oakes WJ. Central nervous system structural lesions causing apnea at birth. J Pediatr 1987; 111: 163–175.
Brouillette RT, Fernbach SK, Hunt CE. Obstructive sleep apnea in infants and children. J Pediatr 1982; 100: 31–40.
Durand M, Cabal LA, Gonzalez F, Georgie S, Barberis C, Hoppenbrouwers T, Hodgman JE. Ventilatory control and carbon dioxide response in preterm infants with idiopathic apnea. Am J Dis Child 1985; 139: 717–720.
Guilleminault C, Souquet M, Ariagno RL, Korobkin R, Simmons FB. Five cases of near-miss sudden infant death syndrome and development of obstructive sleep apnea syndrome. Pediatrics 1984; 73: 71–78.
Henderson-Smart DJ. The effect of gestational age on the incidence and duration of recurrent apnoea in newborn babies. Aust Paediatr J 1985; 17: 273–276.
Krongrad E, O'Neill L. Near miss sudden infant death syndrome episodes? A clinical and electrocardiographic correlation. Pediatrics 1986; 77: 811–815.
Martin RJ, Miller MJ, Carlo WA. Pathogenesis of apnea in preterm infants. J Pediatr 1986; 109: 733–741.
NIH. Infantile apnea and home monitoring: Report of a consensus development conference. NIH Publication #87–2905, 1987.
Oren J, Kelly D, Shannon DC. Identification of a high-risk group for sudden infant death syndrome among infants who were resuscitated for sleep apnea. Pediatrics 1986; 77: 495–499.
Perlman JM, Volpe JJ. Episodes of apnea and bradycardia in the preterm newborn: Impact on cerebral circulation. Pediatrics 1985; 76: 333–338.

Congenital Central Hypoventilation Syndrome (770.81)

Synonyms and Key Words: Congenital central hypoventilation syndrome, central alveolar hypoventilation syndrome, central hypoventilation syndrome, primary alveolar hypoventilation syndrome, Ondine's curse.

Essential Features:

Congenital central hypoventilation syndrome (CCHS) is characterized by hypoventilation, which is worse during sleep than wakefulness and is unexplained by primary pulmonary disease or ventilatory muscle weakness.

Central alveolar hypoventilation (CAHS) is defined as the failure of the automatic control of breathing. Hypoventilation, in the absence of any lung disease or ventilatory muscle dysfunction, is worse during sleep but may also occur during wakefulness.

The CCHS presents in an otherwise normal-appearing infant who does not breathe spontaneously or breathes erratically. In most infants, a problem is evident at birth. The infant cannot be weaned from mechanically assisted ventilation. Other infants may appear to breathe adequately by clinical examination but experience hypoventilation (not necessarily apnea) that is characterized by hypoxia and hypercapnia, resulting in progressive pulmonary hypertension, cor pulmonale, and central nervous system hypoxic damage.

Associated Features: The CCHS is associated with absent or diminished ventilatory responses to both hypoxia and hypercapnia, especially during quiet sleep. During the first few months of life, infants may not yet show greater hypoventilation during sleep; the pattern may only emerge as the infant matures. Blood-gas parameters during wakefulness may be normal. Some infants have a more severe form of the disorder, resulting in hypoventilation during both sleep and wakefulness, regardless of the level of ventilatory support during sleep.

Infants with CCHS may present with apneic episodes. Infants who present at a few months of age can have cyanosis and pulmonary hypertension as the predominant signs. Central alveolar hypoventilation can be seen in infants with myelomeningocele, the Arnold-Chiari malformation, and other neurologic syndromes due to neuroectodermal malformations involving the brain stem or craniocervical junction.

There is a higher than expected frequency of neuroblastoma and Hirschsprung's disease associated with CCHS.

Course: The physiologic abnormalities of CCHS remain for life. The clinical consequences of hypoventilation can be improved or alleviated by providing full ventilatory support only during sleep, or full-time in some children. If the CCHS is untreated, pulmonary hypertension, cor pulmonale, and death may result. Some children may die from apnea or complications of severe hypoventilation.

When treated, infants diagnosed with CCHS may improve over the first 6 to 12 months of life. Infants who present with hypoventilation during both sleep and wakefulness may progress to being able to sustain adequate spontaneous ventilation during wakefulness, but others who initially need only sleep-related support may worsen over time and may require 24-hour ventilatory support.

Even with treatment, these patients often require close monitoring during infancy. Frequent respiratory infections and other physical stresses increase the work of breathing, and full-time ventilatory support coupled with hospitalization to monitor the adequacy of the treatment may be necessary. The ability of these patients to tolerate infections without substantial deterioration in the control of breathing improves with age. By four to five years of age, the children may not require hospitalization with every respiratory infection.

Predisposing Factors: Not known.

Prevalence: Not known, but rare.

Age of Onset: By definition, CCHS is present from birth, although it is not always recognized at birth. Even when the diagnosis is made later in infancy, signs and symptoms can usually be traced back to birth.

Sex Ratio: No difference.

Familial Pattern: None known.

Pathology: The most likely site of pathology is in the respiratory centers of the brain stem, where input from both central and peripheral chemoreceptors is integrated. Unless central alveolar hypoventilation is caused by a major brain stem malformation, such as an Arnold-Chiari malformation, no gross brain stem pathology is evident.

Complications: The clinical signs of hypoxia and hypercapnia can be quite subtle, and children may not look distressed. They do not develop inspiratory retractions, nasal flaring, or other signs of increased respiratory effort in response to hypoxia. As a result, blood gas derangements may progress for quite some time without notice until the child appears to deteriorate suddenly, with a cardiopulmonary arrest or severe decompensation. Thus, physicians and caretakers must be sensitive to very subtle signs of hypoxia, such as lethargy and slight edema.

Children may also show other signs of brain stem dysfunction, such as esophageal dysmotility, which are likely to improve with age. Developmental delay and intellectual impairment, with IQ scores in the 70 to 80 range, are not uncommon sequelae of CCHS. Seizures can occur in some patients.

Polysomnographic Features: Gas exchange can be measured by continuous and noninvasive end-tidal carbon-dioxide measurements, transcutaneous oxygen and carbon-dioxide tensions, arterial oxygen saturation by pulse oximetry, or arterial line with intermittent blood gas measurements. There is a spectrum of severity, but generally, the hypercapnia or hypoxia will worsen as the length of the sleep episode increases. Hypercapnia is usually the first sign of hypoventilation, but hypoxia can be the initial abnormality.

Other Laboratory Test Features: Arterial blood gases obtained through arterial puncture may not give a reliable assessment of gas exchange; blood gases can best be obtained through an indwelling arterial catheter. In severe or untreated patients who are in a steady state, arterial blood gases may demonstrate a compensated respiratory acidosis (high $PaCO_2$ with normal pH). However, in an acute hypoxic episode, such as that caused by a respiratory infection, the metabolic acidosis produced by the hypoxia may eliminate any compensatory metabolic alkalosis that would otherwise be diagnostic of chronic hypoventilation.

In CCHS, brain stem scans obtained by computed axial tomography and magnetic resonance imaging tend to be normal but may reveal a cause, such as Arnold-Chiari malformation, in some patients. Electrocardiogram (ECG) and echocardiogram (right-ventricular dimensions, pulmonic-valve systolic time intervals, septal morphology, pulmonic-valve "a" dip, pulmonic-valve early systolic closure, and acceleration time of pulmonary-artery flow [Doppler]) may show evidence of pulmonary hypertension. Elevated hemoglobin and hematocrit levels may indicate polycythemia from chronic intermittent hypoxia. Pneumograms are unsuited for making the diagnosis of CCHS.

Differential Diagnosis: Acquired central hypoventilation syndrome can be caused by brain stem damage from infection, brain tumors, brain stem trauma, hemorrhage, vascular accidents, and neurologic operations. The clinical and physiologic manifestations are similar to those of the congenital form. Leigh's disease and other inborn errors of metabolism can also cause central hypoventilation syndrome.

A chest radiograph is usually sufficient to rule out lung disease, and fluoroscopy of the diaphragm or normal measurements of ventilatory muscle strength (maximal inspiratory [mouth] pressure or maximal transdiaphragmatic pressures) that are generally rule out ventilatory muscle dysfunction. The subjective response of the patient to being taken off the ventilator is of clinical significance: infants with primary lung or ventilatory muscle disease will usually appear distressed when removed from a ventilator and when hypoxia or hypercapnia set in. In contrast, infants with CCHS do not appear hypoxic, as evidenced by a lack of distress or efforts to increase ventilation.

CCHS with associated pulmonary hypertension has features similar to those of cyanotic congenital heart disease and can be distinguished by ECG, echocardiogram, or cardiac catheterization. Hypothyroidism can cause hypoventilation.

Diagnostic Criteria: Congenital Central Hypoventilation Syndrome (770.81)

A. The patient exhibits shallow breathing, or cyanosis and apnea, that is worse during sleep than in wakefulness and has a perinatal onset.
B. Hypoventilation is worse during sleep than in wakefulness.
C. Ventilatory response to hypoxia and hypercapnia is absent or diminished.
D. Polysomnographic monitoring during sleep demonstrates hypercapnia and hypoxia, predominantly without apnea.
E. No primary lung disease or ventilatory muscle dysfunction can explain the hypoventilation.
F. The symptoms are not due to any other sleep disorder, such as infant sleep apnea.

Minimal Criteria: A plus B plus E plus F.

Severity Criteria:

Mild: Hypoventilation during sleep without any hypoventilation during wakefulness and without pulmonary hypertension or complications.
Moderate: Hypoventilation during sleep with intermittent daytime hypoventilation; pulmonary hypertension and other complications can be controlled or alleviated by ventilatory assistance during sleep only.
Severe: Hypoventilation during both sleep and wakefulness, necessitating full-time chronic ventilatory support.

Duration Criteria:

Acute: 14 days or less.
Subacute: More than 14 days but less than 30 days.
Chronic: 30 days or longer.

Bibliography:

Fleming PJ, Cade D, Bryan MH, Bryan AC. Congenital central hypoventilation and sleep state. Pediatrics 1980; 66: 425–428.

Mellins RB, Balfour HH Jr, Turino GM, Winters RW. Failure of automatic control of ventilation (Ondine's curse). Report of an infant born with this syndrome and review of the literature. Medicine 1970; 49: 487–504.

Oren J, Kelly DH, Shannon DC. Long-term follow-up of children with congenital central hypoventilation syndrome. Pediatrics 1987; 80: 375–380.

Paton JY, Swaminathan S, Sargent CW, Keens TG. Hypoxic and hypercapneic ventilatory responses in awake children with congenital central hypoventilation syndrome. Am Rev Respir Dis 1989; 140: 368–372.

Sudden Infant Death Syndrome (798.0)

Synonyms and Key Words: Sudden infant death syndrome, crib death, cot death.

Essential Features:

Sudden infant death syndrome (SIDS) is unexpected sudden death in which a thorough postmortem investigation fails to demonstrate an adequate cause for death.

At least 80% of SIDS deaths occur at a time when infants were assumed to be asleep. It has not been unequivocally established whether the primary cause of death is cardiac or respiratory failure.

Associated Features: Generally, SIDS victims are believed to have been healthy immediately before death. Temporal association with a mild upper-respiratory infection has been observed in about 60% of SIDS cases, but this finding cannot explain the death.

Course: Usually, death is the first sign of any problem. Between 2% and 6% of SIDS victims had an apparent life-threatening event (ALTE) or apnea of infancy (AOI) for which the parents had sought medical advice before the infant's death.

Predisposing Factors: Although infants who die of SIDS appear ostensibly healthy before death, there is reason to believe that some infants have sustained mild chronic hypoxia either in utero or during their first months of life. To date, however, no physiologic studies or other tests permit identification of infants at increased risk for having SIDS. Only epidemiologic studies have delineated groups of infants at increased risk. These include:

1. *Sleeping Position:* Recent data from the Centers for Disease Control indicate that the rate of SIDS in the United States declined approximately 20% between the early 1990s and 1994. Most of the decline in the SIDS rate has occurred since 1992, and has been attributed to changes in infant sleeping position following the April 1992 statement from the American Academy of

Pediatrics (AAP) that healthy infants be placed on their sides or backs for sleep. In other countries, much larger reductions in the SIDS rate have been observed and attributed largely to information campaigns recommending the non-prone sleeping position for infants. A recent update (1997) from the AAP Task Force on Infant Positioning and SIDS indicates that, for healthy infants, the supine sleeping position is associated with the lowest risk (compared to side and prone positions) and is preferred. The side sleeping positions for infants is also associated with a lower risk of SIDS compared to the prone position.

2. *Tobacco Smoke Exposure:* Numerous studies demonstrate that both prenatal exposure to the effects of maternal cigarette smoking and postnatal tobacco smoke exposure are associated with an increased risk of SIDS. Several studies have shown that the enhancement of risk is proportional to the degree of tobacco smoke exposure.

3. *Preterm Birth:* Infants whose birth weight is below 1,500 grams have a SIDS occurrence rate of 11/1,000 live births. The risk is enhanced in proportion to immaturity.

4. Compared to a singleton birth, a twin or triple birth causes a doubling of risk in infants below 2,500 grams, even after correction for birth weight. After the death due to SIDS of one member of a multiple birth, which is not necessarily the smallest member, the surviving infant or infants are at higher risk of SIDS than is a singleton birth.

5. *Subsequent Siblings of SIDS Victims:* Recently, better-controlled studies have placed the increased risk for siblings at not more than two to four times the rate of the general population (1-2/1,000 live births). Subsequent siblings of two or more SIDS victims have a substantially increased SIDS risk.

6. For infants born to substance-abusing mothers, especially those using opiates and cocaine, the SIDS rate is substantially elevated, to as much as 10 times that of the general population.

7. *AOI:* Two percent to 6% of infants who experienced AOI are estimated to die from SIDS, especially if positive-pressure resuscitation was required to revive the infants from their apneic event.

8. *Ethnicity and Socioeconomic Status:* The SIDS rate is elevated in lower-socioeconomic groups. Black and Eskimo babies are at four to six times increased risk for SIDS; the rate is lower when a correction is made for socioeconomic status.

The following factors also contribute to increased risk: teenage pregnancy, especially if coupled with high parity; short interpregnancy interval; and winter, spring, and fall births. None of the described factors, either singly or in combination, permits accurate prediction of which infant will die of SIDS.

Prevalence: SIDS is estimated to occur in 0.85/1000 live births, with significant variations depending on the items outlined above.

Age of Onset: SIDS is rarely seen during the first week of life; the rate increases sharply after that time and reaches a peak between 10 and 12 weeks of age. Ninety percent of SIDS deaths occur before six months of age. Not more than 1%

of all SIDS deaths occur past the infant's first birthday. Preterm infants die from SIDS later after birth than do their full-term counterparts, yet their corrected post-conceptional age has not reached that of full-term infants. In other words, both immaturity and postnatal experience play a role in deaths from SIDS.

Sex Ratio: The male to female ratio varies from 3:2 to 11:9.

Familial Patterns: Risk in subsequent siblings is two to four times enhanced compared to siblings of infants who did not die from SIDS. This rate is not high enough to postulate a genetic origin of SIDS in most infants.

Pathology: By definition, the postmortem examination of SIDS victims fails to reveal a cause of death. Nonspecific findings may include intrathoracic petechiae, mild pulmonary congestion and edema, minor airway inflammation, empty urinary bladder, and negligible stress effects in the thymus and adrenal gland. In general, SIDS is associated with normal nutrition and development, and none of these minor findings can explain the death.

Research studies have revealed gliosis and other subtle brain-stem changes in some infants, suggesting the possible involvement of breathing or arousal disorders in SIDS. This finding remains a matter of speculation.

Polysomnographic Features: Despite extensive polygraphic recordings of infants at risk for developing SIDS as outlined above, no abnormal polygraphic patterns have been identified that reliably identify the infant who will die of SIDS.

Other Laboratory Test Features: Approximately 100 to 150 tracings, such as pneumograms or fetal heart-rate tracings, have been collected in a number of centers across the world from infants who have subsequently died of SIDS. Together, these results have not revealed conclusive information about either the mechanism of SIDS or death. No specific features of the tracings reliably predict which infants will die of SIDS.

Differential Diagnosis: The cause of SIDS is a matter of speculation, but most investigators agree that the pathophysiology of SIDS will probably be varied. Thus far, a small proportion of infants believed to have died from SIDS probably died from infant botulism. The more common causes of death that must be differentiated are pneumonia, meningitis, myocarditis, intracranial hemorrhage, and child abuse.

Diagnostic Criteria: Sudden Infant Death Syndrome (798.0)

A. Death, which usually occurs during sleep, is unexpected by history.
B. The cause of death is unexplained following a postmortem examination.
C. The infant is under one year of age; rare cases occur between 12 and 24 months of age.
D. The infant appeared to be healthy or in the usual state of health immediately before death.

Minimal Criteria: A plus B plus C plus D.

Severity Criteria: Not applicable.

Duration Criteria: Not applicable.

Bibliography:

CDC. Sudden Infant Death Syndrome - United States, 1983-1994. MMWR 1996;45:859–863.

DiFranza JR, Lew RA. Effect of maternal cigarette smoking on pregnancy complications and sudden infant death syndrome. J Fam Pract 1995;40:385–394.

Fleming PJ, Blair PS, Bacon C, et al. Environment of infants during sleep and risk of the sudden infant death syndrome: Results of 1993-5 case-control study for confidential inquiry into stillbirths and deaths in infancy. Confidential Enquiry into Stillbirths and Deaths Regional Coordinators and Researchers. BMJ 1996;313:191–195.

Hoppenbrouwers T, Hodgman JE. Sudden infant death syndrome (SIDS): An integration of ontogenetic, pathologic, physiologic and epidemiologic factors. Neuropediatrics 1982; 13: 36–51.

Hoppenbrouwers T, Hodgman JE. Sudden infant death syndrome (SIDS). Public Health Rev 1983; 11: 363–390.

Merritt TA, Valdes-Dapena M. SIDS research update. Pediatr Ann 1984; 13: 193–207.

Naeye RL. Sudden infant death. Sci Am 1980; 242: 56–62.

Peterson DR, Sabotta EE, Daling JR. Infant mortality among subsequent siblings of infants who died of sudden infant death syndrome. J Pediatr 1986; 108: 911–914.

NCHS. Advance report of final natality statistics, 1994. Hyattsville, MD: US Department of Health and Human Services, Public Health Service, CDC, 1996. (Monthly vital statistics report; Vol. 44, no. 11 suppl).

Kattwinkel J (Chair), Brooks J, Keenan ME< and Mally M: Positioning and Sudden Infant Death Syndrome (SIDS): Update. Task Force on Infant Positioning and SIDS, American Academy of Pediatrics. Pediatrics 98(6):1216-1218, 1996.

Benign Neonatal Sleep Myoclonus (780.59-5)

Synonyms and Key Words: Twitching, partial myoclonus, sleep myoclonus.

Essential Features:

Benign neonatal sleep myoclonus is characterized by asynchronous jerking of the limbs and trunk that occurs during quiet sleep in neonates.

The jerks usually occur in clusters of four or five, with a frequency of approximately one per second, and are very brief, lasting 40 to 300 milliseconds. The jerks can occur in any part of the body but most often involve the arms or legs, sometimes being most prominent in distal muscle groups. The pattern of movements tends to vary between affected individuals and can consist of flexion and extension or abduction and adduction.

Associated Features: None.

Course: The course is self-limited and benign. The disorder may be present for only a few days or may last for several months.

Predisposing Factors: None known.

Prevalence: Not known, but apparently rare.
Age of Onset: Onset usually occurs within the first week of life.

Sex Ratio: No difference.

Familial Pattern: A family history of the disorder can be present. No genetic studies have been performed.

Pathology: No known biochemical or anatomic pathology.

Complications: None known. The disorder appears to be benign.

Polysomnographic Features: Polysomnography demonstrates paroxysmal muscle activity, predominantly during quiet sleep, with sporadic movements during active sleep. The muscle jerks last from 40 to 300 milliseconds. The activity occurs with the same frequency in both the tracé-alternant patterns of quiet sleep in neonates and the high-voltage slow-wave sleep of older infants. The myoclonus is not associated with sleep-stage transitions or awakenings.

Other Laboratory Test Features: Brain imaging and electroencephalographic (EEG) studies are normal.

Differential Diagnosis: The main diagnosis to exclude is neonatal seizures. Neonatal seizures are usually seen in the context of perinatal disorders such as asphyxia, infection, or metabolic abnormalities. Drug withdrawal can also produce jerking movements.

Infantile spasms are most often seen after the first month of life but sometimes occur earlier. Infantile spasms occur during wakefulness as well as during sleep and are associated with a hypsarrhythmic EEG pattern.

Benign infantile myoclonus of Lombroso and Fejerman usually occurs after the third month of life and only occurs during wakefulness.

Periodic limb movement disorder can occur in infants but typically begins in older age groups. It can be associated with EEG changes of arousal. The muscle activity is of longer duration and recurs at a greater interval (30–40 seconds).

Fragmentary myoclonus consists of similar brief twitchlike muscle jerks, which occur in adults and are often associated with excessive daytime sleepiness. The jerks of fragmentary myoclonus persist during REM sleep and do not show clustering, as seen in the neonatal form of myoclonus.

Diagnostic Criteria: Benign Neonatal Sleep Myoclonus (780.59-5)

A. The infant exhibits muscle jerking during sleep.
B. The disorder occurs in early infancy.
C. Polysomnography demonstrates asynchronous brief (40–300 millisecond) jerks of the limbs or trunk, predominantly during quiet sleep.

D. The infant has no other medical disorder that accounts for the activity.
E. The findings do not meet the diagnostic criteria for other sleep disorders that produce muscle jerking during sleep.

Minimal Criteria: A plus B plus D plus E.

Severity Criteria:

Mild: Muscle activity that produces muscle fasciculations only.
Moderate: Muscle activity that produces limb movements only.
Severe: Muscle activity that produces whole-body movement.

Duration Criteria:

Acute: 7 days or less.
Moderate: More than 7 days but less than 3 months.
Chronic: 3 months or longer.

Bibliography:

Coulter DL, Allen RJ. Benign neonatal sleep myoclonus. Arch Neurol 1982; 39: 191–192.
Dooley JM. Myoclonus in children. Arch Neurol 1984; 41: 138.
Resnick TJ, Moshe SL, Perotta L, Chambers HJ. Benign neonatal sleep myoclonus. Relationship to sleep states. Arch Neurol 1986; 43: 266–268.

SLEEP DISORDERS ASSOCIATED WITH MENTAL, NEUROLOGIC, AND OTHER MEDICAL DISORDERS

A large number of mental and medical disorders are associated with disturbances of sleep and wakefulness. The division into mental and medical categories is somewhat arbitrary and is used here to highlight the less usual association with medical disorders. Mental disorders are very common causes of sleep disturbance. This section is divided into three subsections. The first is a listing of the mental disorders that are more commonly seen and associated with disturbed sleep or wakefulness. The second subsection indicates the importance of neurologic disorders and their effect upon sleep and wake states. The third subsection is a listing of disorders that fall into other medical specialty areas but are insufficient in number to warrant separate subsections.

Only those medical disorders that are commonly seen in the practice of sleep-disorders medicine are listed here or described in the text. A large number of medical and mental disorders are associated with disturbances of sleep and wakefulness, but an exhaustive list is not provided here. As additional important associations with medical disorders become recognized, they will be added to this list if considered appropriate.

Because these disorders are not primary sleep disorders, their *ICD-9-CM* code number is that of the medical or mental disorder. The specific sleep-related symptom should be stated along with the diagnosis (e.g., dysthymia associated with insomnia, *ICD-9-CM* #300.40).

SLEEP DISORDERS ASSOCIATED WITH MENTAL, NEUROLOGIC, AND OTHER MEDICAL DISORDERS

ASSOCIATED WITH MENTAL DISORDERS

1. Psychoses (292-299). 216
2. Mood Disorders (296, 300, 301, 311) 219
3. Anxiety Disorders (300, 308, 309) 224
4. Panic Disorder (300). 227
5. Alcoholism (303, 305) 230

Sleep Disorders Associated with Mental Disorders

Although most mental disorders can have an associated sleep disturbance, the psychoses, mood disorders, anxiety disorders, panic disorder, and alcoholism are presented here because they are commonly seen in patients presenting with sleep complaints and need to be considered in differential diagnoses. Panic disorder, one of the anxiety disorders, has a separate text because this disorder can produce only a sleep complaint. Included under the general mental disorder heading in each text is a listing of the disorders to which the text applies. For example, schizophrenia is listed under the heading of psychoses. Disorders that otherwise would be included under the general heading, such as panic disorder in the anxiety disorders sections, are included under a different *ICD-9-CM* code number to which the text also is relevant. For example, adjustment disorder, *ICD-9-CM* code number 309.24, is included under the description of anxiety disorders, *ICD-9-CM* code number 300.

Psychoses (292-299)

Synonyms and Key Words: Schizophrenia (295), schizophreniform disorder (295.4), drug psychoses (292), other organic psychoses (294), delusional (paranoid) disorder (297), other psychotic disorders (298), childhood psychoses (299), psychotic decompensation, unspecified functional psychosis. (Excludes schizoaffective disorder [295.7], affective psychoses [296], dementia [290], alcoholic psychoses [291].)

Essential Features:

Psychoses are mental disorders characterized by the occurrence of delusions, hallucinations, incoherence, catatonic behavior, or inappropriate affect that causes impaired social or work functioning. Insomnia or excessive sleepiness is a common feature of the psychoses.

Acute psychotic decompensation or the waxing phase of chronic schizophrenia is often associated with significant sleep disruption and is generally characterized by severe difficulty in initiating sleep. Extreme anxiety and preoccupation with delusional material and hallucinatory phenomena may result in motor hyperactivity. Agitated patients may remain awake until exhaustion supervenes. A partial or complete inversion of the day-night cycle or reversion to a polyphasic sleep pattern may be seen. Some patients with chronic or remitted disease may have normal sleep efficiency but show persistent abnormalities in sleep architecture such as a deficit in slow-wave sleep.

Associated Features: Because of major disruptions of sleep-wake timing, there may be other rhythm disturbances (e.g., meals may be taken at odd times).

Course: Reduced sleep efficiency may precede psychotic decompensation and may accompany the acute exacerbation of psychotic symptoms. Patients with residual schizophrenia, as compared to patients in the waxing phase of the illness, may have an associated higher sleep efficiency. The use of adequate antipsychotic medication may increase sleep efficiency and may normalize sleep-wake cycles. Insomnia may alternate with hypersomnia in some patients.

Predisposing Factors: Any medical illness or psychosocial situation that increases stress and anxiety may be a predisposing factor.

Prevalence: Most psychotic patients experience some degree of sleep disruption during exacerbations of their illness.

Sex Ratio: Both sexes are equally likely to have sleep disturbance during an exacerbation of their illness.

Familial Pattern: To date, there are no studies of the familial pattern of sleep disorders among patients with psychosis.

Pathology: Slow-wave sleep deficits in schizophrenia may be associated with intracranial ventricular enlargement.

Complications: Severe sleep disruption may complicate schizophrenia to the degree that patients can become suicidal.

Polysomnographic Features: The sleep patterns of psychotic patients vary widely, with some patients showing almost normal sleep patterns. The specific findings depend on whether the patient has been chronically ill or is experiencing an acute exacerbation. In patients with disrupted sleep, the following might be seen: increased sleep latency, waking after sleep onset, sleep fragmentation, and REM density; decreased total sleep time and slow-wave sleep; shortened REM latency; and variability in REM time.

Other Laboratory Test Features: Recent research suggests that elevations in central norepinephrine levels may be associated with psychotic relapse and reduced sleep efficiency.

Differential Diagnosis: Sleep disturbance due to the psychoses must be distinguished from:

1. Insomnia and hypersomnia due to the mood disorders
2. Insomnia and hypersomnia due to disorders of organic etiology such as periodic limb movement disorder or the sleep apnea syndromes
3. Sedation or akathisia associated with antipsychotic medication
4. Sleep disturbance due to drug-induced psychosis
5. Sleep disturbance due to drug and alcohol withdrawal syndromes
6. Sleep disturbance due to dementia and acute neurologic disorders
7. Sleep disturbance due to post-traumatic stress disorder with paranoia

Diagnostic Criteria: Psychoses Associated with Sleep Disturbance (292-299)

A. The patient has a complaint of insomnia or excessive sleepiness.
B. The patient has a clinical diagnosis of schizophrenia, schizophreniform disorder, or other functional psychosis.
C. Polysomnographic monitoring demonstrates an increased sleep latency, reduced sleep efficiency, an increased number and duration of awakenings, and often a reversed first-night effect.
D. The sleep disturbance is not associated with other medical or mental disorders (e.g., dementia).
E. The complaint does not meet diagnostic criteria for other sleep disorders.

Note: State and code the mental disorder and its predominant symptom on axis A (e.g., brief reactive psychosis associated with insomnia [298.80]). If a psychosis is not associated with a sleep symptom, state and code the psychosis on axis C.

Minimal Criteria: A plus B.

Severity Criteria:

Mild: Mild insomnia or mild excessive sleepiness, as defined on page 23.
Moderate: Moderate insomnia or moderate excessive sleepiness, as defined on page 23.
Severe: Severe insomnia or severe excessive sleepiness, as defined on page 23

Duration Criteria:

Acute: 4 weeks or less.
Subacute: More than 4 weeks but less than 2 years.
Chronic: 2 years or longer.

Bibliography:

Feinberg I, Braun M, Koresko RL, Gottlieb F. Stage 4 sleep in schizophrenia. Arch Gen Psychiatry 1969; 21: 262–266.

Ganguli R, Reynolds CF 3d, Kupfer DJ. Electroencephalographic sleep in young, never-medicated, schizophrenics. A comparison with delusional and nondelusional depressives and with healthy controls. Arch Gen Psychiatry 1987; 44: 36–44.

Kupfer DJ, Wyatt RJ, Scott J, Snyder F. Sleep disturbance in acute schizophrenic patients. Am J Psychiatry 1970; 126: 1213–1223.

van Kammen DP, van Kammen WB, Peters JL, et al. CSF MHPG, sleep and psychosis in schizophrenia. Clin Neuropharmacol 1986; 9(Suppl 4): 575–577.

van Kammen WB, Peters JL, Goetz KL, Neylan TC, van Kammen DP. Diminished slow wave sleep and ventricular enlargement in schizophrenia. Schizophrenia Res 1988; 1: 164–165.

Zarcone VP. Sleep and schizophrenia. In: Williams RL, Karacan I, Moore CA, eds. Sleep disorders; diagnosis and treatment. New York: John Wiley, 1988; 165–188.

Zarcone VP Jr, Benson KL, Berger PA. Abnormal REM latencies in schizophrenia. Arch Gen Psychiatry 1987; 44: 45–48.

Mood Disorders (296, 300, 301, 311)

Synonyms and Key Words: Depressive disorders, major depression–single episode (296.2), major depression recurrent (296.3), dysthymia (300.40), depressive disorder–unspecified (311.00), bipolar disorder–manic type (296.4), bipolar disorder–depressed type (296.5), bipolar disorder–mixed type (296.6), manic-depressive illness (296.7), cyclothymia (301.13), seasonal affective disorder, manic-depressive illness, primary and secondary depression, psychotic depression, depressed mood, mania, hypomania, "masked" depression, "early morning" (premature) arousal, shortened REM sleep latency, increased first REM period density, sleep-onset REM period. (Excludes paranoid states [297], childhood psychoses [299], anxiety disorder [300], somatoform disorders [300].)

Essential Features:

Mood disorders are mental disorders characterized by either one or more episodes of depression or partial or full manic or hypomanic episodes. Typically insomnia and, occasionally, excessive sleepiness, are features of mood disorders.

Mood disorders include bipolar disorder, cyclothymia, major depressive disorder, or dysthymia. Patients with bipolar disorders may show cycling between periods of depression, normal mood, mania, or hypomania. Patients with major depression only, have depressive episodes; therefore, their disorder is described as unipolar. Some patients may show a seasonal pattern, with episodes frequently occurring during the winter months; this finding is more common in patients with bipolar disorders.

Dysthymia (a less severe form of depression formerly referred to as reactive or neurotic depression), cyclothymia (mild bipolar mood swings), and depressed mood reactions are also included here because the insomnia seen with these disorders tends to follow the form related to major depression and bipolar disorder. Another group within the mood disorders is secondary depression, which is defined as depression occurring in connection with other mental or medical disorders; the sleep findings here are usually different from those associated with other mood disorders.

A major, and usually recurrent, disturbance in mood, either of a depressive or manic nature, typically occurs. Although such mood episodes may develop within the context of a life stress, many episodes have no obvious precipitating factors.

The sleep disturbance associated with mood disorders is comprised of two patterns of insomnia that are a part of the diagnostic criteria of the mental disorders. In depression, the insomnia is characterized by difficulty in falling asleep, which is inversely related to age, sleep maintenance disturbance, and "early morning" (premature) awakening; in mania, sleep-onset insomnia occurs and the sleep duration is short.

The most characteristic feature of the insomnia seen in major depression is the repeated awakenings, leading to the so-called "early morning" (or premature) awakening that foreshortens sleep. Waking up too early and not being able to return to sleep is the cardinal complaint. A complaint of excessive sleepiness or frequent napping is most commonly associated with milder bipolar depression; some dysthymic patients also exhibit these features.

Most depressed patients complain of nocturnal restlessness and tired feelings, whereas patients with hypomania or mania, despite abbreviated sleep, do not complain about the lack of sleep and feel refreshed. Despite the "achy," "washed-out" feelings associated with the profound insomnia, most depressed patients are not objectively sleepy during the day. This finding probably relates to their high degree of psychophysiologic arousal, making it difficult for them to sleep at any time.

Associated Features: The severity of the insomnia is correlated with the severity of the mood disturbance, culminating with the most severe insomnia in association with psychotic depression. In general, sleep-onset difficulty is more prominent for younger patients, whereas sleep continuity is more prominent for older patients.

Course: The characteristic insomnia associated with depression is frequently a very early sign of the mood change, often beginning before the clinical depression has become clearly established. The typical course of the untreated mood disorder is to gradually resolve over a period of 6 to 18 months. This illness course can be considerably shortened with the institution of appropriate mental treatment. With the initiation of antidepressant drug treatment, the subjective complaint of insomnia tends to improve more rapidly than does the mood disturbance itself.

Predisposing Factors: Prior episodes of depression increase the risk of further episodes of depression. Increasing age and greater severity of mood disturbance are associated with more severe sleep disturbances.

Prevalence: At least 90% of patients with mood disorders have sleep disturbances at some time. The point prevalence for major depression is about 6%, with a lifetime risk for major depression of 15% to 20%. The lifetime risk for bipolar disorder is approximately 1%.

Age of Onset: Sleep disturbance can occur with mood disorders at any age. Major depression and bipolar depression with concurrent sleep complaints usually start between ages 20 and 40 years and are rarely seen in prepubertal years.

Sex Ratio: The sleep disturbance occurs equally in either sex with mood disorders. Females are more susceptible than males to episodes of major depression and dysthymia, whereas bipolar depression and cyclothymia have more equal representation between the sexes.

Familial Pattern: Major depression is 1.5 to 3 times more common in first-degree relatives of the proband, and bipolar depression is apparently even more heavily represented in families of affected individuals. Sleep-laboratory studies of first-degree relatives of depressed patients have also documented an increased occurrence of some of the abnormalities seen in depressed patients.

Pathology: The disturbed sleep of depressed patients can be associated with a diminished amplitude or with altered phase relationships of circadian rhythms, such as core body temperature rhythm, neuroendocrine secretory patterns, and propensity for REM and slow-wave sleep.

Complications: Depressed or manic patients may engage in self-medication of their sleep disturbance by using alcohol or sedative-hypnotic medication. This treatment may lead to the development of drug tolerance or dependence.

Polysomnographic Features: The sleep tracings of depressed patients show abnormalities in sleep continuity; sleep architecture; and, of particular note, several measures of REM sleep. Sleep latency is typically prolonged in younger depressives; older depressives may fall asleep normally but then experience a continuity disturbance related to frequent awakenings. Sleep-architecture changes consist of reduced delta sleep and increased REM sleep. The delta-sleep abnormality often includes a relative shift of delta waves from the first non-REM (NREM) period to later in the night. This shortened first NREM period results in an earlier onset of the first REM period (i.e., a short REM latency) which constitutes the most characteristic feature of the polysomnographic findings. This finding also occurs in many dysthymic patients, as well as in some patients with other mental disorders.

Other REM sleep alterations include an increase in the density of rapid eye movements, particularly in the first REM period and most commonly in middle-aged or elderly patients with depression. Sleep-onset REM (i.e., REM sleep occurring within 10 minutes of sleep onset) may occur, particularly in older patients. Many acute and agitated depressions (including psychotic depression) are associated with considerable sleep fragmentation and low REM sleep percentage.

The same pattern of sleep disturbance, though less marked, is found to some extent in depressed children and in young adults with depression and depressed mood reactions.

Bipolar depression, in contrast to unipolar depression, may be associated with higher sleep efficiency and complaints of daytime sleepiness, which also may be seen in patients with a seasonal pattern of depressive episodes who meet the criteria for mild bipolar disorder.

The hypomanic or manic patient is distinguished by a profound inability to fall asleep. Once asleep, a patient with severe mania will reawaken and be refreshed after only two to four hours of sleep. In manic conditions, REM sleep latency also may be short, and the length of stages 3 and 4 sleep may be decreased. Sleep disturbances of varying degrees are seen in patients with hypomania or cyclothymia. Patients may also alternate between insomnia with mania and mild daytime sleepiness with depression when an alternating bipolar disorder is the underlying condition.

A different sleep pattern is usually present in patients with secondary depression, which can follow a medical illness. These patients usually also show awakenings and sleep-continuity disturbances but generally have nearly normal REM-sleep latencies and a reduced amount of REM sleep.

Sleep-laboratory assessment is a sensitive means of identifying abnormalities in depressed patients, with at least 90% of depressed patients demonstrating sleep fragmentation; reduction of NREM stages 3 and 4 sleep; shortened REM latency; and increased density of rapid eye movements, particularly in the first REM period.

Polysomnography may be useful in establishing the diagnosis of a mood disorder or in clarifying difficult diagnostic cases. Polysomnographic data suggest the existence a biologic component to the mood disorder and support the inclusion of an appropriate medication or electroconvulsive therapy in the overall treatment regimen.

Other Laboratory Test Features: The circadian temperature rhythm may show a lowered amplitude in the drug-free depressed state, with return to a more normal rhythm with successful somatic treatment. Abnormalities in growth-hormone secretion in depressed patients may include increased secretion during the day but decreased secretion during the night. There is also excess secretion of cortisol and a loss of amplitude in the circadian cortisol pattern.

Differential Diagnosis: Sleep disorders, such as those associated with sleep-induced respiratory impairment and periodic limb movements, must be considered in the differential diagnosis of fatigue and tiredness. The elderly may have few symptoms specifically related to these disorders and can be misdiagnosed as depressed. Conversely, depression may occur in a form that some clinicians refer to as a "masked" depression (i.e., the existence of a depression disguised by denial and somatic symptoms).

In both manic and depressed patients, the effects of drugs and alcohol must be considered in the differential diagnosis of the sleep disturbance. These agents may alter the patient's subjective complaint (particularly in regard to the type and degree of sleep-continuity disturbance) as well as the polysomnographic findings (particularly concerning REM measures).

Although the symptoms of patients with dysthymic disorder overlap clinically with those of patients suffering from chronic anxiety and personality disorders with secondary depression, the shortened REM latency and related circadian-rhythm abnormalities in the distribution of REM sleep are often present in dysthymia but are uncharacteristic of anxiety or personality disorders.

Lability of affect with alterations of depressed and excitable phases may be an early sign of presenile and senile dementia and of other organic mental syndromes that are associated with sleep disturbances.

REM latency may be shortened in certain sleep disorders that may include a depressed mood as part of their presentation. In narcolepsy, patients have other REM features, and their daytime sleepiness is usually more severe than that reported by a patient with a mood disorder. Sleep apnea may cause chronic REM deprivation due to repeated arousals; these patients show other symptoms associated with apnea such as snoring and obstructed breathing. When treated with continuous positive airway pressure, these patients may show a REM rebound. Altered REM sleep features resembling those found in mood disorders may also be seen in patients with acute or chronic sleep deprivation or circadian rhythm sleep disorders such as the delayed sleep-phase syndrome.

Diagnostic Criteria: Mood Disorders Associated with Sleep Disturbance (296-301)

A. The patient has a complaint of insomnia or excessive sleepiness.
B. The complaint is temporally associated with a diagnosis of mood disorder.
C. The complaint is expected to remit if the mood disorder resolves.
D. Polysomnographic monitoring demonstrates at least one of the following:
   1. A shortened REM sleep latency
   2. An increased REM density
   3. Reduced delta sleep
   4. An increased sleep latency, reduced sleep efficiency, and increased number and duration of awakenings
   5. A multiple sleep latency test demonstrates a normal or reduced mean sleep latency.
E. The patient does not have any medical or other mental disorder that can account for the symptom.
F. The symptoms do not meet the diagnostic criteria for other sleep disorders that produce insomnia or excessive sleepiness (e.g., psychophysiologic insomnia).

Note: State and code the specific mood disorder on axis A along with the predominant sleep symptom (e.g., major depressive disorder–recurrent, associated with insomnia [296.3]). If a mood disorder is not associated with the sleep symptom, state and code the mood disorder on axis C.

Minimal Criteria: A plus B.

Severity Criteria: The severity of both the complaint of disturbed sleep and the polysomnographic abnormalities shows a positive correlation with the severity of the mood disorder, as measured by rating scales.

Mild: Mild insomnia or mild excessive sleepiness, as defined on page 23.
Moderate: Moderate insomnia or moderate excessive sleepiness, as defined on page 23.
Severe: Severe insomnia or severe excessive sleepiness, as defined on page 23.

Duration Criteria: The minimum length of the mood disturbance itself is two weeks; however, the polysomnographic changes may precede overt mood changes in patients susceptible to relapse or recurrence of their mood disorder.

Acute: 4 weeks or less.
Subacute: More than 4 weeks but less than 2 years.
Chronic: 2 years or longer.

Bibliography:

Akiskal HS, Lemmi H, Dickson H, King D, Yerevanian B, Van Valkenburg C. Chronic depressions. Part 2. Sleep EEG differentiation of primary dysthymic disorders from anxious depressions. J Affect Dis 1984; 6: 287–295.

Gillin JC, Duncan W, Pettigrew KD, Frankel BL, Snyder F. Successful separation of depressed, normal, and insomniac subjects by EEG sleep data. Arch Gen Psychiatry 1979; 36: 85–90.

Kupfer DJ, Spiker DG, Coble PA, Neil JF, Ulrich R, Shaw DH. Sleep and treatment prediction in endogenous depression. Am J Psychiatry 1981; 138: 429–434.

Kupfer DJ, Thase ME. The use of the sleep laboratory in the diagnosis of affective disorders. Psychiatr Clin North Am 1983; 6: 3–25.

Reynolds CF, Kupfer DJ. Sleep research in affective illness: state of the art circa 1987. Sleep 1987; 10: 199–215.

Rush AJ, Erman MK, Giles DE, et al. Polysomnographic findings in recently drug-free and clinically remitted depressed patients. Arch Gen Psychiatry 1986; 43: 878–884.

Anxiety Disorders (300, 308, 309)

Synonyms and Key Words: Generalized anxiety disorder (300.02), anxiety state unspecified (300.00), social phobia (300.23), simple phobia (300.29), obsessive-compulsive disorder (300.30). (Includes adjustment disorder [309.24], post-traumatic stress disorder [309.89]; excludes panic disorder with agoraphobia [300.21], panic disorder without agoraphobia [300.01].)

Essential Features:

The anxiety disorders are mental disorders that are characterized by symptoms of anxiety and avoidance behavior. The sleep disturbance associated with anxiety disorders is characterized by a sleep-onset or maintenance insomnia due to excessive anxiety and apprehensive expectation about one or more life circumstances.

Frequent awakenings occur either with or without anxiety dreams. Patients may experience ruminative thinking or acute anxiety attacks during periods of wakefulness while lying in bed, not only at sleep onset but also during awakening. They may express intense anxiety during the daytime about the inevitability of each night's poor sleep. Patients in this category display chronic anxiety, with features that include: trembling, muscle tension, restlessness, easy fatigability, shortness of breath, palpitations, tremor, sweating, dry mouth, dizziness, keyed-up feelings, exaggerated startle response, and difficulty concentrating. In addition, they may have superimposed specific phobias or personality traits that are not conducive to personal gratification or coping with stresses in their lives. Psychosis is not evident, and any accompanying affective symptoms are of lower intensity and more chronic duration than are those seen in patients with major depression.

Associated Features: Conditioned qualities due to association of poor sleep with specific sleep environments or worry focused on inability to sleep may also be superimposed but are not the basic process here.

Course: Generalized anxiety disorder is a chronic condition lasting for many years, even lifelong, and the accompanying sleep complaint follows a parallel temporal course.

Predisposing Factors: None known.

Prevalence: Very common.

Age of Onset: Variable, but usually occurs in early adulthood.

Sex Ratio: Generalized anxiety disorder is thought to occur two to three times more commonly in women than in men. This finding may contribute to the generally higher prevalence of insomnia complaints in women; this prevalence has been found in population studies.

Familial Pattern: Generalized anxiety tends to run in families without a clear mode of transmission. Studies of nonclinical populations using the Minnesota Multiphasic Personality Inventory indicate a higher concordance among monozygotic twins in terms of fearfulness and worrying. Such findings strengthen the clinical impression of a higher incidence of anxiety-related sleep disturbance in some families.

Pathology. None known.

Complications: Some patients develop sedative or hypnotic abuse, which can lead to sleep disorders complicating the original condition. Aside from the general epidemiologic association of reduced sleep time and hypnotic use with increased long-term mortality, there are no specific data on complications of the sleep disturbance.

Polysomnographic Features: Polysomnography generally reveals the nonspecific findings of increased sleep latency, decreased sleep efficiency, increased amounts of stage 1 and stage 2 sleep, and decreased slow-wave sleep; these changes are often relatively mild. In general, good concordance exists between the subjective report of sleep and the objective findings. Polygraphic sleep of patients with generalized anxiety has been reported to be similar to that occurring in patients with psychophysiologic insomnia, although sleep efficiency improves in patients with psychophysiologic insomnia when sleep is recorded two nights in a row. Compared to patients with depression, patients with anxiety have been reported to have similar sleep efficiency, diminished REM percent, and longer (relatively normal) REM latencies.

Unlike in patients with major depressive disorder, one night of total sleep deprivation does not ameliorate symptoms of anxiety or dysphoria in patients with anxiety. Except for the more extreme cases of objective nocturnal sleep disturbance among these patients, there is usually little or no physiologic sleepiness seen on the multiple sleep latency test (MSLT).

Other Laboratory Test Features: None.

Differential Diagnosis: The common theme of all of these disturbances is long-standing sleep-onset or maintenance insomnia, which may increase at times of stress but usually has been present for many years.

Anxiety disorders should be contrasted with adjustment sleep disorder, which lasts only a few weeks and occurs in the context of a person with relatively good sleep suddenly experiencing an emotional trauma. In adjustment sleep disorder, there is no premorbid mental history, and sleep has not been impaired before the occurrence of a specific stress. Such stress might include death of a relative, hospitalization, a forthcoming examination, or anticipation of a positive but stimulating event such as a vacation. Although patients with anxiety disorders may initially attribute their poor sleep to such stresses, a more detailed history clearly reveals a long-standing sleep and anxiety disturbance preceding that stress. The disturbance occurs in a person suffering from chronic anxiety or a long-standing personality disorder who has no evidence of a major affective disorder or schizophrenia. Patients with recurrent nightmares (dream anxiety attacks) include a significant number of persons with borderline or schizotypal personality.

Patients with anxiety disorders have some similarities to those with psychophysiologic sleep disturbance. As mentioned earlier, polygraphic measures of sleep are similar, and both groups retrospectively report their nocturnal sleep fairly accurately (in contrast to persons with sleep-state misperception). In patients with anxiety disorders, however, the anxiety is generalized, in contradistinction to patients with psychophysiologic insomnia, in whom the focus of anxiety primarily centers around the sleep complaint. Conditioned anxiety, however, may be superimposed upon the basic process of sleep disturbance in this, as in many other disorders.

Diagnostic Criteria: Anxiety Disorders Associated with Sleep Disturbance (300, 308, 309)

A. The patient has a complaint of insomnia or excessive sleepiness.

B. A long-standing generalized anxiety disorder or other anxiety disorder is present.
C. The sleep disturbance has followed the time course of the anxiety disorder, without significant long periods of remission.
D. Polysomnographic monitoring demonstrates both of the following:
   1. An increased sleep latency, reduced sleep efficiency, increased frequency and duration of awakenings
   2. An MSLT demonstrates a normal or increased sleep latency
E. No medical or other mental disorder accounts for the sleep disturbance.
F. The symptoms do not meet the diagnostic criteria for other sleep disorders producing insomnia (e.g., adjustment sleep disorder, psychophysiologic insomnia).

Note: Specify and code for the type of anxiety disorder and the predominant sleep symptom on axis A (e.g., generalized anxiety disorder associated with insomnia [300.02]). If an anxiety disorder is not the cause of a sleep symptom, state and code the anxiety disorder on axis C.

Minimal Criteria: A plus B plus C.

Severity Criteria:

Mild: Mild insomnia, as defined on page 23.
Moderate: Moderate insomnia, as defined on page 23.
Severe: Severe insomnia, as defined on page 23.

Duration Criteria:

Acute: Less than 1 month.
Subacute: More than 1 month and less than 6 months.
Chronic: 6 months or longer.

Bibliography:

Mendelson WB. Human sleep: research and clinical care. New York: Plenum Publishers, 1987; 323–342.
Reynolds CF 3d, Shaw DM, Newton TF, Coble PA, Kupfer DJ. EEG sleep in outpatients with generalized anxiety: a preliminary comparison with depressed outpatients. Psychiatry Res 1983; 8: 81–89.
Rosa RR, Bonnett MM, Kramer M. The relationship of sleep and anxiety in anxious subjects. Biol Psychol 1983; 16: 119–126.
Sussman N. Anxiety disorders. Psychiatr Ann 1988; 18: 134–189.

Panic Disorder (300)

Synonyms and Key Words: Panic disorder with agoraphobia (300.21), panic disorder without agoraphobia (300.01).

Essential Features:

***Panic disorder** is a mental disorder that is characterized by discrete periods of intense fear or discomfort with several somatic symptoms that occur unexpectedly and without organic precipitation. Panic episodes can be associated with sudden awakenings from sleep.*

The panic attack is characterized by a sudden, intense fear or terror of dying. This feeling of impending doom is a common feature of panic attacks. The symptoms also include dizziness, choking, palpitations, trembling, chest pain or discomfort, sweating, etc. Episodes that occur during sleep are associated with a sudden awakening and the onset of typical symptoms. The patient is subsequently hyperaroused and has difficulty returning to sleep.

Most patients have daytime panic attacks and symptoms of agoraphobia characterized by a fear of being in places or situations from which escape is difficult or embarrassing. Common situations include being alone, in a crowd, on a bridge, or traveling in a bus, train, or car.

Associated Features: The relationship to major depressive disorder is poorly understood, although depressive episodes occur in up to 50% of patients with panic attacks; some family studies suggest significant overlap.

Course: Panic disorder usually begins in young adulthood. It is a chronic condition lasting for many years, and the accompanying sleep complaint follows a parallel temporal course. Many clinicians have the impression that the prevalence of panic disorder declines in old age, suggesting that there has been some decrease in symptomatology.

Predisposing Factors: Adults with panic disorder often have histories of childhood separation anxiety disorder such as refusal to go to school.

Prevalence: Panic disorder has a six-month prevalence of 0.5% to 1.0%.

Age of Onset: The average age of onset is the late 20s.

Sex Ratio: Panic disorder is thought to occur two to three times more commonly in women than in men.

Familial Pattern: Panic disorder tends to run in families without a clear mode of transmission. There is an increased concordance among monozygotic twins by a ratio of roughly five or six to one.

Pathology: None known.

Complications: Panic disorder can be associated with the development of agoraphobia, secondary depressive symptoms, and alcoholism. Some patients develop sedative or hypnotic abuse, which can lead to sleep disorders complicating the original condition.

Polysomnographic Features: As compared to controls, patients with panic disorder may have marginally increased sleep latency and decreased sleep efficiency. Panic episodes tend to occur in non-REM sleep, particularly in stage 2, toward the transition to slow-wave sleep. Although more rare, the panic attack may occur at sleep onset. There is an increase in movement time, but this movement time is not temporally associated with the onset of sleep-related panic attacks. Usually, little or no physiologic sleepiness is seen on the multiple sleep latency test.

Other Laboratory Test Features: None.

Differential Diagnosis: Panic disorder should be differentiated from sleep terror. Sleep-terror episodes commence with a loud scream that occurs out of stage 3 or stage 4 sleep. Patients with sleep terrors do not have daytime panic episodes and do not have agoraphobia. Similarly, panic attacks are not nightmares, which contain much more mental content and cluster around the early morning hours.

Patients with sleep choking syndrome have a focus of complaint on the inability to breathe and do not have daytime panic attacks or agoraphobia. Obstructive sleep apnea may lead to awakenings with panic-type symptoms. Other symptoms of the obstructive sleep apnea syndrome (i.e., snoring, sleepiness) and the absence of daytime anxiety symptoms distinguish apnea from panic disorder.

Diagnostic Criteria: Panic Disorder Associated with Sleep Disturbance (300)

A. The patient has a complaint of an abrupt awakening from sleep or of insomnia.
B. The patient has panic disorder with or without agoraphobia.
C. The sleep disturbance follows the time course of the above mental disturbance, without significant long periods of remission.
D. Polysomnographic monitoring demonstrates an abrupt awakening with a sensation of panic out of stage 2 or stage 3 sleep. More rarely, the attack is triggered at sleep onset.
E. No medical or other mental disorder accounts for the sleep disturbance.
F. The symptoms do not meet the diagnostic criteria for other sleep disorders producing abrupt awakenings from sleep (e.g., sleep terror or nightmare).

Note: State and code the panic disorder and the predominant sleep symptom on axis A (e.g., panic disorder without agoraphobia associated with abrupt awakenings from sleep [300.01]). If the panic disorder is not the cause of a sleep symptom, state and code the panic disorder on axis C.

Minimal Criteria: A plus B plus C.

Severity Criteria:

Mild: Mild insomnia, as defined on page 23.
Moderate: Moderate insomnia, as defined on page 23.
Severe: Severe insomnia, as defined on page 23.

Duration Criteria:

Acute: Less than 1 month.
Subacute: More than 1 month but less than 6 months.
Chronic: 6 months or longer.

Bibliography:

Ballenger JC. Pharmacotherapy of panic attacks. J Clin Psychiatry 1986; 47(Suppl 6): 27–32.
Grunhaus L, Rabin D, Harel Y, Greden JF, Feinberg M, Herman NR. Simultaneous panic and depressive disorders: Clinical and sleep EEG correlates. Psychiatry Res 1986; 17: 251–259.
Hauri PJ, Friedman M, Ravaris CL. Sleep in patients with spontaneous panic attacks. Sleep 1989; 12: 323–337.
Mellman TA, Unde TW. Electroencephalographic sleep in panic disorder. A focus on sleep-related panic attacks. Arch Gen Psychiatry 1989; 46: 178–184.
Raj A, Sheehan DV. Medical evaluation of panic attacks. J Clin Psychiatry 1987; 48: 309–313.
Sussman N. Anxiety disorders. Psychiatr Ann 1988; 18: 134–189.
Uhde TW, Roy-Byrne P, Gillin JC, et al. The sleep of patients with panic disorder: A preliminary report. Psychiatry Res 1985; 12: 251–259.

Alcoholism (303, 305)

Synonyms and Key Words: Chronic alcoholism (303.9), acute alcoholism (303.0), alcohol dependence-intoxication, alcohol withdrawal, alcohol abstinence, REM rebound. (Includes alcohol abuse [305.00], alcoholic psychoses [291], Korsakoff's psychosis [291.1], delirium tremens [291].)

Essential Features:

Alcoholism refers to excessive alcohol intake and applies to both alcohol abuse and dependency. Insomnia or excessive sleepiness is a common feature of alcoholism.

Acute alcohol use produces increased sleepiness, starting about 30 minutes after consumption and lasting for four hours, depending upon the amount of alcohol consumed. Alcohol use before bed reduces the amount of wakefulness for the first three to four hours of sleep, but the amount of wakefulness increases during the last two to three hours of sleep. Sometimes the number of dreams, particularly anxiety dreams, increases.

Chronic, excessive alcohol use may be initially associated with some sleep improvement, with very deep sleep and increased arousal thresholds. The amount of snoring increases. After several days of continued alcohol consumption, sleep becomes fragmented, with short periods of deep sleep interrupted by brief arousals or periods of restlessness. Increasing the alcohol intake temporarily reduces the sleep fragmentation but may also lead to a stuporous state.

Abstinence following chronic excessive alcohol use is first characterized by profound sleep disruption, including occasional nights of very little sleep; during sleep periods, nightmares and other anxiety dreams are sometimes pronounced. Gradually, sleep continuity improves and anxiety dreams decrease over the first two weeks of abstinence (short-term abstinence period). Light sleep with apparent vulnerability to other sleep-disrupting factors (environment or psychologic) is characteristic during short-term abstinence and persists after this two-week period.

Associated Features: Acute alcohol use shortly before sleep onset is associated with an increased incidence of bed-wetting, sleep terrors, and sleepwalking and an exacerbation or even precipitation of loud snoring or sleep apnea. Acute alcohol use in the daytime exacerbates sleepiness that might occur for any other reason, including the usual afternoon sleepiness associated with the circadian rhythm of alertness; this sleepiness disrupts performance and contributes to accidents even when the sleepiness is not associated with significant intoxication.

Toxic conditions, such as Korsakoff's psychosis, alcoholic liver disease, and encephalopathy, can result from chronic alcohol intake. These toxic effects can in themselves disrupt sleep continuity and sleep onset.

During early alcohol abstinence, delirium tremens can occur and are associated with and often preceded by a profound insomnia; the delirium includes apparent intrusion and continuation of anxious "dreamlike" mentation into wakefulness.

Course: Alcohol abuse often begins in adolescence or early adulthood and reaches a peak cause of hospital admissions in persons in the late 30s or 40s. There are often spontaneous remissions of alcohol abuse. The sleep disturbances occur early in the course of excessive alcohol intake, reach a peak when the alcohol abuse peaks, and continue after the alcohol abuse terminates. There is a gradual recovery from the sleep disturbance, which may last as long as two years over the long-term abstinence period. Sleep quality generally improves, with increasing deeper sleep and, possibly, some decrease in the amount of dreaming. Some patients never seem to recover to their normal sleep patterns, even after years of abstinence.

Predisposing Features: A positive family history for alcoholism is often noted, with the patient showing features of insecurity, independence, immaturity, and depression.

Moderate alcohol potentiates the sleepiness caused by other sleep disorders such as insufficient sleep; this potentiation is particularly acute in adolescents and young adults.

Prevalence: Alcohol abuse occurs in about 10% of the population.

Age of Onset: Excessive alcohol use usually begins in late adolescence or early adult life. Although onset can occur at any age, the onset of alcoholism after age 45 years is rare.

Sex Ratio: Alcoholism has a male preponderance of between 2:1 and 5:1.

Familial Pattern: Alcohol abuse has been found to have a strong familial pattern, but no evidence exists that the sleep disturbance associated with alcohol abuse or dependency tends to run in families.

Complications: Acute sleepiness and mental impairment induced by alcohol use in the daytime have been associated with increased accidents, particularly motor vehicle accidents. Even when blood-alcohol levels are too low to indicate significant performance impairment from the alcohol alone, the combination of alcohol intake and sleepiness appears to affect performance.

The early promotion of sleep followed by disruption of sleep later in the sleep period and by rather rapid development of tolerance to the sleep promoting effects of alcohol can lead to an increasing use of alcohol to improve sleep quality. For some individuals, this tolerance represents the early stage of alcohol abuse.

The sleep loss experienced during alcohol withdrawal is one of the major discomforts experienced during alcohol withdrawal; this insomnia contributes to the return or continuation of alcohol use. Profound insomnia on withdrawal often precedes and may be a contributing factor to development of delirium tremens.

Alcohol abuse can often be associated with the use and abuse of other psychoactive drugs.

Polysomnographic Features: Acute alcohol use before bed reduces the amount of awake time and reduces the amount of REM sleep while increasing that of slow-wave sleep for the first three to four hours of sleep. In the last two to three hours of sleep, wakefulness and REM sleep (REM rebound) are increased. After several days of continued excessive alcohol consumption, sleep becomes fragmented and is marked by multiple arousals, increased slow eye movements during stage 2 sleep, and increased alpha electroencephalographic activity during slow-wave sleep. Increasing the alcohol intake temporarily reduces the sleep fragmentation but not the polysomnographic signs of arousal during sleep.

Short-term abstinence following chronic excessive alcohol consumption shows: profound sleep disruption, including occasional nights with very short total sleep time; fluctuations in the amount of REM sleep, which is generally increased (REM rebound) for the first few days; and profound reduction or even absence of slow-wave sleep. Total sleep time and REM sleep characteristics gradually recover to normal values during the first two weeks of abstinence. Slow-wave sleep, however, may not show any significant increase to normal levels during short-term abstinence; instead, slow-wave sleep shows a very gradual recovery that may take as long as two years during long-term abstinence. During long-term abstinence, there also appears to be a general reduction in the number of awakenings from sleep, with some gradual decrease in REM time. Tolerance to the short-term effects of alcohol on sleep and the patient's behavioral experience of desire for alcohol both correlate inversely with the changes in slow-wave sleep. Gradual improvements in sleep and reduced desire for alcohol occur during this protracted abstinence period. Some individuals, however, may never show significant or complete recovery of slow-wave sleep.

Other Laboratory Test Features: Excessive alcohol use is associated with varied laboratory-test abnormalities, particularly those of the liver function test.

Differential Diagnosis: Early morning sleep disruption can occur in depression and circadian rhythm sleep disorders as well as in acute and chronic alcohol use. The numerous sleep disorders that can produce excessive sleepiness need to be differentiated.

The history of alcohol use is essential for the diagnosis. It is important to note that the sleep disrupting effects following chronic excessive alcohol consumption can persist for up to two years and perhaps even longer in some individuals.

Diagnostic Criteria: Alcoholism Associated with Sleep Disturbance (303, 305)

A. The patient has a complaint of insomnia or excessive sleepiness.
B. The patients has a diagnosis of alcoholism.
C. Polysomnographic monitoring during alcohol abuse demonstrates the following:
   1. Increased slow-wave sleep in the first half of the night
   2. Increased REM and wakefulness in the second half of the night and during alcohol withdrawal
   3. Reduced total sleep time and sleep fragmentation
   4. Reduced slow-wave sleep, with only gradual recovery over two years and during abuse or withdrawal
   5. A multiple sleep latency test demonstrates a mean sleep latency of less than 10 minutes.
D. The findings are not associated with any other medical or mental disorder.
E. The findings do not meet the diagnostic criteria for other sleep disorders.

Note: If nightmares are a prominent feature, state and code nightmares on axis A along with the diagnosis of alcoholism. State and code alcoholism on axis A along with the predominant sleep symptom (e.g., alcoholism associated with insomnia [303]).

Minimal Criteria: A plus B.

Severity Criteria:

Mild: Mild insomnia or mild excessive sleepiness, as defined on page 23.
Moderate: Moderate insomnia or moderate excessive sleepiness, as defined on page 23.
Severe: Severe insomnia or severe excessive sleepiness, as defined on page 23.

Duration Criteria:

Acute: 3 months or less.
Subacute: More than 3 months but less than 1 year.
Chronic: 1 year or longer.

Bibliography:

Allen RP, Wagman AM, Faillace L, McIntosh M. EEG sleep recovery following prolonged alcohol intoxication. J Neurol Ment Dis 1971; 153: 6.

Allen RP, Wagman AM, Funderburk FR, Wells DT. Slow wave sleep: A predictor of individual differences in response to drinking? Biol Psychiatry 1980; 15(2): 345–348.

Bates RC. Delirium tremens and sleep deprivation. Mich Med 1972; 71: 941–944.

Gross MM, Hastey JM. A note on REM rebound during experimental alcohol withdrawal in alcoholics. In: Gross MM, ed. Adv Exp Med Biol, 1975; 59: 509–513.

Pokorny AD. Sleep disturbances, alcohol and alcoholism: A review. In: Williams RL, Karacan I, eds. Sleep disorders: Diagnosis and treatment. New York: John Wiley, 1978; 233–260.

Wagman AMI, Allen RP. Effects of alcohol ingestion and abstinence on slow wave sleep of alcoholics. In: Gross MM, ed. Alcohol intoxication and withdrawal. Experimental studies II. New York: Plenum Press, 1975; 453–466.

SLEEP DISORDERS ASSOCIATED WITH MENTAL, NEUROLOGIC, AND OTHER MEDICAL DISORDERS

ASSOCIATED WITH NEUROLOGIC DISORDERS

1. Cerebral Degenerative Disorders (330-337) 234
2. Dementia (331). 237
3. Parkinsonism (332-333) 240
4. Fatal Familial Insomnia (337.9) 245
5. Sleep-Related Epilepsy (345) 247
6. Electrical Status Epilepticus of Sleep (345.8) 252
7. Sleep-Related Headaches (346) 255

Sleep Disorders Associated with Neurologic Disorders

Neurologic disorders that are commonly associated with sleep disturbance are listed and described here. Cerebral degenerative disorders, dementia, and Parkinsonism are commonly recognized neurologic disorders that are associated with sleep disturbance. Epilepsy may be exacerbated by sleep disturbance; epileptic phenomena may occur predominantly during sleep. Therefore, the term *sleep-related epilepsy* is used to denote those forms of epilepsy that are highly associated with the sleep state. Because of its pure association with non-REM (NREM) sleep, electrical status epilepticus of sleep is not included in the sleep-related epilepsy text but is described separately. Headaches, particularly migraine and cluster headaches, can occur predominantly in sleep; therefore, information is presented under the heading of sleep-related headaches.

Cerebral Degenerative Disorders (330-337)

Synonyms and Key Words: Huntington's disease (333.4), torsion dystonia–idiopathic (333.6), torsion dystonia–symptomatic (333.7), musculorum deformans (333.6), spastic torticollis (333.83), blepharospasm (333.81), hereditary progressive dystonia (333.6), segmental dystonias and dyskinesias (333.82), olivopontocerebellar degeneration (333.0), hereditary ataxias (334.2), spinocerebellar degeneration (334.8), Rett syndrome (333.99). (Excludes Parkinsonism [332-333], dementia [331], anterior horn cell disease [335], other spinal cord disease [336], fatal familial insomnia [337.9].)

Essential Features:

Cerebral degenerative disorders are slowly progressive conditions characterized by abnormal behaviors or involuntary movements, often with evidence of other motor system degeneration.

These disorders can produce sleep disturbances and abnormal polysomnographic features. Symptoms can include insomnia, excessive sleepiness, or abnormal movement activity. Circadian sleep-wake cycle disturbances also can occur.

Associated Features: Movements during sleep, particularly during NREM stages 1 and 2, are common. Fragmentary myoclonus, periodic arm or leg movements, dystonic postures, and prolonged tonic contractions of one or more limbs suggest the possibility of a degenerative movement disorder.

Course: Usually slowly progressive.

Predisposing Factors: Variable.

Prevalence: The incidence of sleep disturbance has not been systematically studied in these diseases, but it probably increases over the duration of the disease.

Age of Onset: The onset is variable, depending upon the underlying disorder. Some of the disorders have a specific age of onset (e.g., torsion dystonia commonly presents between ages 6 and 14 years, and Huntington's disease usually occurs in the fourth decade of life).

Sex Ratio: Variable.

Familial Pattern: Variable.

Pathology: Variable, depending on the disease. There usually is evidence of degenerative central nervous system abnormalities; however, with some disorders, such as torsion dystonia, no definite neuropathologic abnormalities have been found.

Complications: Variable.

Polysomnographic Features: Sleep fragmentation is common. Other features that may be present include tonic or phasic limb contractions, isolated electromyographic activity, and periodic leg movements. Respiratory irregularities may be seen if the movement disorder affects the pharynx, larynx, or chest wall.

Depending on the particular disease and its severity, the following additional features may be seen: reduced amounts of REM sleep and stage 3 and stage 4 sleep (olivopontocerebellar degeneration, spinocerebellar degeneration, Huntington's disease) or complete absence of REM sleep (spinocerebellar degeneration), increased muscle tone during some or all of REM sleep (olivopontocerebellar degeneration, spinocerebellar degeneration), slowed REM or reduced

REM density (Huntington's disease, olivopontocerebellar degeneration, spinocerebellar degeneration), low-amplitude electroencephalography (EEG) (Huntington's disease), poorly formed or absent sleep spindles (torsion dystonia, Rett's syndrome), central or obstructive sleep apnea (spinocerebellar degeneration, olivopontocerebellar degeneration), increased numbers of arousals and awakenings, complex behavior during REM sleep, and epileptiform EEG activity (Rett syndrome).

Other Laboratory Test Features: Brain-imaging tests may be indicated. An EEG with appropriate activating procedures may be necessary if a seizure disorder is suspected.

Differential Diagnosis: The differential diagnosis includes drug toxicity, conversion reactions, and various other nonprogressive neurologic and mental disorders. Other movement disorders that may be unassociated with the cerebral degeneration (such as restless legs syndrome, periodic limb movement disorder, REM sleep behavior disorder, nocturnal paroxysmal dystonia, sleep bruxism, and rhythmic movement disorder) need to be differentiated.

Huntington's disease and other degenerative disorders may be accompanied by depression or other mental illnesses that contribute to sleep disturbances. Medications used to treat the disorders also may induce sleep disturbance.

Diagnostic Criteria: Cerebral Degenerative Disorders (330-337)

A. The patient has a complaint of insomnia or excessive sleepiness, or an observer reports that the patient has insomnia. There may be abnormal body movements or an alteration in the number of movements during sleep.
B. The patient has a diagnois of a degenerative nervous system disorder (e.g., Huntington's disease).
C. Polysomnographic monitoring demonstrates one or more of the following:
   1. Reduced sleep efficiency, increased number and duration of awakenings
   2. Abnormal movement activity during the sleep period
   3. A multiple sleep latency test demonstrates a mean sleep latency of less than 10 minutes
D. The symptom is not associated with a mental disorder.
E. Other sleep disorders can be present.

Note: Specify and code the particular degenerative disorder on axis A, followed by the specific symptom (e.g., axis A, Huntington's disease associated with abnormal movements during sleep [333.4]). If a primary sleep disorder such as irregular sleep-wake pattern is the predominant disorder of sleep, specify both the primary sleep disorder and the degenerative cerebral disorder on axis A.

Minimal Criteria: A plus B plus D.

Severity Criteria:

Mild: Mild insomnia or mild sleepiness, as defined on page 23.

Moderate: Moderate insomnia or moderate sleepiness, as defined on page 23, occasionally associated with abnormal movement activity.

Severe: Severe insomnia or severe sleepiness, as defined on page 23, associated with severely abnormal movements during sleep.

Duration Criteria:

Acute: 3 months or less.
Subacute: More than 3 months but less than 1 year.
Chronic: 1 year or longer.

Bibliography:

Hansotia P, Wall R, Berendes J. Sleep disturbances and severity of Huntington's disease. Neurology 1985; 35: 1672–1674.

Jankel WR, Allen RP, Niedermeyer E, Kalsher MJ. Polysomnographic findings in dystonia musculorum deformans. Sleep 1983; 6: 281–285.

Mano T, Shizozawa Z, Sobue I. Extrapyramidal involuntary movements during sleep. Electroencephalogr Clin Neurophysiol 1982; 35(Suppl): 431–442.

Nomura Y, Segawa M, Higurashi M. Rett syndrome–An early catecholamine and indolamine deficient disorder? Brain Dev 1985; 7: 334–341.

Quera-Salva MA, Guilleminault C. Olivopontocerebellar degeneration, abnormal sleep, and REM sleep without atonia. Neurology 1986; 36: 576–577.

Segawa M, Igawa C, Ogiso M, Nomura Y, Kase M. Polysomnographical examination of dystonia syndrome. Electroencephalogr Clin Neurophysiol 1983; 56: 57–58.

Dementia (331)

Synonyms and Key Words: Alzheimer's disease (331.0), Pick's disease (331.1), senile degeneration of brain (331.2), communicating hydrocephalus (331.3), obstructive hydrocephalus (331.4), nonreversible dementia, sundown syndrome, nocturnal delirium, nocturnal confusion, nocturnal wandering, acute brain syndrome, acute confusional state, nocturnal hyperactivity.

Essential Features:

Dementia refers to a loss of memory and other intellectual functions due to a chronic, progressive degenerative disease of the brain. Sleep disturbance in demented patients is characterized by delirium, agitation, combativeness, wandering, and vocalization without ostensible purpose and occuring during early evening or nighttime hours.

Patients with dementia have fragmented sleep with frequent awakenings, and they may have difficulty in initiating sleep or with early morning awakening. The sleep disturbance that is characterized by nocturnal wandering and confusion is often termed the *sundown syndrome*. Patients may become confused or disoriented and may present management problems for care givers or nursing staff. Typical patterns include wandering outside of the house, turning on kitchen appliances, accidentally breaking household items, and shouting inappropriately. These behaviors may also occur during the daylight hours.

Associated Features: Some demented patients present with excessive sleepiness in conjunction with nocturnal sleep disruption, which may be related to the fragmented 24-hour sleep-wake pattern.

Course: The sleep disturbance follows the course of the dementia. The sundown syndrome appears to be present only in the most advanced stage of dementia and may be present intermittently.

Predisposing Factors: The presence of other sleep disorders (such as insomnia due to mental disorders, periodic limb movement disorder, or the sleep apnea syndromes) may predispose the patient to developing more severe sleep disruption. Sundowning may be exacerbated by physical illness in a demented patient. In one recent preliminary study institutionalized elderly, urinary incontinence, increased frequency of bed checks, and better physical health were associated with sundowning. The nocturnal confusion may follow awakenings from REM sleep.

Prevalence: The general prevalence of sleep-related problems is not known, but sleep complaints commonly occur in patients with dementia. Sundown syndrome has been estimated to occur in 12% of a mixed group of demented and nondemented institutionalized patients.

The prevalence of undifferentiated severe dementia has been estimated at approximately 5% of patients over 65 years of age and approximately 15% of those over 85 years of age.

Sex Ratio: After adjusting for life expectancy, there are few differences in the prevalence of dementia.

Familial Pattern: None known. Recent advances in molecular biology indicate that a specific Alzheimer's gene may be present on chromosome 14, 19, or 21 in at least some familial cases.

Pathology: The sleep disturbance and the sundown syndrome may reflect neuropathologic degeneration of the suprachiasmatic nucleus and of other sleep-maintenance systems. Studies suggest the persistence of the circadian temperature rhythm in dementia.

Complications: Sleep disturbance is a common reason for institutionalizing demented patients. Patients with sundown syndrome may inadvertently injure themselves or others. More typically, family life is disrupted.

Polysomnographic Features: Demented patients show increased sleep fragmentation, lower sleep efficiency, decreased stage 3 and stage 4 sleep, and decreased REM sleep as a percentage of total sleep time. REM-latency findings remain equivocal. Fragmentation of the major sleep episode may be present, with excessive sleepiness documented on multiple sleep latency testing. No polysomnographic studies of the sundown syndrome have been reported.

Other Laboratory Test Features: Computed tomographic scanning and magnetic resonance imaging may show evidence of cerebral atrophy. Neuropsychologic testing demonstrates deficits consistent with the diagnosis of dementia.

Differential Diagnosis: Sleepwalking, psychomotor epilepsy, REM sleep behavior disorder, and insomnia due to mental disorders need to be considered in the differential diagnosis.

The diagnosis of Alzheimer's disease should be made only after the exclusion of other reversible causes of dementia such as sepsis, alcoholism, uremia, hepatic failure, electrolyte imbalance, thyroid dysfunction, nocturnal hyperglycemia, acid-base imbalance, or toxic conditions. In addition, during hospitalization, 10% to 15% of patients may show transient periods of nocturnal agitation.

Diagnostic Criteria: Dementia Associated with Sleep Disturbance (331)

A. The patient has a complaint of insomnia, excessive sleepiness, or nocturnal confusion, or the caretaker observes these behaviors.
B. The patient experiences frequent awakenings, daily sleep episodes, or nocturnal confusion.
C. The sleep disturbance is associated with a diagnosis of dementia (e.g., Alzheimer's disease).
D. One or more of the following features may be present:
   1. Nocturnal wandering, with inappropriate activities
   2. Agitation, combativeness
   3. Confusion, disorientation, or frank delirium
E. Polysomnographic monitoring demonstrates both of the following:
   1. Poor sleep efficiency, with an increase in the number and duration of awakenings
   2. A multiple sleep latency test demonstrates increased sleepiness
F. Other medical disorders may be present but do not account for the primary symptoms.
G. Other sleep disorders (e.g., periodic limb movement disorder, obstructive sleep apnea syndrome), may be present but do not account for the primary symptoms.

Note: The diagnosis is stated and coded under the particular form of dementia with the appropriate symptom modifier (e.g., Alzheimer's disease associated with insomnia [331.0]).

Minimal Criteria: B plus C.

Severity:

Mild: The patient has mild memory loss, is oriented, has selected impairment on formal testing (e.g., serial 7s) or in personal life (e.g., balancing checkbook, geographic confusion), has impaired complex reasoning and new learning, has maintained social skills, and is able to provide self care.

Corresponds approximately to Global Deterioration Scale (GDS) (Reisberg et al. 1982) rating of 1 to 4, Clinical Dementia Scale (CDR) (Berg et al. 1984) rating of 0 to 1, and Activities of Daily Living (ADL) (Katz et al. 1963) category A.

Moderate: The patient has a pervasive cognitive decline, is typically disoriented, confuses relevant personal information (e.g., personal phone number), has trouble counting or spelling, retains some overlearned material (e.g., names of children), is likely to have undergone a personality change, and requires some assistance in ADL (e.g., bathing, dressing, toileting). Corresponds to GDS rating of 5-6, CDR rating of 2, and ADL categories of B-D.

Severe: The patient has complete mental confusion, may know only name, has no recognition memory, and cannot provide self care but may be able to feed self with assistance. Speech is virtually absent. Corresponds approximately to GDS rating of 7, CDR rating of 3, and ADL categories E-G.

Duration Criteria:

Acute: Less than 3 months.
Subacute: More than 3 months but less than 1 year.
Chronic: 1 year or longer.

Bibliography:

Evans LK. Sundown syndrome in institutionalized elderly. J Am Geriatr Soc 1987; 35: 101–108.

Feinberg I, Koresko RL, Heller N. EEG sleep patterns as a function of normal and pathological aging in man. J Psychiatr Res 1967; 5: 107–144.

Katzman R, Terry R. The neurology of aging. Philadelphia: Davis FA, 1983.

Lipowski ZJ. Delirium: Acute brain failure in man. Illinois: Springfield, Thomas CC, 1980.

Prinz PN, Vitaliano PP, Vitiello MV, et al. Sleep, EEG and mental function changes in senile dementia of the Alzheimer's type. Neurobiol Aging 1982; 3: 361–370.

Parkinsonism (332-333)

Synonyms and Key Words: Parkinson's disease (332.0), paralysis agitans (332.0), drug-induced parkinsonism (332.1), Shy-Drager syndrome (333.0), multisystem atrophy (330.0), striatonigral degeneration (330.0), progressive supranuclear palsy (333.0), levodopa-induced sleep disturbances (332.1), Parkinson's-ALS-dementia complex, shaking palsy. (Includes postencephalitic parkinsonism [049.8].)

Essential Features:

Parkinsonism *refers to a group of neurologic disorders characterized by hypokinesia, tremor, and muscular rigidity. Insomnia is the most common sleep-related symptom in patients with parkinsonism.*

Apart from insomnia, which is the most common complaint in patients with parkinsonism, other sleep-related difficulties include the inability to get out of bed unaided, the need to arise to go to the bathroom, the inability to turn over in bed, painful leg cramps, vivid dreams and nightmares, back pain, limb jerks, and visual hallucinations.

Characteristic sleep abnormalities include sleep fragmentation, often associated with episodic daytime somnolence; total sleep-wake cycle reversal is sometimes observed. At least six factors contribute to the sleep disturbance in these patients. First, sleep-wake regulation appears to be affected, possibly by the neurochemical changes of the disease, resulting in sleep disruption and reduced amounts of REM and slow-wave sleep. Second, bradykinesia and rigidity can reduce the number of normal body shifts during sleep, leading to discomfort and increased frequency of awakenings. Third, periodic leg movements, tremor, or medication-induced myoclonic movements can produce arousals and can be disruptive to the sleep of bedpartners. Fourth, abnormal upper-airway and chest-wall motor activity can produce disordered breathing, which disturbs sleep. Fifth, circadian rhythms and the sleep-wake schedule can be disrupted by medications or by the disease process itself, leading to nighttime insomnia and daytime fatigue and sleepiness. Sixth, the medications commonly used to treat parkinsonism (dopamine agonists and anticholinergic medications) can produce sleep disruption, including increased numbers of arousals and awakenings and decreased amounts of REM sleep. On the other hand, dopamine agonists can improve sleep by reducing nocturnal rigidity. Dementia occurs in 15% to 30% of patients with Parkinson's disease; in these patients, a breakdown in the sleep-wake cycle is more likely to occur and is characterized by frequent nocturnal awakenings, daytime somnolence, and intermittent confusion that worsens in the evening.

Drug treatment of parkinsonism can (1) improve sleep disturbance due to such symptoms of the disease as rigidity or bradykinesia, (2) alter or exacerbate previously existing sleep disorders, or (3) create new complaints. Ascribing sleep complaints to treatment requires demonstration that symptoms vary with changes in the drug regimen. The symptoms must be differentiable from those ascribable to age or to the severity and duration of disease. Medication-induced sleep complaints are frequently encountered in patients with parkinsonism who are treated with levodopa and bromocriptine; these complaints can occur in up to 80% to 90% of such patients. Vivid dreaming, nocturnal vocalizations, sleep terrors, sleepwalking episodes, nocturnal myoclonic activity, and disorders of the sleep-wake cycle have been reported and appear to be related to the amount and duration of levodopa treatment. Symptoms improve when levodopa administration is restricted to earlier hours of the day and can clear when the drug is discontinued. Symptoms are often exacerbated when other parkinsonism medications are concomitantly employed.

Associated Features: The most severe sleep-related complaints in parkinsonism appear to involve toxicity induced by parkinsonism drugs. Vivid visual hallucinations induced by levodopa are more commonly reported than are auditory, tactile, or olfactory hallucinations. A formal thought disorder is rarely encountered, and hallucinations are frequently recognized as illusions. Other signs of drug toxicity or drug resistance are present in a higher prevalence in patients with sleep complaints, and include nocturnal dystonia (usually of the feet and legs);

choreiform movements of the limbs, face, and axial muscles; and erratic response to medication (on-off phenomenon).

Course: Sleep complaints in patients with parkinsonism generally worsen as the disorder progresses and the duration of treatment lengthens. Prevalence data suggest that sleep fragmentation precedes altered sleep behavior and nocturnal myoclonus. Escalation of levodopa dosage frequently leads to increased sleep-related complaints.

Predisposing Factors: The use of parkinsonism medications is the most common predisposing factor for the development of a sleep disorder. Associated depression or dementia also contributes to an increased likelihood of sleep complaints.

Prevalence: Parkinson's disease affects about 0.1% to 0.3% of the population; the prevalence may be as high as 20% of persons over 60 years of age. Sixty percent to 90% of persons who seek medical treatment for Parkinson's disease have sleep complaints. All ethnic groups are at risk.

Age of Onset: In about two thirds of patients, the onset is between the age of 50 and 60 years. Occasionally, the age of onset may be as early as the third decade.

Sex Ratio: No difference.

Familial Pattern: Parkinson's disease is not genetically transmitted.

Pathology: Accelerated loss of the pigmented, dopaminergic neurons of the substantia nigra, particularly the pars compacta, is a characteristic finding in Parkinson's disease, and some remaining neurons contain Lewy bodies. Pathologic changes are present in the pigmented neurons of the locus coeruleus and the dorsal nucleus of the vagus. Basal ganglia dopaminergic content is reduced, and there are alterations of brain norepinephrine, serotonin, and several neuropeptides. Alterations of dopamine, serotonin, and norepinephrine and metabolism may contribute to the sleep-related complaints.

Complications: Sleep complaints can be exacerbated by drug therapy and toxicity. The onset of dementia is also likely to be associated with increasing sleep disturbance.

Polysomnographic Features: There are no definitive polysomnographic features for the diagnosis of sleep disturbance due to parkinsonism. The following polysomnographic features are commonly seen:

1. *Sleep Fragmentation:* Increased numbers of awakenings and arousals, prolonged sleep latency, increased wake time during sleep, and decreased percentage of REM sleep are characteristic features that generally worsen with increasing disease severity.

2. *Tremor:* Tremor is much less frequent during sleep than during wakefulness and usually disappears at sleep onset. However, tremor may reappear for 5 to 15 seconds during arousals, sleep-stage changes, stage 2 sleep, or just before or after a REM period. Tremor is rarely seen in sleep stages 3 and 4.
3. *Dystonia/Rigidity:* Rarely, prolonged tonic contractions lasting minutes to hours may occur in one or more limbs during sleep.
4. *Movements:* Periodic leg movements, repetitive muscle contractions, isolated twitches, and brief electromyographic (EMG) bursts without associated movement are frequent during REM and non-REM (NREM) sleep. Blepharospasm and repeated blinking may occur at sleep onset.
5. *Atypical Sleep:* REM fragmentation, EMG suppression in the absence of eye movements, electroencephalographic desynchronization, REMs in the absence of characteristic electroencephalographic changes or EMG suppression, REMs during NREM sleep, poorly formed or absent sleep spindles, slowing of waking electroencephalography with poor differentiation of wake and stage 1 sleep may all be present.
6. *Respiration:* Central and obstructive apneas, episodes of hypoventilation, and disorganized patterns of inspiration can occur, particularly in patients with autonomic abnormalities.

Low doses of dopamine agonists tend to improve sleep, whereas higher doses cause sleep disruption. The timing of dopaminergic medication has a marked effect on sleep. Evening doses of levodopa tend to prolong sleep latency, increase REM latency, and shift REM sleep into the second half of the night, while awakenings in the second half of the night are reduced. With sustained treatment, the disruptive effects of the medications on sleep are usually reduced; however, sleep disruption can increase with chronic levodopa therapy. Withdrawal of levodopa is not associated with REM rebound, though normalization of sleep can occur.

Multiple sleep latency testing (MSLT) or daytime polysomnographic recording can show daytime sleepiness. In some patients with daytime sleepiness, background slowing during wakefulness can be seen. Behavioral transitions between apparent wakefulness and sleep can occur with little alteration in polysomnographic features.

Polysomnographic features of related conditions:

Progressive Supranuclear Palsy: Sleep fragmentation, tonic contractions and tonic EMG activity, periodic leg movements, irregular isolated twitches, decreased REM sleep, poorly formed or absent spindles, slowing of waking EEG, poor differentiation of wake from sleep, and poor differentiation of the stages of sleep.

Shy-Drager Syndrome: Sleep fragmentation, decreased REM sleep, respiratory irregularities (central or obstructive sleep apnea, arrhythmic respirations), cardiac arrhythmias, and rapid changes of blood pressure.

Other Laboratory Test Features: Neurologic tests are usually not helpful in diagnosing parkinsonism or the associated sleep alterations, other than to rule out other neurologic disorders.

Differential Diagnosis: Other causes of sleep fragmentation need to be excluded. Periodic movements of sleep, sleep apnea, and circadian rhythm disorders may present with similar findings. Depression may be concomitantly present and may give rise to similar symptoms and findings.

Diagnostic Criteria: Parkinsonism Associated with Sleep Disturbance (332-333)

A. The patient has a complaint of insomnia or excessive sleepiness. The complaint occasionally may be one of altered dreaming or of abnormal motor activity that is disturbing to a bedpartner.
B. Frequent awakenings or daily sleep episodes with or without abnormal motor activity during the sleep period are present.
C. The patient has a diagnosis of parkinsonism.
D. One or more of the following features may be present:
   1. Tremors during arousals or light sleep
   2. Tonic contractions in one or more limbs during sleep
   3. Repetitive muscle contractions or isolated twitches
   4. Relative immobility during sleep
   5. Dystonic movements
E. Polysomnographic monitoring demonstrates both of the following:
   1. A decreased sleep efficiency, with an increase in the number and duration of awakenings
   2. One or more of the following:
      a. Tremors during the sleep period
      b. Tonic contractions
      c. EMG burst activity
      d. Dissociated REM sleep
      e. Reduced spindle activity
   3. A multiple sleep latency test demonstrates increased sleepiness
F. Other medical or mental disorders (e.g., treatable causes of dementia, depression, etc.) may be present but do not account for the primary symptoms.
G. Other sleep disorders (e.g., periodic limb movement disorder, obstructive sleep apnea syndrome) may be present but do not account for the primary symptoms.

Note: The type of parkinsonism should be stated and coded on axis A (e.g., Shy-Drager syndrome [333.0]). The Shy-Drager syndrome may also be associated with obstructive and central sleep apnea syndromes and, if so, should be stated and coded on axis A along with the sleep-related respiratory disorder.

Minimal Criteria: B plus C.

Severity Criteria:

Mild: Mild insomnia or mild excessive sleepiness, as defined on page 23.
Moderate: Moderate insomnia or moderate excessive sleepiness, as defined on page 23.
Severe: Severe insomnia or severe excessive sleepiness, as defined on page 23.

Duration Criteria:

Acute: 3 months or less.
Subacute: More than 3 months but less than 1 year.
Chronic: 1 year or longer.

Bibliography:

Mouret J. Differences in sleep in patients with Parkinson's disease. Electroencephalogr Clin Neurophysiol 1975; 38: 653–657.
Nausieda PA, Weiner WJ, Kaplan LR, Weber S, Klawans HL. Sleep disruption in the course of chronic levodopa therapy: an early feature of the levodopa psychosis. Clin Neuropharmacol 1982; 183–194.
Rabey J, Vardi J, Glaubman H, Streifler M. EEG sleep study in parkinsonian patients under bromocryptine treatment. Eur Neurol 1978; 17: 345–350.
Wyatt RJ, Chase TN, Scott J, Snyder F, Engelman K. Effect of L-dopa on the sleep of man. Nature 1970; 228: 999–1001.

Fatal Familial Insomnia (337.9)

Synonyms and Key Words: Fatal progressive insomnia with dysautonomia, familial thalamic degeneration, anterior and dorsomedial thalamic nuclei, thalamic insomnia.

Essential Features:

Fatal familial insomnia is a progressive disorder that begins with a difficulty in initiating sleep and leads to total lack of sleep within a few months and, later, to spontaneous lapses from quiet wakefulness into a sleep state with enacted dreams (oneiric stupor).

Autonomic hyperactivity, with pyrexia, salivation, hyperhidrosis, tachycardia, and tachydyspnea is present. In the late stages of the disorder, there are somatomotor disturbances, with dysarthria, tremor, spontaneous and reflex myoclonus, dystonic posturing, and a positive Babinski sign. The disorder progresses to an unarousable coma and finally death.

Cognitive function is retained until impaired alertness makes testing impossible.

Associated Features: Extreme body wasting and adrenal insufficiency occur in the terminal stages. Bronchopulmonary infections are also present.

Course: The course is one of relentless worsening of symptoms, especially of autonomic dysfunctions. The disorder is always fatal, usually within 7 to 13 months after onset of symptoms.

Predisposing Factors: Not known.

Prevalence: Not known, but apparently rare.

Age of Onset: Usually in adulthood, especially the fifth or sixth decade of life. Rarely occurs in young adulthood.

Sex Ratio: No difference.

Familial Pattern: The disorder has been found in families in which several generations of family members were affected; fatal familial insomnia is apparently transmitted according to an autosomal-dominant pattern.

Pathology: Severe bilateral loss of neurons, with reactive gliosis restricted to the anterior and dorsomedial thalamic nuclei, with sparing of intervening fibers, and without inflammation or spongiform changes has been described.

Complications: Infections develop in the course of the disease, especially in the late stages.

Polysomnographic Features: In early stages, periods of relaxed wakefulness alternate with episodes of electroencephalographic desynchronization, REM bursts, loss of antigravitary muscle tone, and irregular myoclonic and tremorlike limb-muscle activities associated with vivid dreams. Features of slow-wave sleep are absent throughout the course of illness. In the final stages of the disorder, the electroencephalogram becomes unreactive and progressively flattens until death occurs.

Other Laboratory Test Features: Circadian rhythms of body temperature and heart and respiratory rate may become lost. Endocrine rhythms of growth hormone, prolactin, luteinizing hormone, follicle-stimulating hormone, and adrenocorticotropic hormone are also lost. The functions of the hypothalamus, the pituitary, and their end organs are retained.

Serum and urinary catecholamine and cortisol values are elevated, with undetectable adrenocorticotropic hormone levels.

Differential Diagnosis: This disorder must be differentiated from REM sleep behavior disorder, which is not associated with autonomic hyperactivity or a familial pattern. The differential diagnosis includes dementia, such as Alzheimer's disease and Creutzfeldt-Jakob disease, or even schizophrenia.

Diagnostic Criteria: Fatal Familial Insomnia (337.9)

A. A complaint of insomnia is initially present.
B. Autonomic hyperactivity, with pyrexia, excessive salivation, hyperhidrosis or anhidrosis, and cardiac and respiratory dysfunction is present.
C. Familial pattern is present.
D. Progression to stupor, coma, and death occurs within 24 months.
E. Pathologic examination demonstrates degeneration of anterior and dorsomedial thalamic nuclei.
F. Polysomnographic monitoring demonstrates one or more of the following:
   1. Absence of slow-wave sleep

2. Dissociated REM sleep
3. Myoclonus and tremorlike muscle activity
G. The symptoms are not the result of another medical or mental disorder (e.g., Alzheimer's dementia, Creutzfeldt-Jakob disease, or schizophrenia).
H. The symptoms do not meet the diagnostic criteria for other sleep disorders (e.g., REM sleep behavior disorder).

Minimal Criteria: A plus B plus C plus D plus G.

Severity Criteria:

Mild: Not applicable.
Moderate: Not applicable.
Severe: Always severe.

Duration Criteria:

Acute: 1 month or less.
Subacute: More than 1 month but less than 24 months.
Chronic: Not applicable.

Bibliography:

Lugaresi A, Baruzzi A, Cacciari E, et al. Lack of vegetative and endocrine circadian rhythms in fatal familial thalamic degeneration. Clin Endocrinol 1987; 26: 573–580.

Lugaresi E, Medori R, Montagna P, et al. Fatal familial insomnia and dysautonomia with selective degeneration of thalamic nuclei. N Engl J Med 1986; 315: 997–1003.

Medori R, Gambetti PL, Montagna P, Cortelli P, Baruzzi A, Lugaresi E. Familial progressive insomnia, impairment of the autonomic functions, degeneration of the thalamic nuclei: A new disease? Neurology (NY) 1985; 1: 145(Suppl 35) [Abstract].

Sleep-Related Epilepsy (345)

Synonyms and Key Words: Petit mal epilepsy (345.0), absence seizures (345.0), generalized tonic-clonic epilepsy (345.1), grand mal epilepsy (345.1), complex partial seizures (345.4), temporal lobe epilepsy (345.4), partial (focal) motor seizures (345.5), sleep epilepsy, sleep-related epileptic seizures. Sleep-related epilepsy is not a distinct type of epilepsy, but the term refers to epileptic disorders that are largely restricted to sleep. (Excludes electrical status epilepticus of sleep [345.8].)

Essential Features:

Epilepsy is a disorder characterized by an intermittent, sudden discharge of cerebral neuronal activity. Sleep may have facilitatory effects on epileptic activity.

The influence of the sleep-wake cycle on epilepsy has led to the epilepsies being classified as awakening (diurnal), sleep (nocturnal), and diffuse (random).

Sleep is an important activator of potentially epileptogenic electroencephalographic activity and seizures. Any type of seizure can occur during sleep, but certain types of seizures, such as generalized tonic-clonic (grand mal) seizures, partial seizures with motor symptomatology (partial or focal motor seizures), and partial seizures with complex symptomatology (complex partial seizures), are more likely to occur during sleep. A particular type of idiopathic partial epilepsy, referred to as *benign focal epilepsy of childhood* (Rolandic epilepsy), has a marked tendency to manifest in sleep-related seizures.

Epileptic episodes may cause awakenings from sleep but rarely cause a primary complaint of insomnia. Frequent episodes during sleep may disrupt sleep to the extent that excessive sleepiness may result, and sleepiness may be exacerbated by the sedating effects of anticonvulsant medications. Sleep-related disorders associated with motor activity, such as sleepwalking or sleep terrors, rarely have an epileptic etiology. Epilepsy may also occasionally cause respiratory difficulty during sleep, which should be distinguished from other causes of sleep-related breathing difficulties.

Associated Features: Generalized tonic-clonic seizures are characterized by an abrupt loss of consciousness and an initial brief tonic flexion of the body, with upward deviation of the eyes and pupillary dilatation. This flexion is usually followed by tonic extension, with a forceful expiration producing an "epileptic cry" and diffuse tremor, leading to the clonic phase, which involves the axial and limb musculature. The ictus usually lasts a few minutes. Sweating, urinary incontinence, injuries, and tongue biting may occur. The postictal period is characterized by confusion and then sleep.

Partial (focal) motor seizures are characterized by retention of consciousness, with tonic or clonic jerking movements of the involved body part, usually unilateral face, arm, or leg. There may be a sequential progression of involvement (Jacksonian march) or a secondary generalized tonic-clonic seizure.

In complex partial seizures, the onset sometimes occurs with a blank stare, unresponsiveness, and automatisms consisting of nonpurposeful movements, such as picking and fidgeting of hands or lip smacking. Episodes may be preceded by an aura and are frequently associated with postictal confusion or lethargy. In benign focal epilepsy of childhood, the seizures are usually focal motor, involving the face and arm, as well as generalized tonic-clonic seizures.

Course: In idiopathic generalized tonic-clonic epilepsy, the prognosis is good, with 80% of patients experiencing a five-year remission off anticonvulsant medications in the first 20 years after onset. However, 20% of these patients may relapse within 20 years. The course of the sleep-related symptoms is not known, but most patients who present with a single sleep-related epileptic episode will develop epileptic episodes during wakefulness. Most patients with recurrent sleep-related epileptic seizures continue to have the seizures restricted to sleep. Approximately 20% have a course characterized by seizures occurring during both the sleep and awake states.

The prognosis of partial epilepsy is less favorable. Spontaneous remission does not usually occur, and as many as 35% of cases may prove to be refractory to treatment with anticonvulsant medications. In benign focal epilepsy of childhood, the prognosis is excellent, as virtually all patients have a remission by the age of 15 to 18 years.

Predisposing Factors: In addition to other predisposing factors, irregularities of the sleep-wake cycle (with sleep deprivation) may predispose an individual to developing seizures. Abrupt cessation of anticonvulsant medication in a patient with epilepsy can result in a seizure or status epilepticus.

Prevalence: An estimated 25% of patients with epilepsy have predominantly sleep-related epilepsy.

Age of Onset: Generalized tonic-clonic epilepsy may have its onset at any age; however, about 70% of epileptic patients have the onset during puberty. There is no predilection for a particular age in those patients whose generalized tonic-clonic epilepsy is restricted to sleep.

Partial epilepsy may begin at any age. Complex partial epilepsy usually occurs before the age of 40 years. Benign focal epilepsy of childhood has its onset at age 4 to 12 years in most patients.

Sex Ratio: No difference. In benign focal epilepsy of childhood, there is a slight 3:2 male predominance.

Familial Pattern: Hereditary factors appear to be significant in idiopathic epilepsy. In idiopathic generalized tonic-clonic epilepsy, 7% to 10% of relatives of patients have a history of seizures, which is significantly higher than the general-population incidence of 0.5%.

Heredity does not seem to play a role in symptomatic partial epilepsy. In benign focal epilepsy of childhood, a family history of seizures can be elicited in 10% to 40% of cases.

Pathology: In idiopathic epilepsy (generalized and partial), there are no consistent specific anatomic or biochemical abnormalities. In idiopathic generalized tonic-clonic epilepsy, however, microdysgenesis has been described.

The partial motor epilepsies may occur secondary to many types of localized structural lesions in the central cortex, including neoplasms (benign and malignant, primary and secondary), cysts, infarctions, arteriovenous malformations, etc. In complex partial seizures, hippocampal sclerosis is present in 30% to 50% of patients. A glioma is the next most common discrete lesion. Less common lesions include post-traumatic cicatrix, hematomas, vascular malformations, and residua of cerebral infarcts.

No lesions have been described that are specific to sleep-related epilepsy.

Complications: Acute complications of a generalized tonic-clonic seizure include aspiration pneumonia, limb fractures, vertebral compression, oral trauma, pulmonary edema, and sudden death. Most patients' seizures can be well controlled, but if the seizures are refractory to treatment with anticonvulsant medications, the patient may experience significant psychosocial effects, with education or employment difficulties.

Polysomnographic Features: The characteristic interictal abnormalities on the electroencephalogram (EEG) in generalized tonic-clonic epilepsy are generalized, bilaterally synchronous spike and slow-wave complexes and symmetrical generalized spikes or multiple spike and wave complexes. The spike and slow-wave complex occurs at a frequency of 2.5 to 3.0 or 4 to 5 Hz and usually in bursts of 1 to 4 seconds. Non-REM (NREM) sleep is an activator for such discharges, but the bursts may become fragmented, and multiple spike complexes are more likely to occur. Focal or unilateral spikes also may appear as a partial expression of the generalized seizure disorder. In REM sleep, discharges are markedly suppressed in frequency, or they disappear. The ictal EEG in generalized tonic-clonic seizures is characterized by generalized voltage attenuation with diffuse fast activity. The EEG is then usually obscured by muscle artifact. After the seizure, a diffuse suppression of the EEG activity is followed by generalized slowing.

In partial epilepsy, the characteristic abnormality is a spike or sharp transient that occurs in a localized distribution. The discharges are activated in NREM sleep and suppressed in REM sleep. The ictal EEG pattern is characterized by a localized onset of a paroxysmal rhythmic EEG activity at any frequency. The EEG activity may remain localized or may show spread to adjacent areas or, at times, may become secondarily generalized.

In benign focal epilepsy of childhood, the interictal high-amplitude negative sharp waves have a characteristic and stereotyped morphology. The spikes have a typical distribution in the centrotemporal region and are often bifocal or multifocal. They are markedly activated in NREM sleep.

A daytime 12- to 16-channel EEG with different montages and appropriate activating procedures is the most useful diagnostic test for most patients with epilepsy. An overnight polysomnographic study can be useful in many patients, however, particularly those for whom a daytime EEG that did not demonstrate any abnormalities. When a primary sleep disorder is included in the differential diagnosis of an abnormal nocturnal event, all-night polysomnography can be helpful in determining the exact nature of the episode.

When a limited number of EEG channels are used in polysomnography, little information is obtained on the morphology and site of origin of epileptic discharges. A more extensive EEG array with 12 to 16 EEG channels is often more helpful, especially when the recording speed is increased to the standard EEG rate of 30 mm/second. Additional information can be obtained by simultaneous audiovisual monitoring and polygraphic recording of other physiologic measures.

Other Laboratory Test Features: If epilepsy is suspected, a daytime EEG with full and variable montage is the study of choice. A computed tomographic scan or magnetic resonance imaging scan of the brain is usually indicated in epileptic patients to detect any structural lesion that may be responsible for the epilepsy. Appropriate biochemical testing may be indicated.

Differential Diagnosis: If generalized tonic-clonic seizures are restricted to sleep, a clear description of the event may not be obtained. In the absence of a clonic phase with postictal confusion, a diagnosis of nocturnal paroxysmal dystonia needs to be considered.

An episode of secondary enuresis during sleep should raise the possibility of epilepsy as a cause. Automatic behavior, including sleepwalking, may need to be differentiated from complex partial seizures that occur only during sleep.

Rhythmic movement disorders, such as headbanging, rarely may have an epileptic etiology. In elderly males, a diagnosis of REM sleep behavior disorder with violent motor activity must be considered.

The possibility of psychogenic pseudoseizures should always be kept in mind.

Diagnostic Criteria: Sleep-Related Epilepsy (345)

A. The patient has a complaint of one of the following: abrupt awakenings at night, unexplained urinary incontinence, or abnormal movements during sleep.
B. Greater than 75% of episodes occur during sleep.
C. At least two of the following features are present:
   1. Generalized tonic-clonic movements of the limbs
   2. Focal limb movement
   3. Automatisms (lip smacking, picking at bedcovers, etc.)
   4. Urinary incontinence
   5. Tongue biting
   6. Forceful expiratory "epileptic cry"
   7. Postictal confusion and lethargy
D. Polysomnographic monitoring demonstrates either of the foloowing:
   1. An epileptic EEG discharge in association with the symptom
   2. Interictal epileptiform features in any stage of sleep
E. No medical or mental disorder accounts for the symptom
F. The symptoms do not meet the diagnostic criteria for any other sleep disorder (e.g., nocturnal paroxysmal dystonia, REM sleep behavior disorder, sleep terror).

Note: The specific seizure-disorder type is specified and coded (e.g., sleep-related epilepsy–partial complex type [345.4]).

Minimal Criteria: A plus B plus C.

Severity Criteria:

Mild: Episodes of sleep-related seizures occur up to once per month and are not associated with physical injury.
Moderate: Sleep-related seizures occur more than once per month but not nightly.
Severe: Sleep-related seizures occur almost nightly, often associated with physical injury.

Duration Criteria:

Acute: 1 month or less.
Subacute: More than 1 month but less than 6 months.
Chronic: 6 months or longer.

Bibliography:

Degan R, Niedermeyer E, eds. Epilepsy, sleep and sleep deprivation. Amsterdam: Elsevier, 1984.
Fisch BJ, Pedley TA. Generalized tonic-clonic epilepsies. In: Luders H, Lesser RP, eds. Epilepsy: Electro-clinical syndromes. New York: Springer-Verlag, 1987; 151–185.
Janz D. The grand mal epilepsies and the sleep-waking cycle. Epilepsia 1962; 3: 69–109.
Luders H, Lesser RP, Dinner DS, Morris HH. Benign focal epilepsy of childhood. In: Luders H, Lesser R, eds. Epilepsy: Electro-clinical syndromes. New York: Springer-Verlag, 1987; 303–346.
Sterman MB, Shouse MW, Passouant P, eds. Sleep and epilepsy. New York: Academic Press, 1982.

Electrical Status Epilepticus of Sleep (345.8)

Synonyms and Key Words: Electrical status of sleep, subclinical electrical status epilepticus induced by sleep in children, continuous spikes and waves during sleep, nonconvulsive status epilepticus. The term *electrical status epilepticus of sleep* is preferred; however, the term is not ideal for a disorder that does not have simultaneous clinical features, and this disorder can be seen in patients without clinical epilepsy.

Essential Features:

Electrical status epilepticus of sleep (ESES) is characterized by continuous and diffuse spike and slow-wave complexes persisting through non-REM (NREM) sleep.

The disorder is typically present in children and is not directly associated with clinical features. The complexes are continuous and occupy no less than 85% of the time of NREM sleep. The disorder persists for months and often for more than one year.

Associated Features: Most patients with ESES have underlying epilepsy. The epilepsy is usually of the motor type, either unilateral or generalized tonic-clonic, and usually begins 4.5 years before the discovery of the ESES. Three types of presentation are usually seen in those patients who have epilepsy: (1) only motor seizures throughout the course; (2) initial unilateral partial motor seizures or generalized tonic-clonic seizures in which absences, similar to typical petit mal absences, are present; (3) or rare motor nocturnal seizures with atypical absences, frequently with atonic and clonic components.

Tonic seizures rarely occur, and the epileptic seizures, if present, are usually self-limited, infrequent, and disappear around 10 to 15 years of age.

Course: ESES resolves with increasing age. The exact duration is difficult to establish but ranges between several months and a few years.

Predisposing Factors: None known.

Prevalence: Rare.

Age of Onset: The average age of discovery of ESES is around eight years (range 4.5–14 years).

Sex Ratio: No difference.

Familial Pattern: Genetic factors for ESES have not been established. Sleep studies of siblings and parents have not been reported. Moreover, because the condition has only been recognized since 1971 and because it exists only in childhood, no information is yet available concerning the offspring of patients.

Pathology: Not known.

Complications: There is increasing evidence that the persistence of spike and slow-wave complexes during sleep is responsible for the appearance of severe neurologic impairment, mainly of language function but also with mental impairment and mental disturbances. Two groups of patients can be distinguished:

1. *Patients with normal psychomotor development* before the occurrence of ESES may develop a severe decrease in intellectual function; a marked reduction of language; severe impairment of memory and temporospatial orientation; behavioral disturbances with reduced attention span, hyperkinesis, aggressiveness, and reduced interpersonal contact; and psychotic states. After resolution of the ESES, a global improvement is noted in performance and behavior.
2. *Patients with an abnormal psychomotor development* before the occurrence of ESES often show a worsening of their mental state.

Polysomnographic Features: Polysomnographic studies performed before sleep onset may show interictal electroencephalographic abnormalities such as focal spikes. As the patient falls asleep, bilateral and diffuse 2- to 2.5-Hz spike and slow-wave complexes appear, persisting throughout the NREM sleep stages. The discharges are continuous, and the spike/wave index (SW index [%] of NREM sleep = total sum of SW [minutes] x 100/total NREM duration [minutes]) ranges from 85% to 100%. Focal abnormalities, with frontal predominance, can be observed in the infrequent few seconds of background activity that occur during the fragmented diffuse spike and slow-wave discharges in NREM sleep. During REM sleep, the electrical status disappears, and the paroxysmal abnormalities consist of infrequent bursts of diffuse spike and slow-wave or focal, predominantly frontal, discharges.

The normal cyclic pattern and percentages of NREM and REM sleep are intact. The spike and slow-wave discharge is so prevalent that spindles, K-complexes, or vertex sharp transients are seldom able to be distinguished.

Other Laboratory Test Features: Routine daytime electroencephalographic recordings can show bursts of generalized spike and slow-wave discharges, often associated with focal spikes, or focal spike and wave, involving the frontotemporal and the centrotemporal regions. A full neuropsychologic assessment may demonstrate mental impairment.

Differential Diagnosis: Three syndromes must be considered in the differential diagnosis:

1. *Benign Epilepsy of Childhood with Rolandic Spikes:* ESES has a characteristic pattern of mental impairment. The interictal features of benign epilepsy of childhood with Rolandic spikes are also characteristic. The sleep of patients with benign epilepsy of childhood with Rolandic spikes does not have a spike-wave index of greater than 85%.
2. *Lennox-Gastaut Syndrome:* The presence of tonic seizures in Lennox-Gastaut syndrome is the main distinguishing factor.

3. *Landau-Kleffner Syndrome:* Acquired aphasia or "developmental dysphasia" can occur in ESES, but the dysphasia is usually part of a more widespread mental impairment. The term *Landau-Kleffner syndrome* should be retained for patients with acquired aphasia without continuous spike and slow-wave discharges in NREM sleep.

Diagnostic Criteria: Electrical Status Epilepticus of Sleep (345.8)

A. The disorder is usually asymptomatic, but there may be a complaint of difficulty in awakening in the morning.
B. ESES is frequently but not always associated with epilepsy, particularly typical absences or infrequent partial or generalized motor seizures.
C. The age of onset is typically in childhood.
D. Polysomnographic monitoring demonstrates:
   1. Continuous, generalized spike and slow-wave discharges persisting through NREM sleep stages
   2. A spike-wave index ranging from 85% to 100%
   3. Disappearance of the electrical status during REM sleep
E. Other medical or mental disorders, particularly other seizure disorders, can be present.
F. The symptoms do not meet the diagnostic criteria for other sleep disorders that occur during sleep.

Minimal Criteria: A plus C plus D.

Severity Criteria:

Mild: ESES with continuous focal spike and slow-wave discharges, usually without neuropsychologic disturbances.
Moderate: ESES with generalized spike and slow-wave discharges that is associated with transitory neuropsychologic disturbances.
Severe: ESES with generalized spike and slow-wave discharges that is associated with severe neuropsychologic disturbances.

Duration Criteria:

Acute: 1 month or less.
Subacute: More than 1 month but less than 1 year.
Chronic: 1 year or longer.

Bibliography:

Billard C, Autret A, Laffont F, Lucas B, Degiovanni E. Electrical status epilepticus during sleep in children: A reappraisal from eight new cases. In: Sterman MB, Shouse MN, Passouant P, eds. Sleep and epilepsy. London: Academic Press, 1982; 481–494.
Dalla Bernardina B, Tassinari CA, Dravet C, Bureau M, Beghini G, Roger J. Epilepsie partielle benigne et etat de mal electroencephalographique pendant le sommeil. Rev Electroencephalogr Neurophysiol Clin 1978; 8: 350–353.
Patry G, Lyagoubi S, Tassinari CA. Subclinical "electrical status epilepticus" induced by sleep in children. A clinical and electroencephalographic study of six cases. Arch Neurol 1971; 24: 242–252.

Tassinari CA, Bureau M, Dravet C, Dalla Bernardina B, Roger J. Epilepsy with continuous spikes and waves during sleep. In: Roger J, Dravet C, Bureau M, Dreifuss FE, Wolf P, eds. Epileptic syndromes in infancy, childhood and adolescence. London: John Libbey Eurotext, 1985; 194–204.

Tassinari CA, Bureau M, Dravet C, Roget J, Daniele Natale O. Electrical status epilepticus during sleep in children (electrical status epilepticus of sleep). In: Sterman MB, Shouse MN, Passouant P, eds. Sleep and epilepsy. London: Academic Press, 1982; 465–479.

Sleep-Related Headaches (346)

Synonyms and Key Words: Classic migraine (346.0), migraine with aura (346.0), common migraine (346.1), migraine without aura (346.1), cluster headache (346.2), chronic paroxysmal hemicrania (346.2), migraine–unspecified (346.9), nocturnal migraine, vascular headaches, early morning headaches. (Excludes tension-type headache [307.81].)

Essential Features:

Sleep-related cluster headache, chronic paroxysmal hemicrania, and migraine are severe, mainly unilateral, headaches that often have their onset during sleep.

The patient is either awakened with pain during the night or is aware of an attack on awakening in the morning. Migraine is a familial disorder characterized by recurrent attacks of headache that are widely variable in intensity, frequency, and duration and are typically unilateral but may be bilateral. Cluster headache is an extremely severe, unilateral headache often accompanied by symptoms of autonomic dysfunction. Chronic paroxysmal hemicrania (CPH) is a variant of cluster headache that is strictly unilateral, with attacks that are more frequent and remarkably regular and shorter than those of typical cluster headache. The usual onset of the attacks is during sleep. The relative frequency of cluster-headache attacks that begin during the night is 2.5 times that of headaches that begin during the day. Daytime attacks often begin during naps or periods of physical relaxation. Laboratory recordings have demonstrated that the attacks are more likely to occur out of REM sleep periods and in the immediate post-REM sleep. In some cases of CPH, the attacks are so closely related to REM sleep that they appear to be virtually "REM sleep locked."

Associated Features: Classic migraine is usually associated with prodromes arising from the visual cortex in the form of scotoma or visual hallucinations, followed by unilateral or bilateral headache or throbbing pain felt deeply behind the eye or the frontotemporal region. The attacks are often accompanied by nausea, loss of appetite, photophobia, and vomiting. The cluster headache occurs predominantly in males; the pain usually begins around or above one eye and usually occurs on the same side of the head during subsequent attacks. Severe, excruciating pain is accompanied by signs and symptoms suggesting autonomic dysfunction. Lacrimation is prominent, with conjunctival injection, nasal stuffiness or rhinorrhea, increased forehead sweating, and cardiac arrhythmias. CPH resembles cluster headache with regard to localization and character of pain but has several differentiating features: in CPH, the duration of the attack is shorter, the frequency is usually very high (exceeding 15 attacks per 24 hours), and there is a female preponderance of 70%.

Course: Sleep-related migraine is a benign condition and, with rare exceptions, has no effect on life span. The frequency and the severity of the attacks determine the degree of the patient's incapacity because of the disease. The attacks may persist throughout life; not infrequently, however, they may cease after menopause in women or in late middle life in men. Remission of the attacks is common during pregnancy. Remissions in sleep-related cluster headache usually last between six months and two years and may also occur during pregnancy. Sleep-related CPH has a chronic course similar to that of migraine.

Precipitating Factors: Migraine can be precipitated by sleep, stress, relaxation after stress, trauma, barometric pressure and weather changes, foods, and eating habits. Small doses of alcohol can trigger attacks in most patients with cluster headache. Hypoxia and sleep apnea (particularly during REM sleep) may be major triggering events in cluster headache.

Prevalence: Not known.

Age of Onset: Most sleep-related migraine, cluster headaches, and CPH start in the second or third decades.

Sex Ratio: The sex ratio for migraine is approximately 1:3 (M:F) and for cluster headache is approximately 9:1 (M:F).

Familial Pattern: About 60% of patients with migraines have a positive family history, whereas it is rare to find a positive family history in cluster headache.

Pathology: In migraine, the focal neurologic symptoms are the result of ischemia of the cerebral cortex; the ischemia is caused by arteriolar and capillary constriction causing shunting of blood from the cortex, or platelet aggregation, or a combination of these factors.

An inherited imbalance of monoamine metabolism may render patients more susceptible to developing headaches. In cluster headache, the autonomic nervous system is likely to be involved. Although the autonomic symptoms and signs that accompany cluster headache and CPH are similar, they are not identical. The temporal relationships of migraine, cluster headaches, and CPH are different, suggesting differences in biologic clocks determining the rhythmicity of these conditions. Cluster headache shows profiles of both circa-annual periods as well as circadian/ultradian timing of the attacks.

Polysomnographic Features: Laboratory recordings have demonstrated that awakening with migraine is more likely to occur out of REM sleep. This relationship is stronger in cluster headache and is almost REM locked in some cases of CPH. An association between cluster headache and sleep apnea has recently been reported. In cluster-headache patients with sleep apnea and hypersomnia, airway obstruction occurrs almost exclusively during REM sleep. Other polysomnographic abnormalities include insomnia with frequent and sometimes prolonged awakening, atypical sleep-stage distribution, and marked decrease in stage REM.

Other Laboratory Test Features: Other diagnostic procedures can include brain imaging or electroencephalography.

Differential Diagnosis: The differential diagnosis of sleep-related vascular headaches must include the group of tension "psychogenic" headaches associated with anxiety, tension, and depression. Tension headaches are extremely common and are usually bilateral or have a midline distribution. Headaches due to increased intracranial pressure, as with tumors, arteriovenous malformations, and hematomas; headaches due to cardiovascular disease and hypertension or inflammatory conditions of bones, nerves, and meninges; and pos-ttraumatic headaches have to be excluded. Obstructive sleep apnea syndrome is a common cause of morning headaches.

Diagnostic Criteria: Sleep-Related Headaches (346)

A. The patient has a complaint of headaches during sleep.
B. More than 75% of headache episodes occur during sleep.
C. The patient has a diagnosis of one or more types of headaches.
D. Polysomnographic monitoring demonstrates:
   1. An awakening associated with a complaint of headache
   2. Onset of the headache in sleep, typically REM sleep
E. The headaches can be associated with other medical disorders.
F. Other sleep disorders can be present.

Note: It is recommended that the headache type be classified according to the diagnostic criteria of the Headache Classification Committee of the International Headache Society and stated in conjunction with the appropriate ICD-9-CM code number (e.g., chronic paroxysmal hemicrania [346.2]). Code and state the particular headache type on axis A, preceded by the words "sleep-related," (e.g., sleep-related cluster headache).

Minimal Criteria: A plus B plus C.

Severity Criteria:

Mild: Mild discomfort, typically associated with only rare (less than monthly) episodes.
Moderate: Moderately severe discomfort, often, but not always, associated with up to four episodes per month.
Severe: Cluster headaches are always severe; discomfort is often, but not always extreme; the headaches are associated with more than one episode per month.

Duration Criteria:
Acute: 3 months or less.
Subacute: More than 3 months but less than 12 months.
Chronic: 12 months or longer.

Bibliography:

Dexter JD, Weitzman ED. The relationship of nocturnal headaches to sleep stage patterns. Neurology 1970; 20: 513–518.

Classification and diagnostic criteria for headache disorders, cranial neuralgias and facial pain. Headache Classification Committee of the International Headache Society. Cephalalgia 1988; Suppl 7: 1–96.

Kayed K, Godtlibsen OB, Sjaastad O. Chronic paroxysmal hemicrania IV: "REM sleep locked" nocturnal headache attacks. Sleep 1978; 1: 91–95.

Kayed K, Sjaastad O. Nocturnal and early morning headaches. Ann Clin Res 1985; 17: 243–246.

Lance JW. The mechanism and management of headache, 4th ed. London: Butterworths, 1982.

SLEEP DISORDERS ASSOCIATED WITH MENTAL, NEUROLOGIC, AND OTHER MEDICAL DISORDERS

ASSOCIATED WITH OTHER MEDICAL DISORDERS

1. Sleeping Sickness (086) 260
2. Nocturnal Cardiac Ischemia (411-114) 263
3. Chronic Obstructive Pulmonary Disease (490-494). 265
4. Sleep-Related Asthma (493) 269
5. Sleep-Related Gastroesophageal Reflux (530.81) 272
6. Peptic Ulcer Disease (531-534) 274
7. Fibromyalgia (729.1) 278

Sleep Disorders Associated with Other Medical Disorders

A variety of other medical disorders that have features occurring during sleep or that cause sleep disturbance are listed here. Though sleeping sickness is rare outside the continent of Africa, the disorder is included here because it is commonly seen in Africa. Other infectious disorders, such as encephalitis lethargica, are not included here because they rarely occur.

Cardiac ischemia during sleep can lead to myocardial infarction or cardiac arrhythmias, and the ischemia may not be symptomatic. A description of nocturnal cardiac ischemia is presented in view of its importance, in the hope of stimulating further research on the factors related to its cause. Although the importance of myocardial infarction during sleep is clear, this diagnosis is rarely seen acutely in the practice of sleep-disorders medicine and rarely needs to be included in the differential diagnosis of a patient presenting with sleep complaints.

Chronic obstructive pulmonary disease and sleep-related asthma are common enough in the population to warrant inclusion here. Other pulmonary disorders can have sleep-related features but rarely present because of the sleep disturbances. Many new respiratory disorders can produce a disturbed pattern of breathing during sleep that leads to the development of the central sleep apnea syndrome.

Two gastrointestinal disorders are included in this section, sleep-related gastroesophageal reflux and peptic ulcer disease. The discomfort associated with peptic ulcer disease commonly occurs during the major sleep episode. This disease may be diagnosed from purely sleep-related symptoms. Although the incidence of peptic ulcer disease appears to be declining in the United States, in some other countries, notably Japan, it is very high.

Fibromyalgia, also known as fibrositis syndrome, is included because it is associated with abnormal electroencephalographic patterns during sleep, called alpha sleep or alpha-delta sleep.

Sleeping Sickness (086)

Synonyms and Key Words: Gambian trypanosomiasis (086.3), Gambian sleeping sickness (086.3), Rhodesian trypanosomiasis (086.4), Rhodesian sleeping sickness (086.4), trypanosomiasis, unspecified (086.9). (Excludes American trypanosomiasis [Chagas' disease] [086.0-086.2].)

Essential Features:

Sleeping sickness is a protozoan-caused illness characterized by an acute febrile lymphadenopathy; after a usual latency period of four to six months, the lymphadenopathy is followed by excessive sleepiness associated with a chronic meningoencephalomyelitis.

The acute phase begins after an incubation period of some two weeks following infection by the causal fusiform protozoan Trypanosoma brucei, usually from inoculation by a tsetse fly bite. During the acute phase, there is high remitting fever, tender lymphadenopathy, and severe headache. A characteristic circinate erythema occurs, with painful subcutaneous edema of the hands, feet, and periorbital tissues. The signs and symptoms reoccur intermittently over months to years. The lymph nodes of the posterior cervical triangle may become prominent. As direct cerebral involvement begins, nocturnal sleep becomes fragmented, and marked excessive sleepiness occurs. There is usually a vacant facial expression, droopy eyelids, and often a droopy lower lip. Spontaneous talk may be minimal, and patients become inactive and torpid. If untreated, sleeping sickness usually results in death.

Associated Features: The associated features are numerous and depend upon the degree of nervous system involvement. Patients may show tremor of the hands and tongue or choreiform movements. Seizures are frequent, particularly during an acute onset of cerebral involvement or during terminal status epilepticus. There may be loss of sphincter control. Ophthalmoplegia is common.

Course: If untreated, the disorder is lethal. The Rhodesian form is the most severe, usually terminating fatally within one year if untreated. Early treatment may produce full recovery; late treatment results in various degrees of neurologic impairment. Death occurs most frequently from coma, status epilepticus, hyperpyrexia, or intercurrent infection.

Predisposing Factors: Living in areas of endemic disease with infected tsetse flies gives a high risk of infection. The risk also increases if any causes of lowered resistance to infection are present.

Prevalence: The precise prevalence is unknown. The disease, however, is extremely common in endemic areas of tropical Africa.

Age of Onset: Occurs from infancy to old age.

Sex Ratio: No difference.

Familial Pattern: None.

Pathology: The tsetse fly inoculates the protozoan *(Trypanosoma brucei)* into the subcutaneous pool of blood that forms during the fly's feeding. The protozoa multiply, and a local chancre is produced. The organisms reach the general circulation via the lymphatic system. Starting two to three weeks after the bite, waves of parasitemia occur, during which the organism is easily detected in the blood. Brain involvement may occur after about one month in Rhodesian sleeping sickness or as late as several years after infection in Gambian sleeping sickness. The disease is first manifested as a diffuse leptomeningitis (when seizures are most common), then as a perivascular cerebritis. In later stages, a demyelinating panencephalitis occurs. Central nervous system lesions predominate in brain stem regions.

Complications: The potential complications are many and depend upon the progression of the disease. Myocarditis can occur.

Polysomnographic Features: In the early stages of sleeping sickness, there is loss of all the transient features of stage 1 and stage 2 non-REM (NREM) sleep, including vertex sharp transients, spindles, and K-complexes. Subsequently, all stages of NREM sleep become indistinguishable. The electroencephalogram (EEG) throughout NREM sleep becomes homogeneous, with either diffuse high-amplitude slow waves or diffuse theta and lower-amplitude delta activity. Patients can show pseudorhythmic EEG delta bursts in wakefulness and in NREM sleep. In the advanced stage of the disease, some 50% of patients show characteristic recurrent three- to seven-second-duration periods of lower-amplitude waves in the beta and alpha frequencies (or occasionally theta activity) associated with transient tachycardia, respiratory changes, and increased muscle tone. These findings appear to represent recurrent "microarousals." Epileptiform discharges may be recorded during these events. Relatively normal REM sleep patterns are maintained until death. Multiple sleep latency tests have not been reported but are expected to demonstrate evidence of pathologic sleepiness.

Other Laboratory Test Features: The diagnosis is confirmed by demonstration of trypanosomes in blood, lymphatic fluid, tissue taken from lymph nodes, or cerebrospinal fluid or in laboratory rats or mice that have been injected with fluids from infected humans. Anemia, hypermacroglobulinemia, spontaneous clumping of erythrocytes, and an elevated sedimentation rate are usually present. The cerebrospinal fluid may show mononuclear pleocytosis, increased protein levels, or increased IgM. The usual sevenfold or more elevation in cerebrospinal-fluid IgM levels is typical of trypanosomiasis. Specific trypanosomal antibodies are diagnostically useful.

Routine EEGs show a normal or only slightly slowed alpha rhythm until very late in the disease. Marked sleepiness and increased numbers of sleep-wake transitions are characteristic early signs, as is an increase in delta activity. The latter consists of bilaterally synchronous and symmetrical delta bursts that are maximum anteriorly or multifocal delta waves. Late in the disease, the delta bursts occur periodically and may be superimposed upon an otherwise essentially flat (isoelectric) recording in the final stages.

Differential Diagnosis: American trypanosomiasis (Chagas' disease) is caused by *Trypanosoma cruzi* and does not produce excessive sleepiness as a major feature. The main diagnostic problem consists of separating African sleeping sickness (due to *Trypanosoma brucei*) from other forms of symptomatic hypersomnia, particularly other forms with an infectious origin; these other forms include hypersomnia related to encephalopathies of viral, bacterial, or parasitic origin other than trypanosomas. Idiopathic hypersomnia, narcolepsy, and disorders of excessive sleepiness due to sleep apnea syndromes, periodic limb movement disorder, or other etiologies seldom pose diagnostic difficulties.

Diagnostic Criteria: Sleeping Sickness (086)

A. The patient has a complaint of severe sleepiness.
B. The complaint is associated with a diagnosis of trypanosomiasis.
C. Polysomnographic monitoring demonstrates all of the following:
   1. Loss of NREM sleep EEG transients (vertex sharp transients, sleep spindles, K-complexes) plus recurrent microarousals
   2. Bursts of delta activity
   3. A mean sleep latency of less than 10 minutes on the multiple sleep latency test
D. The complaint is not associated with other medical or mental disorders (e.g., viral meningoencephalitis).
E. Other sleep disorders can be present but do not account for the primary sleep complaint.

Note: Specify and code the type of sleeping sickness known (e.g., Gambian sleeping sickness [086.3]).

Minimal Criteria: A plus B.

Severity Criteria:

Mild: Mild excessive sleepiness, as defined on page 23.
Moderate: Moderate excessive sleepiness, as defined on page 23, and moderate disruption of the major sleep episode, with loss of recognizable NREM sleep stages and frequent microarousals.
Severe: Severe excessive sleepiness, as defined on page 23, and severe disruption of the major sleep episode, with diffuse theta activity and delta bursts.

Duration Criteria:

Acute: 1 month or less.
Subacute: More than 1 month but less than 1 year.
Chronic: 1 year or longer.

Bibliography:

Bert J, Collomb H, Fressy J, Gastaut H. Etude electrographique du sommeil nocturne. In: Fischgold H, ed. Le sommeil de nuit normal et pathologique. Paris: Masson, 1965; 334–352.

Gallais P et al. Etude electroencephalographique de la trypanosomaise humaine africaine. Rev Neurol 1957; 85: 95–104.

Mulligan HW, ed. The African trypanosomiasis. London: Allen and Irvin, 1970.

Plourde JJ. Trypanosomiasis. In: Winthrobe MW et al., eds. Harrison's principles of internal medicine. New York: McGraw-Hill, 1972; 1026–1028.

Radermacker J. Systematique et electroencephalographique des encephalites et encephalopathies. Paris: Masson et Cie, 1956.

Schwartz BA, Escande C. Sleeping sickness: Sleep study of a case. Electroencephalogr Clin Neurophysiol 1970; 3: 83–87.

Nocturnal Cardiac Ischemia (411-414)

Synonyms and Key Words: Unstable angina (411.1), coronary insufficiency–acute (411.8), nocturnal angina (413.0), angina decubitus (413.0), Prinzmetal's angina (413.1), angina pectoris (413.9), atherosclerotic heart disease (414.0), asymptomatic cardiac ischemia (412), silent ischemia (412).

Essential Features:

Nocturnal cardiac ischemia is characterized by ischemia of the myocardium that occurs during the major sleep episode.

Nocturnal cardiac ischemia can produce a feeling of pressure during sleep, which may be "viselike" in the center of the chest or described as a "clenched fist." This pressure or pain may radiate upward to the chin and jaw and to the arms, especially the left arm. These features may also be present during the waking hours and may be associated with activity at that time. Electrocardiographic monitoring during sleep reveals horizontal ST-segment depression or ST-segment elevation of 1 mm or more. The ischemia noted on the electrocardiogram (ECG) may not be associated with chest pain.

Associated Features: Typical features of angina with exertion may occur during the day, and silent ischemia may occur during the nighttime or sleeping hours or when the individual lies down. Electrocardiographic changes of ischemia occur more frequently in the early morning hours, at a time when REM sleep occurs. Ischemia can also occur during the initial hours of sleep and at that time may be related to a fall in blood pressure and heart rate.

Course: The course depends on the underlying cardiac disorder, be it coronary-artery disease, valvular disease, or coronary artery spasm. The presence of ischemia on the ECG during rest, whether or not the ischemia is symptomatic, is usually a manifestation of coronary artery disease.

Predisposing Factors: Predisposing factors are the presence of coronary artery disease or valvular disease such as aortic stenosis. Other risk factors include hypertension, cigarette smoking, elevated blood cholesterol levels and low-density lipoprotein levels, obesity, and sleep-induced hypoxemia. Patients with obstructive sleep apnea syndrome appear to have a higher prevalence of nocturnal cardiac ischemia than does the general population.

Prevalence: Unknown.

Age of Onset: Seen most commonly in middle-aged males but can occur in women, especially postmenopausal women.

Sex Ratio: There is a strong male preponderance of coronary artery disease; this preponderance is especially strong before age 60.

Familial Pattern: There is a strong familial tendency for coronary artery disease and aortic stenosis secondary to a bicuspid aortic valve.

Pathology: Nocturnal cardiac ischemia may be due to either coronary artery spasm or an intrinsic coronary artery disease, such as atherosclerosis.

Complications: Complications can include significant ventricular cardiac arrhythmias, left-ventricular failure, acute myocardial infarction, and sudden death.

Polysomnographic Features: Polysomnography demonstrates ST-wave changes, characterized by at least a 1-mm horizontal depression in the ST segment. There may be ST-segment elevation during coronary artery spasm, especially in the presence of Prinzmetal's variant angina. REM sleep with tachycardia as well as slow-wave sleep with a fall in blood pressure and heart rate can lead to ischemia. Sleep-related breathing disorders, especially obstructive sleep apnea syndrome, are often associated with oxygen desaturation that can lead to cardiac ischemia.

Other Laboratory Test Features: Baseline ECGs may be normal or abnormal. Cardiac exercise testing with thallium is usually positive for ischemic heart disease. Echocardiography will demonstrate aortic stenosis if present. Cardiac catheterization with coronary angiography may be indicated.

Differential Diagnosis: Nocturnal chest pain and pressure may be produced by left-ventricular failure (paroxysmal nocturnal dyspnea), sleep-related gastroesophageal reflux, peptic ulcer disease, or primary pulmonary disease.

Diagnostic Criteria: Nocturnal Cardiac Ischemia (411-414)

A. The patient may have a complaint of chest pain, or the disorder may be asymptomatic.
B. Electrocardiography demonstrates the features of cardiac ischemia.
C. Polysomnography demonstrates electrocardiographic evidence of cardiac ischemia during sleep, with ST-segment elevation or depression of 1 mm or more.
D. The primary complaint is not due to other medical disorders such as pulmonary disease.
E. Other sleep disorders (e.g., obstructive sleep apnea syndrome) may be present and may precipitate the disorder.

Note: If obstructive sleep apnea syndrome produces nocturnal cardiac ischemia, state and code both diagnoses on axis A.

Minimal Criteria: A plus B.

Severity Criteria:

Mild: Not applicable.
Moderate: Not applicable.
Severe: Always severe.

Duration Criteria:

Acute: Less than 24 hours.
Subacute: More than 1 day but less than 7 days.
Chronic: 7 days or longer.

Bibliography:

Burack B. The hypersomnia-sleep apnea syndrome: Its recognition in clinical cardiology. Am Heart J 1984; 107: 543–548.

Muller JE, Ludmer PL, Willich SN, et al. Circadian variation in the frequency of sudden cardiac death. Circulation 1987; 75: 131–138.

Nowlin JB, Troyer WG Jr, Collins WS, et al. The association of nocturnal angina pectoris with dreaming. Ann Intern Med 1965; 63: 1040–1046.

Schroeder JS, Motta J, Guilleminault C. Hemodynamic studies in sleep apnea. In: Guilleminault C, Dement WC, eds. Sleep apnea syndromes. New York: Alan R. Liss, 1978; 177–196.

Chronic Obstructive Pulmonary Disease (490-494)

Synonyms and Key Words: Chronic obstructive pulmonary disease (491.2), chronic obstructive lung disease (491.2), chronic obstructive airway disease (491.2), chronic bronchitis (491.2), blue bloaters–Type B (491.2), emphysema (492), pink puffers–Type A (492.8), bronchiectasis (494), bronchitis–unspecified (490). (Includes chronic airway obstruction–unspecified [496], cystic fibrosis [277.0], bronchopulmonary dysplasia [770.7]. Excludes asthma [493].)

Essential Features:

Chronic obstructive pulmonary disease is characterized by a chronic impairment of airflow through the respiratory tract between the atmosphere and the gas-exchange portion of the lung. Altered cardiorespiratory physiology during sleep or a complaint of insomnia can occur.

The respiratory disturbance in chronic obstructive pulmonary disease is more fixed than is that of asthma, which is characterized by a spontaneous or therapeutically induced reversibility of airflow limitation.

Sleep disturbance commonly occurs in patients with chronic obstructive pulmonary disease and is characterized by difficulty initiating sleep, frequent awakenings with respiratory distress, shortness of breath or nocturnal cough, frequent brief arousals throughout the night, and a feeling of being unrested upon awakening (occasionally with morning headaches). Oxygen desaturation can occur, particularly in association with REM sleep. The sleep disturbance may be exacerbated by the medication used for the treatment of chronic obstructive pulmonary disease, particularly the xanthine derivatives such as theophylline.

Patients with chronic obstructive pulmonary disease have been subdivided into two groups: '*pink puffers*'–who typically have shortness of breath associated with increased lung volumes, mild hypoxemia, and normal or low arterial PCO_2 levels and '*blue bloaters*'–who also have shortness of breath and hypoxemia but are hypercapnic, with evidence of pulmonary hypertension, cor pulmonale, and secondary polycythemia. Sleep-related exacerbation of hypoxemia is more likely to occur in patients who are blue bloaters.

Associated Features: Short periods of central apnea may occur in patients who have chronic obstructive pulmonary disease with oxygen desaturation. The episodes of hypoxemia during sleep are more likely to occur during REM sleep and can last from one or two minutes up to one hour or longer. Chronic subjective and objective sleep disturbances, such as prolonged sleep latency, frequent awakenings, reduced sleep efficiency, and early morning awakenings, are often seen in patients with chronic lung disease and respiratory insufficiency but do not necessarily correlate with the presence of oxygen desaturation.

Obstructive sleep apnea syndrome may coexist with chronic obstructive pulmonary disease and may contribute to the sleep-related symptoms. The presence of obstructive sleep apnea syndrome with chronic obstructive pulmonary disease is sometimes called the "overlap syndrome" and may be more likely to predispose the patient to the development of awake alveolar hypoventilation and right-heart failure.

Predisposing Factors: Chronic obstructive pulmonary disease is typically seen in adult individuals who are cigarette smokers. Obesity appears to be an aggravating factor in the development of the sleep disturbance and sleep-related oxygen desaturation. In children, respiratory infections, bronchopulmonary dysplasia, cystic fibrosis, and ciliary anomalies are often the cause.

Prevalence: Most patients with chronic obstructive pulmonary disease will develop some disturbance of nocturnal sleep quality. About 25% of patients who have an awake arterial oxygen tension of greater than 60mmHg will show a 5% or greater drop in oxygen saturation during REM sleep. A greater prevalence of oxygen desaturation during sleep can be expected in those patients with daytime resting hypoxemia below 55mmHg.

Age of Onset: The sleep disturbance related to chronic obstructive pulmonary disease can occur at any age with the development of the underlying disease. The respiratory disorder occurs most often in individuals over the age of 50 years, but it can occur in children at any age from infancy.

Sex Ratio: The prevalence of chronic obstructive pulmonary disease is higher in males, and there does not appear to be any sex difference in the tendency to develop associated sleep disturbance.

Familial Pattern: Not known.

Pathology: Mucus and inflammation of the airway walls, destruction of the lung parenchyma, narrowed airways due to thickened mucosa, or constriction of the airway smooth muscle are typical features.

Complications: The complications include disturbed sleep, nocturnal arrhythmias, and the development of cor pulmonale and death.

The sleep disturbance can produce significant psychologic effects of anxiety and depression and can produce a tendency for excessive sleepiness. Nocturnal arrhythmias, especially supraventricular events, are very common in patients with advanced respiratory disease. Ventricular arrhythmias may be more liable to occur when the oxygen saturation values fall below 60% during sleep. The oxygen desaturation causes pulmonary vascular constriction, with an elevated pulmonary-artery pressure. Destruction of the pulmonary vascular bed may also contribute to the development of pulmonary hypertension.

Course: The sleep disturbance appears to correlate with the progression of the underlying pulmonary disease. With decreasing pulmonary function, the sleep disturbance, oxygen desaturation, and cardiac complications progress.

Polysomnographic Features: Sleep is characterized by a difficulty in initiating sleep. These difficulties are often concurrent with symptoms of shortness of breath in the recumbent position; the shortness of breath may be exacerbated by obesity and the associated basal lung-field compression. Total inability to lie flat during sleep may necessitate that polysomnographic monitoring be performed with the patient in a semirecumbent position. Mucus accumulation will cause disturbed sleep, with frequent episodes of coughing and expectoration. During acute exacerbations of chronic obstructive pulmonary disease, the performance of polysomnography may not be possible due to the patient's intense shortness of breath and restlessness. The sleep shows a reduction in the amount of slow-wave sleep and REM sleep, with frequent sleep-stage changes, arousals, and awakenings. Arterial oxygen desaturation may occur independent of apneic events, particularly during REM sleep. Concurrent obstructive apneic events may be present in some patients, particularly in those who are obese. Cardiac arrhythmias that are not necessarily related to the episodes of hypoxemia may be present during polysomnographic monitoring.

Daytime multiple sleep latency tests may demonstrate a reduced mean sleep latency that usually correlates with the degree of nocturnal sleep disruption.

Other Laboratory Test Features: Pulmonary-function testing indicates obstructive airway disease. The findings of chest radiography are variable, depending upon the predominance of either emphysema or bronchitis. A deficiency in alpha-antitrypsin may be found.

Differential Diagnosis: Patients with chronic obstructive pulmonary disease are liable to have sleep disturbance that may be due to other causes of insomnia. Insomnia due to anxiety or depression is not uncommon in patients with chronic obstructive pulmonary disease, and psychophysiologic insomnia may also occur as a result of the chronically disturbed sleep patterns. Acute exacerbations of chronic obstructive pulmonary disease may produce an adjustment sleep disorder.

Respiratory disturbance during sleep occurs with the obstructive sleep apnea syndrome. If disorders such as kyphoscoliosis, poliomyelitis, muscular dystrophy, or other neurologic disorders are present concurrently, they may contribute to the development of central sleep apnea syndrome.

It may not be possible to clinically distinguish patients with central alveolar hypoventilation syndrome and chronic obstructive pulmonary disease from patients who have the blue bloater form of chronic obstructive pulmonary disease. The only distinguishing feature may be evidence of alveolar hypoventilation prior to the development of chronic obstructive pulmonary disease.

Patients with sleep-related asthma will have reversible bronchospasm.

Diagnostic Criteria: Chronic Obstructive Pulmonary Disease (490-496)

A. The patient has a complaint of insomnia or excessive sleepiness.
B. The sleep disturbance is temporally related to the presence of chronic obstructive pulmonary disease.
C. Polysomnographic monitoring demonstrates all of the following:
   1. Reduced sleep efficiency, with an increase in sleep latency and number of awakenings; reduced total sleep time, with frequent sleep-stage changes; reduced stage 3 and stage 4 sleep; and reduced REM sleep
   2. Oxygen desaturation during sleep
D. The respiratory disturbance is not due to other medical disorders (e.g., asthma).
E. Other sleep disorders can be present but do not account for the primary complaint.

Note: State and code chronic obstructive pulmonary disease on axis A along with the primary symptom (e.g., chronic obstructive lung disease associated with insomnia [491.2]).

Minimal Criteria: A plus B.

Severity Criteria:

Mild: Usually associated with mild insomnia or mild sleepiness, as defined on page 23, and chronic obstructive pulmonary disease of mild severity is present.
Moderate: Usually associated with moderate insomnia or moderate sleepiness, as defined on page 23, and usually associated with a diagnosis of moderately severe chronic obstructive pulmonary disease.
Severe: Usually associated with severe insomnia or severe sleepiness, as defined on page 23, and usually associated with a diagnosis of severe chronic obstructive pulmonary disease.

Duration Criteria:

Acute: 1 month or less.
Subacute: More than 1 month but less than 6 months.
Chronic: 6 months or longer.

Bibliography:

Calverley PMA, Brezinova V, Douglas NJ, Catterall JR, Flenley DC. The effect of oxygenation on sleep quality in chronic bronchitis and emphysema. Am Rev Respir Dis 1982; 126: 206–210.

Fleetham J, West P, Mezon B, Conway W, Roth T, Kryger M. Sleep, arousals and oxygen desaturation in chronic obstructive pulmonary disease. The effect of oxygen therapy. Am Rev Respir Dis 1982; 126: 429–433.

Flenley DC. Chronic obstructive pulmonary disease. In: Kryger MH, Roth T, Dement WC, eds. Principles and practice of sleep medicine. Philadelphia: WB Saunders, 1989; 601–610.

Guilleminault C, Cummiskey J, Motta J. Chronic obstructive airflow disease and sleep studies. Am Rev Respir Dis 1980; 122: 397–406.

Sleep-Related Asthma (493)

Synonyms and Key Words: Extrinsic asthma (493.0), intrinsic asthma (493.1), asthma–unspecified (493.9), sleep-related asthma, nocturnal asthma, nighttime asthma, night awakening with asthma.

Essential Features:

Sleep-related asthma refers to asthma attacks that occur during sleep.

Patients awaken with dyspnea, wheezing, coughing, air hunger, or chest tightness. The symptoms usually improve with the administration of bronchodilating medications.

Associated Features: Patients may awaken with coughing that continues until they expectorate thick secretions or mucus plugs. Mild nocturnal hypoxemia of 5% to 6% is usually associated with asthma. In children, the hypoxemia is generally more severe and is proportional to the severity of the airway obstruction.

Sleep disruption due to nocturnal episodes of asthma commonly leads to complaints of poor sleep, daytime fatigue, and, less frequently, daytime sleepiness.

Predisposing Factors: A good correlation exists between the severity of asthma and the frequency of sleep-related asthmatic episodes. In patients with chronic asthma, the onset of sleep-related asthma often indicates a general deterioration of the asthma, but persons with relatively mild daytime asthmatic symptoms may also experience sleep-related asthma. Esophageal reflux during sleep, with or without aspiration of gastric contents, may occasionally be a provoking factor.

Course: Episodes of sleep-related asthma decrease in frequency and severity with effective treatment. The use of medications such as the xanthines, however, may lead to insomnia.

Prevalence: Sixty-one percent to 74% of patients with asthma report nighttime awakenings due to sleep-related asthma. Up to 40% of patients on routine asthma treatment have reported awakening every night with episodes of asthma.

Age of Onset: Variable, depending on the type of asthma.

Sex Ratio: No difference.

Familial Pattern: Not known.

Pathology: Several factors involving circadian variations in physiology or hormonal function may underlie sleep-related asthma. Bronchial resistance is increased during early morning hours in normal subjects, and this process appears to be accentuated in asthmatic individuals. Asthmatics have demonstrated a 20% to 50% decrease in airflow throughout the night. Nighttime exposure to allergens or delayed response to allergen exposure during the waking hours may induce sleep-related asthma. The airway-inflammatory response may be increased at night due to the circadian nadir in plasma epinephrine and cortisol concentrations and a corresponding increase in eosinophil concentrations. Another factor is the relatively rapid metabolism of most antiasthmatic medications, with substantially reduced drug levels during early morning hours.

Complications: The complications are those of sleep disturbance and impaired ventilation. Insomnia and excessive sleepiness may result. Asthmatic episodes can result in nocturnal death.

Polysomnographic Features: Asthmatic attacks rarely occur in the first hour of sleep or in stage 3 or stage 4 sleep. Attacks tend to cluster later in the sleep period but appear to be randomly distributed throughout all sleep stages. Awakenings occur when the patient experiences an asthmatic attack. Esophageal pressure monitoring demonstrates increasing negative intrathoracic pressures immediately preceding and during an attack.

Other Laboratory Test Features: Pulmonary function testing demonstrates reversible obstructive airway disease. A chest radiograph may demonstrate lung hyperinflation. Sputum and blood eosinophilia and high serum IgE levels may indicate an allergic component.

Differential Diagnosis: Sleep-related asthma must be differentiated from congestive heart failure with paroxysmal nocturnal dyspnea, sleep-related gastroesophageal reflux, abnormal sleep-related swallowing syndrome, nocturnal cardiac ischemia, central alveolar hypoventilation syndrome, sleep-related laryngospasm, sleep choking syndrome, or obstructive sleep apnea syndrome.

Diagnostic Criteria: Sleep-related Asthma (493)

A. The patient has a complaint of insomnia or excessive sleepiness, and cough or dyspnea.
B. The complaint is temporally related to the presence of asthma.
C. Associated features include one or more of the following:
   1. Dyspnea and wheezing
   2. Expectoration of thick sputum
   3. Improvement with the use of bronchodilating medications
D. Polysomnographic monitoring demonstrates asthmatic episodes occurring randomly during sleep but not in slow-wave sleep.
E. Other medical or mental disorders (e.g., paroxysmal nocturnal dyspnea) are not the cause of the symptoms.
F. Other sleep disorders (e.g., obstructive sleep apnea syndrome, sleep-related swallowing syndrome, sleep-related gastroesophageal reflux) can be present but are not the cause of the symptom producing ventilatory difficulties during sleep.

Minimal Criteria: A plus B.

Severity Criteria:

Mild: Mild insomnia or excessive sleepiness, as defined on page 23. Episodes usually occur less frequently than once per week and resolve spontaneously.
Moderate: Moderate insomnia or excessive sleepiness, as defined on page 23, with episodes usually occuring on an almost nightly basis and resolving only after the individual takes prescribed medication.
Severe: Severe insomnia and excessive sleepiness, as defined on page 23, with episodes occurring more than once per night and resolving only after the individual takes prescribed medication. On at least one occasion, physician intervention has been required.

Duration Criteria:

Acute: 7 days or less.
Subacute: More than 7 days but less than 6 months.
Chronic: 6 months or longer.

Bibliography:

Catterall JR, Rhind GB, Stewart IC, Whyte KF, Shapiro CM, Douglas NJ. Effect of sleep deprivation on overnight bronchoconstriction in nocturnal asthma. Thorax 1986; 41: 676–680.

Clark TJH. The Philip Elleman lecture. The circadian rhythm of asthma. Br J Dis Chest 1985; 79: 115–124.

Douglas NJ. Asthma. In: Kryger MH, Roth T, Dement WC, eds. Principles and practice of sleep medicine. Philadelphia: WB Saunders, 1989; 591–600.

Montplaisir J, Walsh J, Malo JL. Nocturnal asthma: features of attacks, sleep and breathing patterns. Am Rev Respir Dis 1982; 125: 18–22

Sleep-Related Gastroesophageal Reflux (530.81)

Synonyms and Key Words: Reflux esophagitis, esophagitis, heartburn, gastroesophageal reflux disease (GERD).

Essential Features:

Sleep-related gastroesophageal reflux is characterized by regurgitation of stomach contents into the esophagus during sleep.

This is a disorder in which the patient can awaken from sleep with a sour taste in the mouth or a burning discomfort or pain in the chest (heartburn). The pain is usually substernal, with a feeling of general chest pain or tightness similar to that due to angina. The pain appears to be caused by gastric fluid or contents that have been regurgitated from the stomach into the esophagus and pharynx. Awakenings from sleep associated with the discomfort can lead to a complaint of insomnia. The gastroesophageal reflux often is asymptomatic during sleep.

Associated Features Associated features of this disorder can include symptoms of dysphagia, odynophagia, laryngopharyngitis, laryngospasm, and epigastric burning similar to that associated with a duodenal ulcer.

Course: GERD is a chronic, unrelenting disease that is rarely cured. If untreated, the course of the disease may progress over a period of years to worsening heartburn that will occur postprandially, between meals, and during sleep. Over a number of years, this symptom may become associated with changes such as esophageal erosions and ulcers that can progress to a stricture of the esophagus. The most serious manifestation of GERD is the development of Barrett's esophagus, which is the formation of gastric columnar epithelium that replaces the normal squamous epithelium of the esophagus. Barrett's esophagus may be a premalignant condition.

Predisposing Factors: Lower-esophageal-sphincter pressures below 10 mmHg predispose the patient to the development of GERD. Obesity or pregnancy may also be predisposing conditions, though these conditions are of less etiologic importance than are low sphincter pressure, gastric emptying, and peristaltic efficiency of the esophagus.

Prevalence: Unknown. It is estimated, however, that approximately 7% to 10% of the general population has daily heartburn. Heartburn on a weekly basis is thought to occur in as much as one third of the normal population.

Age of Onset: The incidence of this disorder increases with age. The disorder is substantially more common in individuals over 40 years old.

Sex Ratio: When mild, the disease occurs equally in males and females. In Barrett's esophagus, there appears to be a male predominance.

Familial Pattern: None.

Pathology: Pathology can be described in three categories: histologic, endoscopic, and manometric. The classic histologic changes associated with chronic GERD relate to basal-zone hyperplasia and papillary elongation. Other less specific changes are the presence of neutrophilic or eosinophilic infiltration. Endoscopic changes range from mild erythema, erosions, and ulcerations to severe erosions with stricture. The most severe complication that is identified primarily by histology is Barrett's esophagus, which is the presence of columnar epithelium in the esophagus. The manometric abnormalities associated with chronic GERD include both decreased lower esophageal sphincter pressure (generally below 10 mmHg) and decreased esophageal peristaltic amplitude.

Complications: The complications of GERD include: erosive esophagitis with stricture, resulting in chronic dysphagia and weight loss; Barrett's esophagus; laryngopharyngitis; pulmonary aspiration, with lung abcess; bronchiectasis; and exacerbation of bronchial asthma.

Polysomnographic Features: Polysomnography with continuous pH monitoring demonstrates an episode of reflux during sleep; the reflux is often associated with an awakening.

Other Laboratory Test Features: Endoscopic examination of the esophagus with or without biopsy may be indicated. Histologic examination of altered esophageal mucosa may reveal ulcerative changes or Barrett's esophagus.

Differential Diagnosis: The differential diagnosis includes primarily peptic ulcer disease. The chest pain can be similar to that associated with angina. Awakenings from sleep with coughing and choking may lead to consideration of sleep-related breathing disorders, abnormal swallowing syndrome, sleep choking syndrome, sleep-related laryngospasm, and paroxysmal nocturnal dyspnea. Polysomnographic evaluation with respiratory and pH monitoring can differentiate these disorders.

Diagnostic Criteria: Sleep-Related Gastroesophageal Reflux (530.81)

A. The patient has a complaint of recurrent awakenings from sleep. The disorder occasionally can be asymptomatic.
B. Episodes of chest discomfort or burning substernal pain occur during sleep.
C. Other features that occur during sleep include one or more of the following:
   1. A sour or bitter taste in the mouth

2. Coughing or choking
   3. Heartburn
D. Polysomnographic monitoring demonstrates either of the following:
   1. Arousals from sleep
   2. Gastroesophageal acid reflux on pH monitoring during sleep
E. No other medical or mental disorder (e.g., angina, monilial esophagitis, etc.) accounts for the symptom.
F. Other sleep disorders (e.g., obstructive sleep apnea syndrome, may be present but do not account for the symptom).

Minimal Criteria: A plus B plus C, or A plus D.

Severity Criteria:

Mild: Symptomatic episodes occur no more than once per week or asymptomatic episodes are detected by pH monitoring; usually not associated with, or mild evidence of, esophageal irritation.
Moderate: Episodes occur almost nightly, and are typically associated with evidence of esophageal irritation.
Severe: Episodes occur every night and more than once per night and are often associated with evidence of moderate or severe esophageal irritation.

Duration Criteria:

Acute: 7 days or less.
Subacute: More than 7 days but less than 1 month.
Chronic: 1 month or longer.

Bibliography:

Castell DO, Johnson LF, eds. Esophageal function in health and disease. New York: Elsevier Biomedical, 1983.
Castell DO, Wu W, Ott D, eds. Gastroesophageal reflux disease: Pathogenesis, diagnosis, therapy. Mt. Kisco, New York: Futura Publishing, 1985.
Orr WC. Gastrointesinal disorders. In: Kryger MH, Roth T, Dement WC, eds. Principles and practice of sleep medicine. Philadelphia: WB Saunders, 1989; 622–629.
Orr WC, Johnson LF, Robinson MG. Effect of sleep on swallowing, esophageal peristalsis, and acid clearance. Gastroenterology 1984; 86: 814–819.
Orr WC, Robinson MG. The sleeping gut. Med Clin North Am 1981; 65: 1359–1376.
Orr WC, Robinson MG, Johnson LF. Acid clearance during sleep in the pathogenesis of reflux esophagitis. Dig Dis Sci 1981; 26: 423–427.

Peptic Ulcer Disease (531-534)

Synonyms and Key Words: Gastric ulcer (531), duodenal ulcer (532), gastrojejunal ulcer (534), peptic ulcer disease, epigastric night pain, nocturnal pH monitoring. (Includes, if associated with ulceration, dyspepsia [536.8], hyperacidity [536.8], hyperchlorhydria [536.8].)

Essential Features:

Peptic ulcer disease is characterized by gastric or duodenal ulceration by acid and pepsin that can produce awakenings from sleep with pain or discomfort in the abdomen.

The main sleep-related feature of this disorder is a spontaneous epigastric pain (primarily duodenal) that occurs at night. The pain is usually a dull, steady ache rather than colicky and it appears most often within one to four hours after sleep onset. Tenderness or muscular rigidity occurs in the epigastrium. The pain usually is intermittent; with acute or subacute perforation, however, the pain is intense and constant. The pain can produce arousals and awakenings from sleep, leading to a complaint of insomnia.

Associated Features: Associated features of this disorder may include symptoms of acid indigestion. Epigastric burning sensation, heartburn, or an unpleasant taste in the mouth can occur and are similar to the symptoms associated with sleep-related gastroesophageal reflux. The pain sometimes radiates to the chest, substernum, or back. The characteristic hungerlike pain often changes to a sensation of fullness, nausea, or cramping pain if pyloric obstruction occurs. Pain relief commonly follows food ingestion or the onset of gastrointestinal bleeding.

Course: Peptic ulcer disease is a chronic, self-limiting disease that is easily cured but frequently relapsing. The most serious complication of peptic ulcer disease is perforation with bleeding, which may lead to death.

Predisposing Factors: Hereditary factors are involved in the etiology of peptic ulceration. Relatives of patients with peptic ulcers also tend to develop peptic ulcers. Cigarette smoking is known to be associated with a greater risk of developing duodenal ulceration. Drug ingestion can be a causative factor; corticosteroids, aspirin, indomethacin, phenylbutazone, nonsteroidal anti-inflammatory drugs, and analgesics have all been implicated. Although an increased incidence of peptic ulcer disease has been noted in shift workers, other studies have failed to document a similar increase in other groups with presumed high-stress work environments such as air traffic controllers. There is an increased incidence of peptic ulceration in patients with "stressful" occupations, mental patients, alcoholics, and patients with liver cirrhosis. In addition, gastric ulceration is more prevalent in excessive burns (Curling's ulcer), shock, major medical illness, acute brain damage (Cushing's ulcers), following an operation, and in the terminal stages of any fatal illness.

Prevalence: The incidence of peptic ulceration varies between countries and is high in the Japanese population (approximately 1% incidence). The incidence of duodenal ulceration is decreasing in the United States. Duodenal ulcers are three times more common than gastric ulcers in the western countries.

Age of Onset: The occurrence of duodenal ulceration peaks at 20 years of age, and as age advances, the incidence declines, possibly related to the age-dependent decrease of gastric acid secretion. The occurrence of gastric ulcer, however, peaks between 50 and 60 years of age.

Sex Ratio: There is a male preponderance of about 2.5:1.

Familial Pattern: Peptic ulceration occurs two to three times as frequently in first-degree relatives of individuals with peptic ulcer disease as in relatives of controls or in the general population.

Pathology: In acute peptic ulceration, penetration occurs into the full mucosal depth or muscularis mucosae. Circular and small lesions, usually less than 1 cm in diameter, are found. In chronic peptic ulcers, the histologic appearance varies with the activity, chronicity, and degree of healing. Characteristically, there is a superficial thin layer of necrotic fibrinoid debris, an acute, nonspecific, cellular-infiltrating zone with neutrophils, and an active granulation tissue layer infiltrated with mononuclear leukocytes in the base.

Complications: The three most common complications of peptic ulcer disease are (1) hemorrhage, (2) perforation, and (3) impairment of gastric emptying due to deformity and scarring of the stomach and duodenum. When bleeding from a peptic ulcer is pronounced, anemia, hematemesis, melena, or hematochezia appears. Perforation is the abrupt extension of the ulcer through all layers of the intestinal wall, permitting the free escape of intraluminal contents into the peritoneal cavity. Death from peritonitis and septicemia usually will occur unless the perforation is closed surgically or is induced to seal off by intensive medical therapy. Peptic ulcer disease is a common cause of pyloric obstruction and gastric stasis.

Polysomnographic Features: Polysomnography demonstrates an awakening followed by abdominal pain. Intragastric pH measurements show that the intragastric pH level, which is higher in gastric ulcer disease than in duodenal ulcer disease, is lower during awakenings and wakefulness than in slow-wave sleep. Several studies have demonstrated a pronounced circadian rhythm in basal acid secretion, with peaks generally occurring between 9 p.m. and midnight in most individuals.

Other Laboratory Test Features: A diagnosis of peptic ulcer disease is usually made by the demonstration of an ulcer crater on radiographic studies. Endoscopy with simultaneous biopsy is essential to rule out malignancy and to establish a definitive diagnosis. Recently, endoscopic ultrasonography has been performed to estimate the depth of gastric ulceration and to confirm healing.

Differential Diagnosis: The differential diagnosis includes disorders that produce nocturnal abdominal pain. Other diseases such as gastric cancer, cholelithiasis, pancreatitis, parasitic diseases, reflux esophagitis, and irritable bowel syndrome should be considered. Because the pain of the peptic ulceration occurs late after meals, a diagnosis of hypoglycemia or hyperinsulinemia must be excluded. Diabetic radiculopathy and syphylitic neuralgia are rare causes. Nocturnal angina must also be included in the differential diagnosis of epigastric pain.

Diagnostic Criteria: Peptic Ulcer Disease (531-534)

A. The patient has a complaint of recurrent awakenings from sleep.
B. Episodes of epigastric night pain occur within one to four hours after sleep onset.
C. Other features that occur during sleep include one or more of the following:
   1. Radiating pain in the chest, substernum, or back
   2. Heartburn or burning sensation, with gastroesophageal reflux
   3. Fullness, nausea, or cramping pain, with the occurrence of pyloric obstruction
D. Peptic ulcer disease is associated with "stressful" occupations, shift workers, mental patients with insomnia, or hereditary preponderance.
E. The patient has a diagnosis of peptic ulcer disease.
F. Polysomnographic monitoring demonstrates both of the following:
   1. Arousals from sleep
   2. High acidity of gastric and duodenal fluids (as detected by gastric-acidity or pH monitoring) in the acute or subacute stage of peptic ulcer disease during sleep
G. No other medical or mental disorder (e.g., nocturnal angina, cholelithiasis, pancreatitis, accounts for the symptom).
H. No other sleep disorder (e.g., sleep-related gastroesophageal disease, causes the abdominal pain during sleep).

Minimal Criteria: A plus B plus E.

Severity Criteria:

Mild: Symptomatic episodes occur no more than once per week.
Moderate: Symptomatic episodes occur almost nightly, typically associated with evidence of highly acidic intragastric pH.
Severe: Symptomatic episodes occur every night and more than once per night.

Duration Criteria:

Acute: 2 months or less.
Subacute: More than 2 months but less than 1 year.
Chronic: 1 year or longer.

Bibliography:

Orr WC. Gastrointestinal disorders. In: Kryger MH, Roth T, Dement WC, eds. Principles and practice of sleep medicine. Philadelphia: WB Saunders, 1989; 622–629.

Segawa K, Mabuchi C, Shiozawa Z, Nakazawa S. The nocturnal intragastric pH in EEG sleep stages in peptic ulcer patients. Gastroenterol (Jpn) 1977; 12: 1–6.

Segawa K, Nakazawa S, Tsukamoto Y, et al. Peptic ulcer is prevalent among shift workers. Dig Dis Sci 1987; 32: 449–453.

Stacher G, Presslich B, Starker H. Gastric acid secretion and sleep stages during natural night sleep. Gastroenterology 1975; 68: 1449–1455.

Fibromyalgia (729.1)

Synonyms and Key Words: Rheumatic pain modulation disorder, fibrositis syndrome.

Essential Features:

Fibrmyalgia is characterized by diffuse musculoskeletal pain, chronic fatigue, unrefreshing sleep, and increased tenderness in specific localized anatomic regions, without laboratory evidence of contributing articular, nonarticular, or metabolic disease.

Patients with the fibromyalgia typically complain of light sleep that is characterized by physical discomfort, and these patients awaken feeling tired and lethargic with discomfort and stiffness in the joints. The daytime tiredness and fatigue, at times characterized by more specific complaints of excessive sleepiness, persist throughout the day.

The muscles or groups of muscles, especially those of the neck and shoulder muscles, are painful and tender. Particularly sensitive muscles and regions include the mid-upper border of the trapezius, the erector spinae muscle in the neck, the lateral sternal border over the pectoralis major, just below the occipital crest, the lumbar erector spinae muscles, the lumbar triangle, the anterior superior spine, the mid-gluteus maximus, the mid-lateral thigh, and the medial knee superior to the adductor tubercle. Minor trauma or changes in the weather, particularly cold or dampness, appear to exacerbate the muscle discomfort. The local application of heat and massage and the use of anti-inflammatory agents often bring about some relief.

The onset of the muscle discomfort is usually rapid and develops over a period of days. The discomfort generally will become most noticeable during the nocturnal hours.

Associated Features: Some patients with the fibromyalgia have associated periodic limb movements; these patients generally are older and have a later onset of illness.

The chronicity and diffuseness of the symptoms often lead to a delayed diagnosis, resulting in features of an anxiety disorder or depression.

Course: Fibromyalgia generally has a chronic relapsing course that lasts months or years. Treatment generally induces only minor or temporary improvement. The sleep complaints may be improved by specific treatment even though the muscle discomfort can persist.

Predisposing Factors: A history of prior "flulike" febrile illness is reported in approximately 50% of patients with fibromyalgia.

Prevalence: Not known, but apparently not rare.

Age of Onset: Onset usually occurs in early adulthood, although fibromyalgia may occur for the first time in the elderly.

Sex Ratio: Fibromyalgia appears to be more common in females, in the ratio of 8:1.

Familial Pattern: None known.

Pathology: None known.

Complications: Complications are due to the muscle discomfort and sleep disturbance, which often may lead to anxiety and depression.

Polysomnographic Features: Characteristic polysomnographic features have been reported in fibromyalgia. Patients with fibromyalgia characteristically will show alpha (7.5-11 Hz) electroencephalographic activity occurring during non-REM (NREM) sleep. The occurrence of alpha activity during slow-wave sleep is particularly characteristic and is termed alpha-delta activity. Sleep stages otherwise appear to be normal in percentage.

Patients with fibromyalgia may demonstrate associated periodic limb movements on nocturnal polysomnography.

Multiple sleep latency testing has not been reported in this disorder, but objective daytime sleepiness is not believed to be a feature of fibromyalgia.

Other Laboratory Test Features: Laboratory investigations for rheumatic disorders are normal.

Differential Diagnosis: The sleep disturbance needs to be differentiated from that due to other causes of nonrestorative sleep. Obstructive sleep apnea syndrome, central sleep apnea syndrome, insomnia due to mental disorders, and psychophysiologic insomnia need to be considered in the differential diagnosis.

Fibromyalgia needs to be differentiated from other disorders that produce myalgia. Polymyalgia rheumatica is a disorder that mainly affects the elderly and is characterized by myalgia but can be excluded by the presence of more severe muscle stiffness and the elevated sedimentation rate that is seen in polymyalgia. Other rheumatic disorders, such as rheumatoid arthritis or osteoarthritis, can be excluded by the characteristic clinical, serologic, and radiologic features.

Sleep disturbance related to a dysthymic disorder needs to be differentiated from that due to fibromyalgia. Compared to patients with dysthymia, patients with fibromyalgia report more muscle pain upon awakening as well as discomfort during sleep. Alpha activity during NREM sleep is not a feature of dysthymic disorder.

Patients with the chronic fatigue syndrome (postinfectious neuromyasthenia) have similar findings to patients who report the onset of fibromyalgia following a febrile illness. Compared to normal controls, patients with the fibromyalgia do not have elevated Epstein-Barr antibody titer levels.

Diagnostic Criteria: Fibromyalgia (729.1)

A. The patient has a complaint of unrefreshing sleep and myalgia.
B. The myalgia is not associated with other musculoskeletal disorders.

C. Firm, tender zones are found within the muscles, particularly those of the neck and shoulders.
D. Polysomnography demonstrates both of the following:
   1. Alpha activity (7.5-11-Hz) during NREM sleep, particularly stage 3 and stage 4 sleep
   2. A normal mean sleep latency on multiple sleep latency test
E. No other medical disorder, particularly rheumatic disorders, accounts for the symptoms.
F. Other sleep disorders can be present but are not the cause of the myalgia.

Minimal Criteria: A plus B plus C.

Severity Criteria:

Mild: Muscle discomfort that does not occur daily.
Moderate: Muscle discomfort that occurs on a daily basis but is not severe enough to require analgesic therapy.
Severe: Muscle discomfort that requires treatment with analgesic medications.

Duration Criteria:

Acute: 7 days or less.
Subacute: More than 7 days but less than 3 months.
Chronic: 3 months or longer.

Bibliography:

Moldofsky H, Saskin P, Lue FA. Sleep and symptoms in fibrositis syndrome after a febrile illness. J Rheumatol 1988; 15: 1701–1704.

Moldofsky H, Tullis C, Lue FA. Sleep related myoclonus in rheumatic pain modulation disorder (fibrositis syndrome). J Rheumatol 1986; 13: 614–617.

Moldofsky H, Tullis C, Lue FA, Quance G, Davidson J. Sleep-related myoclonus in rheumatic pain modulation disorder (fibrositis syndrome) and in excessive daytime somnolence. Psychosomatic Med 1984; 46: 145–151.

Saskin P, Moldofsky H, Lue FA. Sleep and post-traumatic rheumatic pain modulation disorder (fibrositis syndrome). Psychosomatic Med 1986; 48: 319–323.

PROPOSED SLEEP DISORDERS

1. Short Sleeper (307.49-0).................................... 282
2. Long Sleeper (307.49-2)..................................... 285
3. Subwakefulness Syndrome (307.47-1) 288
4. Fragmentary Myoclonus (780.59-7) 291
5. Sleep Hyperhidrosis (780.8)................................. 293
6. Menstrual-Associated Sleep Disorder (780.54-3) 295
7. Pregnancy-Associated Sleep Disorder (780.59-6) 297
8. Terrifying Hypnagogic Hallucinations (307.47-4)................ 300
9. Sleep-Related Neurogenic Tachypnea (780.53-2) 302
10. Sleep-Related Laryngospasm (780.59-4)....................... 304
11. Sleep Choking Syndrome (307.42-1) 307

Proposed Sleep Disorders

This fourth section of the *International Classification of Sleep Disorders* includes those sleep disorders for which insufficient or inadequate information is available to substantiate the unequivocal existence of the disorder. Some of these disorders, such as sleep-related laryngospasm, are newly described and some disorders, such as short sleeper, may be controversial as to whether they are disorders in their own right or are at the extreme end of the range of normal physiology.

A short sleeper or long sleeper is a person who has either a shorter or longer sleep episode than is considered normal but has sleep that is not pathologic. People with these sleep-duration features can present with a complaint of either inability to sleep or excessive sleepiness, and, therefore, these two disorders are important in differential diagnoses. Their descriptions are necessary to provide appropriate diagnostic information for clinical purposes.

The subwakefulness syndrome, also known as the subvigilance syndrome, has been described for many years. It is unclear, however, whether this is a variant of another disorder of excessive sleepiness, such as idiopathic hypersomnia, or represents a manifestation of a psychologic state. Therefore, subwakefulness syndrome is included in the this section.

Fragmentary myoclonus is a newly described disorder that has been associated with excessive sleepiness. It consists of frequent brief myoclonic jerks occurring at random in many muscle groups. Fragmentary myoclonus could be a variant of the normal phasic muscle activity that typically is seen at sleep onset. Insufficient published information is currently available on this disorder.

Sleep hyperhidrosis, also known as night sweats, can be due to a variety of underlying disorders such as neurologic disorders and the obstructive sleep apnea syndrome. An idiopathic form of this disorder occurs but has rarely been described in the literature.

Sleep disturbance that is characterized by either insomnia or excessive sleepiness is commonly seen in relation to the menstrual cycle, menopause, or pregnancy. Although it is well recognized that these disturbances occur, reports of the sleep characteristics are rare, and the underlying cause of these sleep disturbances is unclear. Whether these disorders are due to a specific and primary effect upon the sleep mechanisms or another disorder (e.g., premenstrual stress syndrome or back pain related to pregnancy) is not known.

Terrifying hypnagogic hallucinations are intensely frightening hallucinatory phenomena that occur at sleep onset. Although they may be associated with other sleep disorders, such as narcolepsy, they can occur in an idiopathic form. Terrifying hypnagogic hallucinations have rarely been described, and their differentiation from unpleasant sleep-onset dreams has not been clearly established.

Sleep-related neurogenic tachypnea has been reported to occur in an idiopathic form, although it is associated more commonly with underlying neurologic disorders. This rarely described disorder is presented here to encourage recognition of the features to prompt further research.

Sleep-related laryngospasm and the sleep choking syndrome are two disorders that occur with a complaint of sleep-related breathing difficulties. Patients with these disorders are likely to present to sleep-disorders clinicians particularly because the symptoms are similar to those of the obstructive sleep apnea syndrome. Although the exact cause of the underlying disorders is unknown, the inclusion of the disorders in this text should allow the clinical features to be recognized more easily and the nature of the disorders to be clarified.

All the proposed sleep disorders are described in the anticipation that additional information will be forthcoming in the medical literature to more clearly establish the nature of these disorders. It is to be expected that if this aim is achieved, the list of proposed sleep disorders will change in future editions of the *International Classification of Sleep Disorders*.

Short Sleeper (307.49-0)

Synonyms and Key Words: Short sleeper, "healthy" hyposomnia, asymptomatic, extreme low end of normal sleep-duration continuum.

Essential Features:

*A **short sleeper** is an individual who habitually sleeps substantially less during a 24-hour period than is expected for a person in his or her age group.*

The short sleeper is neither subjectively nor objectively somnolent in the daytime (the short sleep is restorative) and is unable to sleep longer despite opportunities and attempts to do so. Sleep is unbroken, and the short sleeper has no complaints about the quality of sleep or difficulties with mood, motivation, or performance during wakefulness. The constricted sleep is not on a voluntary basis, and there are no weekend or holiday reversions to conventional or long-sleep patterns.

A reasonable criterion for this diagnosis is a regular daily pattern of total sleep time that is less than 75% of the lowest normal quantity for age. In absolute terms, a regular sleep duration averaging less than 5 hours per 24 hours before the age of 60 years is an unusually short sleep pattern. After the age of 60, there is an apparent increase in prevalence of a short-sleep pattern in the absence of pathology. Some short sleepers sleep for periods of only 45 minutes to 3 hours each day without compromise of waking faculties.

Associated Features: Psychologically, short sleepers have been described as basically normal, with a tendency to hypomanic behavior. They are also described as smooth, efficient persons who are distinct "nonworriers." They may seek assistance because of the concerns of family or referring physicians that the short-sleep behavior represents a psychologic or medical abnormality or because the short sleep creates awkward family and social situations.

Demographic data have suggested a correlation between short sleep and reduced life expectancy. The main source of this relationship is probably the shortening of total sleep time resulting from medical pathologies. The survey studies from which such correlations were derived were not able to explore the probability that one or several root pathologic causes are responsible for both the higher mortality ratios and short sleep. The question of a causal connection between unconventional sleep durations in the absence of sleep or medical pathology and reduced life expectancy is not answerable at the present time.

Course: Apparently lifelong in typical cases. In individuals under age 60 years, the development of a short-sleep pattern may signal the presence of underlying sleep disorder or other medical pathology.

Predisposing Factors: None.

Prevalence: Apparently rare.

Age of Onset: The pattern usually begins in early adolescence or young adulthood and endures throughout life, without the development of known impairment or complications.

Sex Ratio: Predominantly male.

Familial Pattern: A tendency to run in families has been described, but clear genetic data are not available.

Pathology: Short sleepers presumably represent the extreme end of the normal sleep-duration continuum.

Complications: There is a potential for complications from misguided attempts to increase the patient's sleep time by pharmacologic intervention with hypnotics.

Polysomnographic Features: The polysomnogram shows a short sleep latency and very few arousals after sleep onset. Absolute amounts of sleep stages 3 and

4 are normal for age, whereas stage 2 and REM sleep are lower in amount than in conventionally sleeping individuals. Increased absolute amounts of either stage 3 and stage 4 or REM sleep suggest recovery sleep in a sleep-deprived individual rather than true short sleep. No intrasleep pathology (e.g., sleep apnea or periodic limb movements) is present. If given the opportunity to continue sleep, the patient is consistently unable to do so. The patient is not aware of any time distortion and is accurate about both the qualitative and quantitative aspects of the recorded sleep. Multiple sleep latency testing (MSLT) shows no evidence of pathologic sleepiness.

Other Laboratory Test Features: None helpful.

Differential Diagnosis: It is important to differentiate the short sleeper from patients with underlying medical or mental causes of shortened sleep. In most of the latter, the patient complains of difficulty in falling asleep, frequent awakenings, or both, and these historic features are accompanied by complaints concerning daytime functioning, exhaustion, fatigue, and altered mood. Patients with bipolar affective disorder who are in the hypomanic or manic phase of their illness often sleep only a few hours per night and feel quite well in the daytime. The histories of such patients, however, typically include periods of major depression during which complaints of insomnia or hypersomnia have been present.

A sleep-wake log in short sleepers should show consistently short sleep at approximately the same clock times on a daily basis and no substantial differences between sleep amounts on work nights compared to weekends, holidays, and vacations.

Diagnostic Criteria: Short Sleeper (307.49-0)

A. The patient can have a complaint of insomnia.
B. The patient has a daily total sleep time of less than 75% of the age-related norm.
C. The sleep pattern must have been present for at least six months.
D. The patient does not have excessive sleepiness.
E. Polysomnographic monitoring demonstrates both of the following:
   1. A short total sleep time with a spontaneous final awakening
   2. The mean sleep latency is within normal limits on the multiple sleep latency test
F. No other significant underlying medical or mental disorder accounts for the findings.
G. The findings do not meet the diagnostic criteria for any other disorder causing insomnia.

Minimal Criteria: A plus B plus C plus D.

Severity Criteria:

Mild: Mild short sleep or insomnia, as defined on page 23. An adult has a total sleep time of less than six hours but more than four hours.

Moderate: Moderate short sleep or insomnia, as defined on page 23. An adult has a total sleep time of less than four hours but more than three hours.
Severe: Extreme short sleep or insomnia, as defined on page 23. An adult has a total sleep time of less than three hours.

Duration Criteria:

Acute: Not applicable.
Subacute: Not applicable.
Chronic: 6 months or longer.

Bibliography:

Hartmann E, Baekeland F, Zwilling GR. Psychological differences between long and short sleepers. Arch Gen Psychiatry 1972; 26: 463–468.

Jones H, Oswald I. Two cases of healthy insomnia. Electroencephalogr Clin Neurophysiol 1968; 24: 378–380.

Kripke DF, Simons RN, Garfinkel L, Hammond EC. Short and long sleep and sleeping pills: Is increased mortality associated? Arch Gen Psychiatry 1979; 36: 103–116.

Webb WB. Are short and long sleepers different? Psychol Rep 1979; 44: 259–264.

Long Sleeper (307.49-2)

Synonyms and Key Words: Long sleeper, "healthy" hypersomnia, extreme high end of normal sleep-duration continuum.

Essential Features:

*A **long sleeper** is an individual who consistently sleeps substantially more in 24 hours than does the typical person of his or her age group. Sleep, although long, is basically normal in architecture and physiology.*

Individuals who are long sleepers have normal sleep efficiency and timing of sleep. In uncomplicated cases, there are no complaints about quality of sleep, daytime sleepiness, or difficulties with awake mood, motivation, or performance, as long as sufficient sleep is obtained routinely to fulfill the apparent increased sleep "need."

A chronic, regular daily pattern of total sleep time of more than 10 hours per 24 hours in young adults is a reasonable criterion for this diagnosis. Many long sleepers, because of occupation or education demands, function with reasonable success on 9 hours of sleep per night during the work or school week, with increases to 12 to 15 hours per 24 hours on weekends and holidays. Obtaining less than this amount of sleep leads to daytime symptoms of insufficient sleep (e.g., sleepiness, reduction in alert cognitive efficiency).

Associated Features: Although they generally function within the normal range of psychologic functioning, long sleepers who have been studied psychologically (mostly males) appear to have characteristic personality features. They are higher on most scales of the Minnesota Multiphasic Personality Inventory (particularly and significantly the social introversion scale) than are short sleepers. On interview, long sleepers appear either depressed or anxious, but mildly so, and are described as worriers.

Long sleepers seek clinical evaluation and assistance because of awkwardness in family and social relationships related to the increased amount of sleep they obtain and because they or their referring physicians believe that they are psychologically or medically ill. The history, however, reveals that the pattern is quite long standing and stable, with no suggestion of either major medical or mental disease. Usually, the long-sleep pattern began in childhood, is well established by early adolescence, and endures throughout life without evidence of early conditioning, later impairments, or complications. Some long sleepers present with complaints of excessive sleepiness. In these patients, the history typically reveals a lifelong pattern of long sleep, and the daytime sleepiness is associated with more recent curtailment of sleep due to attempts to meet social or occupation obligations.

Demographic data from several population studies appear to link long and short sleep to reduced life expectancy. With long sleep, this relationship may have its source mainly in acquired increases in total sleep times associated with medical and sleep pathologies, not in long sleep as represented by the long sleeper. The surveys from which the above correlations were drawn were not able to explore the likelihood that root pathologic causes are responsible for both the higher mortality rates and protracted sleep.

Course: Apparently lifelong in typical cases. In the absence of a childhood history of long sleep, the development of a long-sleep pattern may signal underlying sleep or other medical or mental pathology.

Predisposing Factors: None.

Prevalence: Apparently rare.

Age of Onset: Childhood.

Sex Ratio: Predominantly female.

Familial Pattern: A tendency to occur in families has been described, but clear genetic data are lacking.

Pathology: Long sleepers presumably represent the extreme high end of the normal sleep-duration continuum.

Complications: A potential exists for the development of complications from misguided attempts on the part of the patient or well-meaning physicians to decrease the patient's total sleep time by pharmacologic intervention with stimulants.

Polysomnographic Features: Like short sleepers, long sleepers have normal absolute amounts of sleep stages 3 and 4, but amounts of stage 2 and REM sleep are somewhat higher than normal. The patient has no problem with time distortion or ability to be accurate about the quantity or quality of sleep. No intrasleep pathology (e.g., sleep apnea or periodic limb movements) is present. If given the opportunity, the patient is consistently able to sleep 10 or more hours per day. If the multiple sleep latency test (MSLT) is performed, no evidence of pathologic sleepiness is present, assuming that the patient has obtained the usual sleep amounts for several nights before the procedure.

Other Laboratory Test Features: Brain imaging may be indicated to rule out the presence of intracerebral pathology.

Differential Diagnosis: It is important to differentiate the long sleeper from patients with underlying medical or mental causes of long sleep. In most of the latter, the history indicates that the condition is an acquired one (i.e., there is a history of previously conventional and normal sleep durations during childhood). Many pathologic causes of increased sleep have an acute or subacute onset and rarely show the stable duration of the long sleeper. In addition, most of these causes show a demonstrable polysomnographic abnormality. Nevertheless, differentiation from pathologic conditions of hypersomnia may be difficult in the adolescent or child because the normal continuum of sleep duration is somewhat higher in these age groups than in adults. The correct diagnosis is often made chiefly by exclusion of specific diagnostic features associated with other conditions (e.g., cataplexy in early cases of narcolepsy or loud snoring in obstructive sleep apnea syndrome) and by requirement of few or no complaints concerning the quality of the individual's awake-state functioning.

Essential to the diagnosis of long sleeper is the consistency of the pattern, documented by a carefully kept sleep log, which should try to show a daily pattern of 10 to 12 hours sleep over a 2- to 4-week span. In general, the long sleeper's decision to consult a sleep clinician has little to do with symptoms of nonrestorative or disturbed sleep or with complaints about napping or daytime sleepiness. Rather, the complaint usually focuses on the curtailment of the awake period by the apparent increased need for sleep. Nevertheless, it is plausible that complaints of excessive sleepiness may occur in a naturally long sleeper who curtails sleep for social or occupation reasons. In such cases, a dual diagnosis of insufficient sleep syndrome and long sleeper may be the most appropriate classification.

It is rare that a natural long sleeper temporarily or persistently develops insomnia. Under such circumstances, a difficult situation may confront the clinician who is asked to evaluate a complaint of insomnia, with or without daytime symptoms, in an individual who is sleeping seven to eight hours nightly. A preceding life history of long sleep in a patient with an intercurrent medical or mental illness and polysomnographic evidence of sleep fragmentation, despite aggregate sleep amounts of seven to eight hours, may validly lead to a diagnosis of long sleeper. Such patients should not be confused with those without sleep disorders who, by definition, should not have prior histories of long sleep. In addition, the long sleeper with an intercurrent insomnia accurately reports the quality and quantity of sleep compared with polysomnographically defined sleep.

Diagnostic Criteria: Long Sleeper (307.49-2)

A. The patient has habitually prolonged sleep periods or excessive sleepiness.
B. The daily total sleep time is 10 hours or greater.
C. The sleep pattern typically has been present since childhood.
D. Polysomnographic monitoring demonstrates both of the following:
   1. A total sleep time of 10 hours or greater
   2. The mean sleep latency is within normal limits on the MSLT
E. No significant underlying medical or major mental disorder accounts for the symptoms.
F. The symptoms do not meet the diagnostic criteria for any other sleep disorder producing a prolonged sleep period or excessive sleepiness.

Minimal Criteria: A plus B plus C plus E plus F.

Severity Criteria:

Mild: The patient has an almost daily complaint of requiring too much sleep to feel rested on awakening, often associated with mild feelings of fatigue or tiredness. The need for sleep does not produce any impairment of social or occupation functioning.
Moderate: The patient has a daily complaint of requiring too much sleep to feel rested on awakening, associated with mild to moderate feelings of fatigue or tiredness. The need for sleep produces a mild impairment of social or occupation functioning.
Severe: The patient has a daily complaint of requiring too much sleep to feel rested on awakening, associated with moderate to severe feelings of fatigue or tiredness. The need for sleep produces a moderate to severe impairment of social or occupation functioning.

Duration Criteria:

Acute: Not applicable.
Subacute: Not applicable.
Chronic: 6 months or longer.

Bibliography:

Hartmann E, Baekeland F, Zwilling GR. Psychological differences between long and short sleepers. Arch Gen Psychiatry 1972; 26: 463–468.
Kripke DF, Simons RN, Garfinkel L, Hammond EC. Short and long sleep and sleeping pills: Is increased mortality associated? Arch Gen Psychiatry 1979; 36: 103–116.
Webb WB. Are short and long sleepers different? Psychol Rep 1979; 44: 259–264.

Subwakefulness Syndrome (307.47-1)

Synonyms and Key Words: Subvigilance syndrome.

Essential Features:

Subwakefulness syndrome *consists of a complaint of an inability to sustain* *daytime alertness without polysomnographic evidence of nocturnal sleep disruption or severe excessive sleepiness.*

Although the patient has a sensation of sleepiness, frequent naps or irresistible sleepiness do not occur. Polysomnography demonstrates a normal quality and duration of the major sleep episode. There is no objective evidence of severe excessive sleepiness; however, there may be evidence of drowsiness or the lightest stages of sleep.

Associated Features: The daytime drowsiness can have secondary effects upon concentration, attentive abilities, memory, fatigability, and other cognitive functions.

Course: The course is usually chronic, with unrelenting subjective sleepiness.

Predisposing Factors: Unknown.

Prevalence: Rare, fewer than 50 cases are documented in the literature.

Sex Ratio: No difference.

Familial Pattern: None known.

Pathology: None known. An abnormality of the mechanisms sustaining full alertness is postulated.

Complications: There may be associated impaired psychosocial functioning, depending upon the intensity and persistence of the daytime drowsiness.

Polysomnographic Features: Continuous daytime polysomnographic recordings show recurrent or persistent signs of drowsiness, with either a slow and diffuse alpha rhythm or stage 1 drowsiness and occasional stage 2 patterns. These patterns tend to "wax and wane," with episodes of "microsleeps" alternating with normal wakefulness. REM sleep does not occur in the daytime recording.

Nocturnal polysomnographic recordings are normal. Multiple sleep latency testing demonstrates mainly stage 1 and occasionally stage 2 sleep on some or all naps, but the mean sleep latency is always greater than five minutes.

Other Laboratory Test Features: Tests to exclude the presence of chronic medical illness may be necessary.

Differential Diagnosis: The subwakefulness syndrome must be distinguished from other causes of excessive sleepiness, such as idiopathic hypersomnia, narcolepsy, recurrent hypersomnia, and menstrual-associated sleep disorder. The disorder must also be differentiated from insufficient sleep syndrome and circadian-rhythm sleep disorders. The daytime fatigue and sleepiness must be differentiated from those due to other causes of nocturnal sleep disruption such as psychophysiologic insomnia, insomnia associated with depression, obstructive sleep apnea syndrome, or periodic limb movement disorder.

Diagnostic Criteria: Subwakefulness Syndrome (307.47-1)

A. The patient has a complaint of drowsiness or excessive sleepiness.
B. The complaint is present for at least six months.
C. The sleepiness is mild and is not frequent or irresistible.
D. The sleepiness does not occur within 18 months of head trauma.
E. Polysomnographic monitoring demonstrates both of the following:
   1. A normal major sleep episode
   2. A mean sleep latency of greater than five minutes on the multiple sleep latency test
F. Continuous 24-hour polysomnography demonstrates intermittent drowsiness, with stage 1 sleep occurring in a "waxing and waning" pattern across the daytime.
G. No other medical or mental disorder (e.g., hypothyroidism, diabetes, depression, accounts for the symptom).
F. The symptoms do not meet the diagnostic criteria of any other sleep disorder (e.g., idiopathic hypersomnia, narcolepsy, post-traumatic hypersomnia, causing excessive sleepiness).

Minimal Criteria: A plus B plus C plus D.

Severity Criteria:

Mild: Mild excessive sleepiness, as described on page 23.
Moderate: Moderate excessive sleepiness, as described on page 23.
Severe: Severe excessive sleepiness, as described on page 23.

Duration Criteria:

Acute: 1 year or less.
Subacute: More than 1 year but less than 2 years.
Chronic: 2 years or longer.

Bibliography:

Jouvet M, Pujol JF. Role des monoamines dans la regulation de la vigilance. Etude neurophysiologique et biochimique. Rev Neurol 1972; 127: 115–138.
Mouret JR, Renaud B, Quenin P, Michel D, Schott B. Monoamines et regulation de la vigilance. I. Apport et interpretation biochimique des donnees polygraphiques. Rev Neurol 1972; 127: 139–155.
Roth B. L'activite de sommeil dans l'EEG comme indicateur d'une insuffisance chronique de l'etat vigil. Electroencephalogr Clin Neurophysiol 1957; 7: 309–311 (Suppl).
Roth B. Narcolepsy and hypersomnia. Basel: Karger, 1980.

Fragmentary Myoclonus (780.59-7)

Synonyms and Key Words: Fragmentary non-REM (NREM) myoclonus, twitching, partial myoclonus, sleep myoclonus.

Essential Features:

Fragmentary myoclonus is characterized by jerks that consist of brief involuntary "twitchlike" local contractions that involve various areas of both sides of the body in an asynchronous and asymmetrical manner during sleep.

Muscles of the arms, legs, and face may all be involved. The twitches persist irregularly for about 10 minutes or up to an hour or more; they do not occur in brief clusters. The muscle activity occurs predominantly in NREM sleep and may be associated with the symptom of excessive sleepiness.

Associated Features: Awareness of the twitchlike movements is usually not present. The affected person rarely may notice the jerks, especially when the jerks are particularly intense at sleep onset. Patients with prolonged episodes of twitching may have coexistent excessive sleepiness along with secondary effects of sleepiness upon concentration, memory, fatigability, and other cognitive functions.

Course: Usually benign. There is no evidence for progressive intensification of the condition.

Predisposing Factors: It appears that any cause of chronic sleep fragmentation may be associated with marked fragmentary myoclonus. This disorder has been described with obstructive and central sleep apnea syndromes, central alveolar hypoventilation syndrome, narcolepsy, periodic limb movement disorder, and different causes of insomnia. In apneic patients, the twitching intensifies during periods of increased hypoxemia.

Prevalence: Unlike the normal myoclonus that occurs at sleep onset and in REM sleep and is a universal physiologic phenomenon, persistent fragmentary myoclonus appears to be quite rare. Fragmentary myoclonus occurs in 5% to 10% of patients suffering from excessive sleepiness.

Age of Onset: Adulthood.

Sex Ratio: Strong male predominance has been described.

Familial Pattern: None known.

Pathology: None known.

Complications: The disorder may be the sole abnormality in some cases of excessive sleepiness. No other serious consequences are known.

Polysomnographic Features: The jerks are associated with brief (usually 75- to 150-millisecond), asymmetrical, asynchronous electromyographic (EMG) potentials in various muscles of the face, arms, and legs. The amplitude varies from about 50 to several hundred microvolts; the larger amplitudes are usually associated with visible movement. Episodes of myoclonic potentials last from 10 minutes to several hours. They often appear at sleep onset, continue through NREM sleep stages, including slow-wave sleep, and persist during REM sleep, in which they appear superimposed upon the normal phasic clusters of physiologic REM myoclonus. They are electromyographically similar to those that occur during REM sleep. The EMG activity occasionally also persists during electroencephalographic periods of wakefulness within the sleep period or is present in drowsiness before sleep onset. The electroencephalogram usually shows no changes at the time of the jerks, although high-amplitude EMG potentials may be associated with a K-complex or even with transient electroencephalographic arousal. There are no ocular or autonomic accompaniments.

Other Laboratory Test Features: None.

Differential Diagnosis: Periodic limb movements can be differentiated from fragmentary myoclonus by the longer duration (2.5-10 seconds) and stereotyped pattern of occurrence of periodic limb movements. Periodic limb movements in sleep occasionally consist of bursts of multiple brief jerks (polymyoclonus).

Intense sleep-related fragmentary myoclonus must also be differentiated from sleep-onset myoclonus, which is similar, and from transient REM-sleep myoclonus, which is limited to the REM state and typically occurs in 5- to 15-second clusters, usually associated with other transient phenomena such as bursts of rapid eye movements or cardiorespiratory irregularities. Multifocal myoclonus may occur with severe degenerative central nervous system diseases and encephalopathies such as the Unverricht-Lundborg syndrome. In degenerative and encephalopathic cases, the myoclonus is maximal in wakefulness, diminishes during drowsiness, and is rare or disappears entirely during sleep. Brief bilaterally synchronous movements, such as sleep starts, startle responses in sleep, and generalized forms of myoclonic muscle activity during epileptic seizures, are readily distinguishable, as are slower movements such as those of restless legs syndrome, dystonias, and tonic spasms.

Diagnostic Criteria: Fragmentary Myoclonus (780.59-7)

A. The patient has a complaint of excessive sleepiness or twitch-like limb movements during sleep.
B. Involuntary, brief, local contractions in varied muscle groups occur asynchronously and asymmetrically.
C. Polysomnographic monitoring demonstrates recurrent brief (75-150-millisecond) EMG potentials in various muscles; the potentials occur asynchronously in a sustained manner without clustering.
D. No other medical disorder accounts for the muscle activity.
E. The findings may be seen in association with other sleep disorders such as obstructive sleep apnea syndrome.

Minimal Criteria: B plus C.

Severity Criteria:

Mild: Asymptomatic or associated with mild sleepiness, as defined on page 23.
Moderate: Associated with moderate sleepiness, as defined on page 23.
Severe: Associated with severe sleepiness, as defined on page 23.

Duration Criteria:

Acute: 3 months or less.
Subacute: More than 3 months but less than 1 year.
Chronic: 1 year or longer.

Bibliography:

Broughton R, Tolentino MA. Fragmentary pathological myoclonus in NREM sleep. Electroencephalogr Clin Neurophysiol 1984; 57: 303–309.

Broughton R, Tolentino MA, Krelina M. Excessive fragmentary myoclonus in NREM sleep: A report of 38 cases. Electroencephalogr Clin Neurophysiol 1985; 61: 123–133.

Sleep Hyperhidrosis (780.8)

Synonyms and Key Words: Night sweats, excessive sweating.

Essential Features:

Sleep hyperhidrosis is characterized by profuse sweating that occurs during sleep.

The patient may or may not have excessive sweating during waking hours.

Associated Features: The sweating can cause an awakening because of discomfort due to wet sleepwear, and the patient may have to arise to change into another set of sleepwear.

Course: Some patients may have a lifelong tendency to sweat excessively during sleep; in other patients, the disorder appears to be self-limited.

Predisposing Factors: Excessive night sweats can be due to a chronic or febrile illness. Other patients appear to be healthy but can have a subtle and unrecognized autonomic disorder.

Prevalence: Unknown.

Age of Onset: Can occur at any age, but most commonly seen in early adulthood.

Sex Ratio: No difference.

Familial Pattern: None known.

Pathology: None known.

Complications: See associated features.

Polysomnographic Features: Polysomnographic features have not been reported.

Other Laboratory Test Features: Quinizarin powder, which turns purple on contact with sweat, can be used to demonstrate localized areas of excessive sweating.

Differential Diagnosis: Underlying chronic disorders and illnesses that can cause fever need to be excluded. Sleep hyperhidrosis has been reported in association with diabetes insipidus, hyperthyroidism, pheochromocytoma, hypothalamic lesions, epilepsy, cerebral and brain stem strokes, cerebral palsy, chronic paroxysmal hemicrania, spinal cord infarction, head injury, and familial dysautonomia. Sleep hyperhidrosis can occur in pregnancy and can be produced by the use of antipyretic medications.

Excessive sweating can be seen in patients with obstructive sleep apnea syndrome, presumably because of the associated autonomic disturbance.

Diagnostic Criteria: Sleep Hyperhidrosis (780.8)

A. The patient has a complaint of excessive sweating during sleep.
B. Polysomnography with quinizarin powder dusted on affected areas is expected to demonstrate excessive sweating during sleep.
C. The primary complaint can be due to other medical disorders, such as febrile illness or diabetes insipidus.
D. Other sleep disorders (e.g., obstructive sleep apnea syndrome) may be present and can precipitate the disorder.

Note: If the hyperhidrosis is without cause, state the diagnosis as sleep hyperhidrosis–essential type. If a sleep disorder such as obstructive sleep apnea syndrome produces sleep hyperhidrosis, state and code both diagnoses on axis A. If associated with a nonsleep medical diagnosis, state sleep hyperhidrosis on axis A and the medical diagnosis on axis C.

Minimal Criterion: A.

Severity Criteria:

Mild: No bathing or change of clothing is required; the patient may have to turn the pillow or remove blankets.
Moderate: Sleep is disturbed by the need to arise and wash the face or other affected body areas, but no clothing change is necessary.
Severe: A bath or change of clothing is required.

Duration Criteria:

Acute: 1 month or less.
Subacute: More than 1 month but less than 6 months.
Chronic: 6 months or longer.

Bibliography:

Cunliffe WJ, Johnson CE, Burton JL. Generalized hyperhidrosis following epilepsy. Br J Dermatol 1971; 85: 186–188.
Geschickter EH, Andrews PA, Bullard RW. Nocturnal body temperature regulation in man: A rationale for sweating in sleep. J Appl Physiol 1966; 21: 623–630.
Lea MJ, Aber RC. Descriptive epidemiology of night sweats upon admission to a university hospital. South Med J 1985; 78: 1065–1067.
Raff SB, Gershberg H. Night sweats. A dominant symptom in diabetes insipidus. JAMA 1975; 234: 1252–1253.

Menstrual-Associated Sleep Disorder (780.54-3)

Synonyms and Key Words: Menstruation-associated insomnia, premenstrual insomnia, premenstrual hypersomnia, climacteric insomnia, menopausal insomnia (627.2), recurrent hypersomnia.

Essential Features:

Menstrual-associated sleep disorder is a disorder of unknown cause, characterized by a complaint of either insomnia or excessive sleepiness, that is temporally related to the menses or menopause.

The three forms of menstrual-associated sleep disorder include (1) premenstrual insomnia, (2) premenstrual hypersomnia, and (3) menopausal insomnia.

Premenstrual insomnia is characterized by difficulty in falling asleep or remaining asleep in temporal association with the menstrual cycle. This form of insomnia commonly occurs in the week before the onset of the menses. The insomnia occurs on a recurrent basis for at least three consecutive months.

Premenstrual hypersomnia is characterized by sleepiness occurring in association with the menstrual cycle. The patient has no complaints of persistent, excessive sleepiness at other times in the menstrual cycle.

The primary feature of menopausal insomnia is the presence of repeated nocturnal awakenings, associated with "hot flashes" or "night sweats" in a woman with other signs and symptoms of menopausal status. A sleep-onset disturbance is not a prominent feature.

Menstrual-associated sleep disorder is diagnosed only if the patient with premenstrual symptoms does not meet the criteria for a mental diagnosis of premenstrual disorder.

Associated Features: None known.

Course: The course of menstrual-associated sleep disorder is not known. Menopausal insomnia appears to resolve spontaneously over months or several years.

Predisposing Factors: Unknown.

Prevalence: Not known.

Age of Onset: Not known.

Sex Ratio: Only occurs in females.

Familial Pattern: None known.

Pathology: None known.

Complications: Chronic anxiety and depression may result from the prolonged sleep disturbances.

Polysomnographic Features:

Premenstrual Insomnia: Polysomnography during the sleep disturbance may show frequent sleep-stage transitions, prolonged awakenings, decreased sleep efficiency, or abnormal sleep-stage distribution. Polysomnographic evaluation at other times of the menstrual cycle will show normal sleep architecture.

Premenstrual Excessive Sleepiness: Polysomnography demonstrates normal duration and quality of nocturnal sleep. The multiple sleep latency test can demonstrate sleepiness during the symptomatic episode.

Menopausal Insomnia: Polysomnography demonstrates spontaneous awakenings, often associated with subjective complaints of "hot flashes" or "night sweats."

Other Laboratory Test Features: Hormone assays may show changes in levels of hormones consistent with a specific phase of the menstrual cycle or menopause.

Differential Diagnosis: Other disorders that produce difficulty in initiating and maintaining sleep, such as psychophysiologic insomnia or insomnia associated with mental disorders, need to be differentiated. Disorders of excessive sleepiness, such as recurrent hypersomnia, sleep deprivation, or an irregular sleep-wake pattern, should be considered in the differential diagnosis of premenstrual hypersomnia.

Diagnostic Criteria: Menstrual-Associated Sleep Disorder (780.54-3)

A. The patient has a complaint of insomnia or episodes of excessive sleepiness.
B. The complaint of insomnia or excessive sleepiness is temporally related to the menstrual cycle, or the complaint of insomnia is temporally associated with the menopause.
C. The disorder is present for at least three months.
D. Polysomnographic monitoring demonstrates both of the following:
   1. Reduced sleep efficiency and reduced total sleep time, with frequent awakenings during the symptomatic time

2. A sleep latency of less than 10 minutes on the multiple sleep latency test obtained during the time that symptoms of excessive sleepiness are present
E. Other medical or mental disorders, except premenstrual syndrome, can be present.
F. No other sleep disorder accounts for the symptom.

Note: The particular type of sleep disorder (i.e., premenstrual insomnia, premenstrual hypersomnia, or menopausal insomnia) can be stated on axis A (e.g., menstrual-associated sleep disorder–premenstrual insomnia type). If the patient meets the criteria for a mental diagnosis of premenstrual syndrome, state and code premenstrual syndrome on axis A.

Minimal Criteria: A plus B plus C.

Severity Criteria:

Mild: Usually associated with mild insomnia or mild excessive sleepiness, as defined on page 23.
Moderate: Usually associated with moderate insomnia or moderate excessive sleepiness, as defined on page 23.
Severe: Usually associated with severe insomnia or severe excessive sleepiness, as defined on page 23.

Duration Criteria:

Acute: 6 months or less.
Subacute: More than 6 months but less than 12 months.
Chronic: 12 months or longer.

Bibliography:

Billiard M, Guilleminault C, Dement WC. A menstruation-linked periodic hypersomnia. Kleine-Levin syndrome or new clinical entity? Neurology 1975; 25: 436–443.
Billiard M, Passouant P. Hormones sexuelles et sommeil chez la femme. Rev Electroencephalogr Neurophysiol Clin 1974; 4: 89–106.
Ho A. Sex hormones and the sleep of women. In: Chase MH, Stern WC, Walter PL, eds. Sleep and research. Brain information service/brain research institute, Volume 1. Los Angeles: UCLA, 1972; 184.

Pregnancy-Associated Sleep Disorder (780.59-6)

Synonyms and Key Words: Pregnancy-associated excessive sleepiness, pregnancy-associated insomnia.

Essential Features:

***Pregnancy-associated sleep disorder** is characterized by the occurrence of either insomnia or excessive sleepiness that develops in the course of pregnancy.*

The sleep disorder associated with pregnancy usually is biphasic. It typically begins with excessive sleepiness and can progress to severe insomnia. In rare instances, nightmares, sleep terrors, and postpartum psychosis may occur.

Associated Features: Pregnancy-associated sleep disorder is often associated with lack of concentration, irritability, apathy, and moodiness. Hypertension, proteinuria, glycosuria, ketonuria, anemia, and morning sickness can be associated with pregnancy. Some women also develop lower-back pain, which can exacerbate the sleep problems.

Course: The first trimester is commonly associated with sleepiness and complaints of tiredness that can precede realization of pregnancy. Total sleep time increases during the first trimester, and patients will frequently nap. Sleep normalizes in the second trimester, but toward the end of the second trimester, the frequency of awakenings increases. The latency to sleep, the number of awakenings, and sleeplessness increase to above normal amounts in the third trimester. These sleep problems may be accounted for by the patient's inability to find a comfortable sleep position, back pain, urinary frequency, and fetal activity. Sleep disruption persists after delivery, with nocturnal childcare being an important contributing factor, but gradually declines in the late postpartum period.

Predisposing Factors: None known.

Prevalence: Occurs in most pregnant women. Sleep terrors and postpartum psychosis are rare.

Age of Onset: Pregnant women of any age.

Sex Ratio: Occurs only in women.

Familial Pattern: None known.

Pathology: None known. The sleepiness that occurs during the first trimester is presumably related to hormonal and biochemical changes of pregnancy. The insomnia during the final trimester, however, is probably due to discomfort, bladder distention, and fetal movement.

Complications: In the initial phase of this disorder, patients may be cognitively impaired due to sleepiness. It has been suggested that postpartum psychosis may be in some way related to the sleep-stage changes that occur in late pregnancy and immediately after delivery. Though sleep-stage fluctuations disappear within a few weeks following delivery in most cases, in some women, the fluctuations may persist for several months or longer.

Various pathologies associated with complications of pregnancy (e.g., toxemia of pregnancy, can increase the severity of the sleep disorder).

Polysomnographic Features: The first trimester of pregnancy is associated with increased sleep time. Towards the end of the second trimester and continuing into the last trimester, the number of awakenings increases. Sleep latency and awake time after sleep onset also increase. As the pregnancy approaches term, stage 4 sleep declines. In one study, four of seven women had a complete loss of stage 4 sleep during late pregnancy.

The excessive sleepiness may be evident on multiple sleep latency testing, with a mean latency below 10 minutes.

Two dramatic changes in sleep occur following delivery: (1) REM sleep decreases markedly, then normalizes over the next two weeks and (2) stage 4 sleep begins to come back to previous levels.

Other Laboratory Test Features: If pregnancy is suspected in a patient presenting with symptoms of excessive sleepiness, pregnancy testing should be performed.

Differential Diagnosis: In its early phase, pregnancy-associated sleep disorder must be differentiated from other disorders of excessive sleepiness. It is not uncommon that the sleep problems are noticed before the patient realizes she is pregnant. Pregnancy testing can provide confirmation. In the third trimester, this condition must be differentiated from other disorders of initiating and maintaining sleep. Polysomnographic evidence of sleep apnea, periodic limb movements, or other abnormal sleep events may be necessary to substantiate sleep disorders other than those associated with normal pregnancy.

Diagnostic Criteria: Pregnancy-Associated Sleep Disorder (780.59-6)

A. The patient has a complaint of either insomnia or excessive sleepiness.
B. The sleep disturbance begins and is present during pregnancy.
C. Polysomnographic monitoring demonstrates either of the following:
   1. Frequent arousals and reduced sleep efficiency
   2. A prolonged habitual sleep period
D. A multiple sleep latency test demonstrates a mean sleep latency of less than 10 minutes.
E. No other medical or mental disorder accounts for the primary symptom.
F. No other sleep disorder is present that could account for the symptoms.

Minimal Criteria: A plus B.

Severity Criteria:

Mild: Mild insomnia or mild sleepiness, as defined on page 23.
Moderate: Moderate insomnia or moderate sleepiness, as defined on page 23.
Severe: Severe insomnia or severe sleepiness, as defined on page 23.
  Parasomnias such as nightmares or sleep terrors may be present.

Duration Criteria:

Acute: 7 days or less.
Subacute: More than 7 days but less than 1 month.
Chronic: 1 month or longer.

Bibliography:

Errante J. Sleep deprivation or postpartum blues? Top Clin Nurs 1985; 6: 9–18.
Fast A, Shapiro D, Ducommun EJ, Friedmann LW, Bouklas T, Floman Y. Low-back pain in pregnancy. Spine 1987; 12: 368–371.
Karacan I, Heine W, Agnew HW, Williams RL, Webb WB, Ross JJ. Characteristics of sleep patterns during late pregnancy and the postpartum periods. Am J Obstet Gynecol 1968; 101: 579–586.
Karacan I, Williams RL, Hursh CJ, McCaulley M, Heine MW. Some implications of the sleep pattern of pregnancy for postpartum emotional disturbances. Br J Psychiatr 1969; 115: 929–935.
Postpartum periods ;obEditorial;cb. Am J Obstet Gynecol 1968; 101: 579–586.

Terrifying Hypnagogic Hallucinations (307.47-4)

Synonyms and Key Words: Sleep-onset nightmares.

Essential Features:

Terrifying hypnagogic hallucinations are terrifying dream experiences that occur at sleep onset and are similar to, or at times indistinguishable from, those dreams that take place within sleep.

During these episodes, the normal reverie of the drowsy state (hypnagogic sensations), such as vague thoughts, illusions, and mild misperceptions of the environment, becomes hallucinatory in nature, with threatening content. The dreamer awakens in an anxious state and recall of a "bad dream" is detailed.

Associated Features: There may be intense and even major body movements in bed, mumbling, vocalizations, or occasional screaming. Awakening may be associated with great fear, although the autonomic activation is typically much less intense than in sleep terrors. Some subjects recall simultaneous perception of terrifying dreams and of the sleeping environment in what has been called "double consciousness."

Course: The course is usually benign, although in some patients, terrifying hypnagogic hallucinations result in deterioration of daytime psychologic functioning.

Predisposing Factors: Any factor that leads to sleep-onset REM periods with intense phasic activity can predispose the patient to developing these attacks. Such factors include, in particular, acute withdrawal from REM-suppressant medication and the presence of narcolepsy. In narcolepsy, the attacks represent intense, vivid hypnagogic hallucinations.

Prevalence: Terrifying hypnagogic hallucinations are extremely rare in the general population, where their exact prevalence is unknown. They are not uncommon, however, in acute recovery from REM suppression and occur in perhaps 4% to 8% of patients with narcolepsy.

Age of Onset: Any age.

Sex Ratio: No difference.

Familial Pattern: Not known.

Pathology: None known.

Complications: None known. Recurrent terrifying hypnagogic hallucinations often lead to sleep-onset insomnia through fear of the events.

Polysomnographic Features: Recordings during terrifying hypnagogic hallucinations are few in number but have confirmed the occurrence of these hallucinations during sleep-onset REM periods.

Other Laboratory Test Features: None reported.

Differential Diagnosis: Normal hypnagogic reverie does not have the nightmarish quality of these attacks. Typical, vivid, hypnagogic hallucinations, as seen in narcolepsy, consist of intense dreaming at sleep onset. These hallucinations, however, do not cause the patient to awaken in an acute anxious state. Nightmares occur during sleep, typically in the second half of the night, when REM sleep is most prevalent and intense. The phenomenology of nightmares is similar or identical to that of terrifying hypnagogic hallucinations.

Sleep terrors usually occur during slow-wave sleep in the first third of the night and are associated with acute terror, a bloodcurdling scream, and autonomic hyperactivity. Sleep terrors are poorly recalled. Sleep-related complex partial epileptic seizures with vivid hallucinations are exceptionally rare and are usually associated with an epileptic discharge, with clinically similar seizures present in the daytime.

Diagnostic Criteria: Terrifying Hypnagogic Hallucinations (307.47-4)

A. The patient complains of a sudden awakening at sleep onset, with immediate recall of frightening hallucinations.
B. Alertness is present immediately upon awakening, with little confusion or disorientation.
C. Polysomnographic monitoring demonstrates all of the following:
   1. An abrupt awakening from at least 10 minutes of REM sleep
   2. Mild tachycardia and tachypnea during the episode
   3. Absence of epileptic activity in association with the disorder
D. Other medical disorders can be present but do not account for the hallucinations.
E. Other sleep disorders, such as nightmares, sleep terrors, or narcolepsy, can be present but do not account for the findings.

Note: If terrifying hypnagogic hallucinations occur in the absence of an underlying disorder, state and code as terrifying hypnagogic hallucinations–idiopathic type. If narcolepsy is present, both narcolepsy and terrifying hypnagogic hallucinations should be stated and coded on axis A.

Minimal Criteria: A plus B.

Severity Criteria:

Mild: Episodes occur less frequently than once per month.
Moderate: Episodes occur between once per month and once per week.
Severe: Episodes occur more often that once per week.

Duration Criteria:

Acute: 7 days or less.
Subacute: Longer than 7 days but less than 3 months.
Chronic: 3 months or longer.

Bibliography:

Broughton R. Human consciousness and sleeping/waking rhythms: A review and some neuropsychological considerations. J Clin Neuropsychol 1982; 4: 193–218.
Broughton R. Neurology and dreaming. Psychiatr J Univ Ottawa 1982; 7: 101–110.
Gastaut H, Broughton R. A clinical and polygraphic study of episodic phenomena in sleep: The Sakel lecture. Recent Adv Biol Psychiatry 1965; 7: 197–221.
Roth B. Narcolepsy and hypersomnia. Basel: Karger, 1980.

Sleep-Related Neurogenic Tachypnea (780.53-2)

Synonyms and Key Words: Sleep-related tachypnea, polypnea during sleep of neurogenic origin.

Essential Features:

Sleep-related neurogenic tachypnea is characterized by a sustained increase in respiratory rate during sleep. The respiratory rate occurs at sleep onset, is maintained throughout sleep, and reverses immediately upon return to wakefulness.

The tachypnea is not directly associated with hypercapnia or hypoxemia. Most patients with sleep-related neurogenic tachypnea present with a complaint of excessive sleepiness.

Associated Features: The associated features depend upon underlying medical conditions. Brain stem signs, pseudotumor cerebri with optic atrophy, explosive arousals, intense nightmares, and other respiratory signs (including snoring and sleep apnea) have been reported in patients with this disorder. An idiopathic form of the disorder can occur.

Course: Chronic or intermittent, dependent upon the course of the underlying disorder.

Predisposing Factors: Lesions of any type involving the brain stem respiratory centers, particularly the medulla.

Prevalence: Very rare.

Age of Onset: Variable.

Sex Ratio: No difference.

Familial Pattern: None known.

Pathology: No known specific autopsy findings. Clinical diagnoses of known pathology include the lateral medullary syndrome, multiple sclerosis, and pseudotumor cerebri. Some patients do not have evidence of any intracerebral lesion.

Complications: None known.

Polysomnographic Features: Polysomnographic monitoring has demonstrated sustained sleep-related tachypnea of 20% to 180% compared to waking levels. Respiratory rates during sleep can be as high as 44 breaths per minute (bpm), as compared with 19 bpm in wakefulness. Sleep efficiency is typically low, with pronounced sleep fragmentation. Multiple sleep latency testing is expected to demonstrate excessive sleepiness.

Other Laboratory Test Features: None.

Differential Diagnosis: Tachypnea can be due to hypoxemia, hypercapnia, or acidemia; however, other features of obstructive sleep apnea syndrome, central sleep apnea syndrome, or central alveolar hypoventilation syndrome are then present.

Diagnostic Criteria: Sleep-Related Neurogenic Tachypnea (780.53-2)

A. The disorder is either asymptomatic or leads to a complaint of excessive sleepiness.
B. Sustained tachypnea is present during sleep only.
C. Polysomnographic monitoring demonstrates both of the following:
   1. A greater than 20% increase in respiratory rate over waking levels that is sustained throughout sleep stages, occurs immediately with sleep onset, and terminates immediately with return to wakefulness
   2. Absence of hypercapnia or hypoxemia during sleep
D. This disorder is not due to medical disorders other than neurologic disorders (e.g., multiple sclerosis).
E. Other sleep disorders producing tachypnea (e.g., central alveolar hypoventilation syndrome) cannot be present.

Note: If there is no evident neurologic cause, state and code the disorder as sleep-related neurogenic tachypnea–idiopathic type. If other neurologic disorders are present, state the primary related diagnosis on axis A along with sleep-related neurogenic tachypnea.

Minimal Criterion: B.

Severity Criteria:

Mild: A 20% to 50% increase in respiratory rate.
Moderate: A 50% to 100% increase in respiratory rate.
Severe: Over 100% increase in respiratory rate.

Duration Criteria:

Acute: 1 month or less.
Subacute: More than 1 month but less than 6 months.
Chronic: 6 months or longer.

Bibliography:

Broughton R, MacLean G, Willmer J, Peloquin A. Polypnea during sleep of neurogenic origin. Sleep Res 1988; 17: 152.

Willmer JP, Broughton RJ. Neurogenic sleep related polypnea–A new disorder? Sleep Res 1989; 18: 322.

Sleep-Related Laryngospasm (780.59-4)

Synonyms and Key Words: Choking, apnea, functional upper-airway obstruction, spasmodic croup, paradoxical vocal cord motion, Munchhausen's stridor, vocal cord spasm, laryngospasm. Sleep-related laryngospasm is the preferred term because it indicates the association with sleep and the implicated mechanism of obstruction.

Essential Features:

Sleep-related laryngospasm refers to episodes of abrupt awakenings from sleep with an intense sensation of inability to breathe and stridor.

Patients with sleep-related laryngospasm typically will immediately jump out of bed, often clutching their throat. Inspiratory efforts are accompanied by a stidorous sound that is often heard by a bedpartner, who is usually awakened by the episode. Episodes typically last from a few seconds to less than five minutes and resolve spontaneously. Patients frequently will indicate that a drink of water speeds the resolution of symptoms.

Sleep-related laryngospasm episodes are infrequent, usually occurring only two or three times per year.

Associated Features: Intense anxiety or panic is present until the obstruction resolves. Temporary hoarseness of the voice occasionally may result. Cyanosis may occasionally occur during an episode.

Course: Unknown. There appears to be a spontaneous resolution of episodes.

Predisposing Factors: None known.

Prevalence: Appears to be rare.

Age of Onset: Most often seen in middle age.

Sex Ratio: Mainly occurs in males.

Familial Pattern: None known.

Pathology: True or false vocal cord spasm appears to be the cause determined in a few patients. No structural abnormality is seen in the upper airway on endoscopic evaluation. Dynamic inspiratory constriction of the cords has been suggested as a possible pathophysiologic mechanism.

Complications: Hoarseness of the voice can occur but appears to always be transient.

Polysomnographic Features: Polysomnographic monitoring demonstrates no evidence of obstructive apneic episodes or other cardiopulmonary abnormalities during sleep. An episode has been documented to occur out of stage 3 sleep, but the episodes typically do not occur in the sleep laboratory. Two nights of polysomnographic monitoring may be required to rule out obstructive sleep apnea as a cause. Monitoring of pH may be necessary to look for gastroesophageal reflux as a cause of the symptom.

Other Laboratory Test Features: Endoscopic evaluation of the upper airway is necessary to determine vocal cord function and to exclude other upper-airway pathology.

Differential Diagnosis: Obstructive sleep apnea is the disorder that usually needs to be distinguished from sleep-related laryngospasm. Sleep-related gastroesophageal reflux, either by itself or in association with obstructive sleep apnea, also needs to be excluded.

Sleep-related abnormal swallowing syndrome can be differentiated by the frequent episodes of gurgling sounds associated with choking that usually are present during polysomnographic monitoring.

The sleep choking syndrome is characterized by the lack of stridor and the frequent occurrence of the episodes.

Sleep terrors can be distinguished by the absence of a full awakening, lack of focus on upper-airway choking, and the return to sleep readily after the event.

Panic disorders can be differentiated by the diurnal presence of episodes; lack of history of agoraphobia, anxiety, or depression; and the absence of both stridor and observed respiratory difficulty.

Sometimes, stridor can be induced voluntarily by the patient which has led to the diagnosis of Munchhausen's stridor. These episodes have been reported to occur during the night and can be difficult to distinguish from vocal cord spasm of an organic and nonvoluntary cause.

Diagnostic Criteria: Sleep-Related Laryngospasm (780.59-4)

A. The patient has a complaint of abrupt awakening during sleep.
B. The patient has a complaint of infrequent (less than once per week) choking episodes during sleep.
C. Stridor is associated with the choking.
D. Associated features include at least two of the following:
   1. Rapid heart rate
   2. Intense anxiety
   3. Sensation of impending death
   4. Residual, temporary hoarseness
E. Polysomnographic monitoring of an episode has not been reported; however, it is expected to demonstrate an apneic episode followed by an abrupt arousal.
F. Interictal polysomnographic monitoring demonstrates normal ventilation during sleep.
G. The symptoms do not meet the criteria for any other medical or mental disorder (e.g., panic disorder).
H. The symptoms do not meet the diagnostic criteria for any other sleep disorder that can account for the symptom (e.g., obstructive sleep apnea syndrome, sleep choking syndrome, sleep terrors).

Note: If sleep-related laryngospasm is associated with a known cause, such as sleep-related gastroesophageal reflux, state and code both diagnoses on axis A.

Minimal Criteria: A plus C.

Severity Criteria:

Mild: Not applicable.
Moderate: Episodes that occur less than once every three months and are usually associated with a moderate autonomic response.
Severe: Episodes that occur more than once every three months and are usually associated with a severe autonomic response.

Duration Criteria:

Acute: 7 days or less.
Subacute: More than 7 days but less than 3 months.
Chronic: 3 months or longer.

Bibliography:

Appelblatt NH, Baker SR. Functional upper airway obstruction. Arch Otolaryngol 1981; 107: 305–306.
Collett PW, Brancatisano T, Engel LA. Spasmodic croup in the adult. Am Rev Respir Dis 1983; 127: 500–504.
Kryger MH, Acres JC, Brownell L. A syndrome of sleep, stridor and panic. Chest 1981; 80: 768.
Thorpy MJ, Aloe F. Sleep-related laryngospasm. Sleep Res 1989; 18: 313.

Sleep Choking Syndrome (307.42-1)

Synonyms and Key Words: Choking, breath holding, psychogenic stridor, emotional laryngospasm, functional abduction paresis, respiratory glottic spasm. The term sleep choking syndrome is preferred because it specifies the predominant complaint.

Essential Features:

Sleep choking syndrome is a disorder of unknown etiology characterized by frequent episodes of awakening with a choking sensation.

The patient awakens suddenly with an intense feeling of inability to breathe due to a choking sensation. Episodes usually occur with an almost nightly frequency and sometimes occur repeatedly throughout the night. The awakening is associated with fear, anxiety, and often a feeling of impending death. The patient is immediately fully awake, and the feelings of fear rapidly subside. The episodes of fear are always associated with a feeling of inability to breathe. Stridor does not occur, and bedpartners do not observe impaired breathing. These patients do not experience nightmares, sleep terrors, or other forms of nocturnal anxiety attacks.

Associated Features: Fear and other features of increased autonomic activity, such as tachycardia, can occur. The disorder rarely may lead to insomnia.

Course: Not known. Sometimes the disorder is resolved after the patient is reassured following objective documentation of the benign nature of the disorder.

Predisposing Factors: May be more likely to occur in individuals with obsessive compulsiveness, hypochondriasis, and anxiety.

Prevalence: Not known, apparently rare.

Age of Onset: Appears to be most prevalent in early to middle adulthood. Not known to occur in children.

Sex Ratio: Appears to be more common in young adult females.

Familial Pattern: Not known.

Pathology: None known.

Complications: The disorder may produce an anxiety disorder.

Polysomnographic Features: The episodes typically do not occur in the laboratory, often despite a reported nightly occurrence at home. Polysomnographic monitoring demonstrates no evidence of cardiopulmonary abnormalities during sleep. Two nights of polysomnographic monitoring are usually required to rule out organic episodes and to accumulate sufficient objective sampling to reassure the patient.

Other Laboratory Test Features: Holter monitoring may be indicated to eliminate a cardiac cause of the episodes.

Differential Diagnosis: The sleep apnea syndromes are the disorders that most commonly need to be distinguished from the sleep choking syndrome. Because of the sensation of upper-airway obstruction, obstructive sleep apnea syndrome is the disorder most likely to be considered. Sleep-related abnormal-swallowing syndrome is distinguished by gurgling sounds that accompany the episodes and the clear physical nature of the choking episodes. Cardiac irregularity that causes respiratory difficulty must be considered.

Sleep terrors can occasionally be confused with sleep choking episodes but can be distinguished by the absence of a full awakening, lack of focus on upper-airway choking, and the easy return to sleep after the event.

Panic disorders can be differentiated by the diurnal presence of panic episodes. To make the diagnosis of sleep choking syndrome, the episodes must occur only during sleep and must not be associated with a history of agoraphobia. A coexisting depressive disorder or anxiety disorder should not be present.

Sleep-related laryngospasm presents in a similar way but is characterized by stridor with choking that is usually witnessed by a bedpartner. The laryngospasm episodes occur infrequently and rarely, if ever, occur more than once per night.

Diagnostic Criteria: Sleep Choking Syndrome (307.42-1)

A. The patient complains of abrupt awakenings during sleep.
B. Choking episodes occur frequently (almost nightly) during sleep.
C. Associated features include at least two of the following:
   1. Rapid heart rate
   2. Intense anxiety
   3. Sensation of impending death
D. Polysomnographic monitoring demonstrates normal ventilation during sleep.
F. No other medical or mental disorder (e.g., panic disorder) can account for the symptoms.
G. The symptoms do not meet the diagnostic criteria for any other sleep disorder (e.g., obstructive sleep apnea syndrome, sleep-related abnormal swallowing syndrome, sleep terrors).

Minimal Criteria: A plus B plus C.

Severity Criteria:

Mild: Episodes occur less than once every night and are usually associated with a mild autonomic response.
Moderate: Episodes occur nightly and are usually associated with a moderate autonomic response.
Severe: Episodes occur more than once per night and are usually associated with a severe autonomic response.

Duration Criteria:
Acute: 7 days or less.
Subacute: More than 7 days but less than 1 month.
Chronic: 1 month or longer.

Bibliography:

Arnold GE. Disorders of laryngeal function. In: Paparella MM, Shumrick DA, eds. Otolaryngology Volume III Head and neck. Philadelphia: WB Saunders, 1973; 3: 638.

Thorpy MJ, Aloe FS. Choking during sleep. Sleep Res 1989; 18: 314.

CLASSIFICATION OF PROCEDURES

Procedures that are commonly used in the diagnosis and treatment of sleep disorders are listed on axis B, along with the appropriate *ICD-9-CM* code number. The name of the procedure and the associated code number should be stated.

To allow for greater specification in the practice of sleep-disorders medicine, the *ICD-9-CM* code numbers for some entries have been expanded to the fifth-digit level (e.g., "Other Sleep Disorder Function Tests"). *ICD-9-CM* #89.18 has been expanded for the Multiple Sleep Latency Test to #89.180. This expansion is not part of the authorized *ICD-9-CM* coding system; however, the first four-digit code numbers are compatible with *ICD-9-CM* codes.

For code numbers of tests not listed here, please refer to the appropriate section of the *International Classification of Diseases*, 9th Revision, Clinical Modification, Volume 3.

Diagnostic and Nonsurgical Procedures (87-99)

SLEEP TESTS

Polysomnogram	89.17
Multiple Sleep Latency Test	89.180
Maintenance of Wakefulness Test	89.181
Actigraphy	89.182
Constant Routine Evaluation	89.183
Other Endogenous Circadian Phase Assessment	89.184
Pupillometry	89.185
Electrophysiologic Performance Testing	89.186
Ambulatory Sleep Monitoring	89.187
Sleep Video Monitoring	89.188
Other Sleep Tests	89.189

RESPIRATORY TESTS

Arterial Blood Gases	89.65
Pulmonary Function Tests	89.38

CARDIOLOGY TESTS

Echocardiography	88.72
Rhythm Electrocardiogram	89.51
Holter Monitoring	89.54

IMAGING TESTS

Computerized Axial Tomography of the Head	87.03
Lateral Head and Neck Soft Tissue X-ray	87.09
Cephalometrics	87.12
Chest X-Ray	87.44
Barium Swallow	87.61
Upper GI Series	87.62
Magnetic Resonance Imaging of Brain and Brain stem	88.91

NEUROLOGIC TESTS

Electroencephalogram	89.14
Other Nonoperative Neurologic Function Tests	89.15
Video Electroencephalographic Monitoring	89.151
Electromyography	93.08

PSYCHOLOGIC TESTS

Administration of Intelligence Tests	94.01
Stanford-Binet	94.010
Wechsler Adult Intelligence Scale	94.011
Wechsler Intelligence Scale for Children	94.012
Other	94.019
Administration of Psychologic Tests	94.02
Bender Visual-Motor Gestalt Test	94.020
Benton Visual Retention Test	94.021
Minnesota Multiphasic Personality Inventory	94.022
Wechsler Memory Scale	94.023
Other	94.029
Character Analysis	94.03
Other Psychologic Evaluation and Testing	94.08
Beck Depression Inventory	94.080
Profile of Mood States	94.081
State Trait Anxiety Inventory	94.082
Structured Interviews (Schedule for affective disorders and schizophrenia, Structured clinical interview DSM III or IV, etc.)	94.083
Neuropsychologic Tests (Halstead, Luria, etc.)	94.084
Sleep Log	94.085
Stanford Sleepiness Scale	94.086
Other Sleep Questionnaires	94.087
Other	94.089
Psychologic Mental Status Determination, Not Otherwise Specified	94.09

OTOLARYNGOLOGIC TESTS

Rhinoscopy	21.21
Pharyngoscopy	29.11
Laryngoscopy	31.42

PSYCHIATRIC THERAPY

Psychiatric Drug Therapy	94.25
Hypnosis	94.32
Behavior Therapy	94.33
Behavior Modification	
Aversion Therapy	
Relaxation Training	
Family Therapy	94.42

RESPIRATORY THERAPY

Intermittent Positive Pressure Breathing (IPPB)	93.91
Other Mechanical Ventilation	93.92
Nasal Continuous Positive Airway Pressure (CPAP)	93.90
Oxygen Therapy	93.96
Other Respiratory Procedures	93.99

DENTAL APPLIANCES AND THERAPY

Orthodontic Device	V58.5
Dental Wiring	93.55

OTHER

Penile Blood Pressure Testing	64.19
Esophageal Manometry	89.32
Gastroesophageal pH Monitoring	89.39
Light Therapy	99.83

Operations (01-86)

Surgical procedures occasionally performed on some patients who undergo sleep medicine evaluation are listed here.

SURGICAL THERAPY

Submucous Resection of Nasal Septum	21.5
Uvuloplasty	27.79
Palatoplasty	27.69
Uvulopalatopharyngoplasty	29.4
Tonsillectomy without Adenoidectomy	28.2
Tonsillectomy with Adenoidectomy	28.3
Temporary Tracheostomy	31.1
Permanent Tracheostomy	31.2
Insertion of Diaphragmatic Pacemaker	34.85
Insertion of Cardiac Pacemaker	37.80
Gastroplasty	44.69
Penile Prosthesis Implantation	
Noninflatable Prosthesis	64.95
Inflatable Prosthesis	64.97
Mandibular Reconstruction	76.43

ICSD CODING SYSTEM

The axial system uses *ICD-9-CM* coding wherever possible. Additional codes are included for procedures and physical signs of particular interest to sleep-disorders clinicians. Modifying information, such as symptom, severity, and duration, also can be specified and coded by a special *ICSD* sleep code.

Coding of the modifiers is optional and is intended primarily for epidemiologic, statistical, and research purposes. However, clinicians are encouraged to use the full system whenever possible. A shorter version of the axial system is described on page 13 for those who wish to state and code a minimum of information.

Axis A

For specifying severity and duration of the disorder, and its associated symptom, the *ICSD* coding system uses an additional four-digit code. The use of the modifiers is discussed in the following sections of this manual, e.g.,

Periodic Limb Movement Disorder, moderate, chronic,
 with excessive sleepiness   780.52-4   Sleep Code [F235]

Axis B

Laboratory procedures, operations, and procedure features are listed on axis B and are derived from the three-digit rubric of the *ICD-9* Classification of Procedures, e.g.,

Palatoplasty   27.6

The three-digit rubric for some procedures has been expanded in the *ICD-9-CM* Procedure Classification to the fourth-digit level for greater specificity, e.g.,

Electroencephalogram   89.14

The *ICSD* coding system has added an alphanumeric sleep code that is also stated on axis B to allow for coding of procedural features that are specific to sleep-disorders medicine, e.g.,

Sleep Efficiency   Sleep Code P5

These new rubrics can be used for specifying the presence, absence, and frequency of the feature by adding an additional alpha character at the third-digit level, e.g.,

Sleep Efficiency, decreased   Sleep Code P5[D]

Axis C

The diagnoses and codes stated on axis C are those of *ICD-9-CM* (or *ICD-9*, if *ICD-9-CM* is not available) that are not sleep-disorders diagnoses, e.g.,

Hypertension   401.0

An *ICSD* code is not necessary for this section. The *ICSD* coding system is described in greater detail in the following pages.

Axis A Modifiers

This portion of the manual describes the modifiers to be used on axis A.

Axis A diagnoses may be qualified by the use of several modifiers that indicate whether a diagnosis is "Provisional" or "Final," whether the disorder was "In Remission" at the time the patient was seen, and whether the disorder had an "Acute Onset." In addition, three modifiers specify the severity and duration of the disorder and the associated main symptom.

Diagnostic Criteria

When a diagnosis is stated on axis A, it will be assumed that the disorder has met the criteria for a final diagnosis. The alpha code "F" is to be stated before the *ICSD* sleep code to indicate that the diagnosis is no longer a working diagnosis but is a "Final" or "Definitive" diagnosis, e.g.,

    Axis A   Narcolepsy   347   *ICSD* Code [F]

This alpha code does not necessarily mean that the criteria listed in the text have all been met, although it is expected that the criteria will have been met in most cases. The decision to use code "F" is to be based on the clinician's judgment of whether or not the diagnosis is considered to be final.

If a final diagnosis cannot be made at the time that the diagnosis is to be stated, then the words "Provisional Diagnosis" will be placed in parentheses after the diagnosis. The alpha character "P" will be placed before the *ICSD* sleep code number, e.g.,

    Axis A   Narcolepsy (Provisional Diagnosis)   347   ICSD Code [P]

Remission

A diagnosis usually will be given if a disorder or disease is present. Occasionally, however, a patient may be seen after the disorder has resolved. In this case, the diagnosis can still be given, but it should be followed by the words "In Remission" or "Resolved" (whichever is more applicable) in parentheses after the diagnosis. No alpha code exists for this modifier, e.g.,

    Axis A   Obstructive Sleep Apnea Syndrome (Resolved)   780.53

Acute Onset

If the onset of a disorder is particularly acute and it is important to convey the acuteness of the onset, the words "Acute Onset" can be placed in parentheses after the diagnosis. No alpha code exists for this modifier, e.g.,

    Axis A   Narcolepsy (Acute Onset)   347

Severity

The first diagnosis modifier, noted at the second sleep-code-digit level, indicates the severity of the condition:

0   indeterminate
1   mild
2   moderate
3   severe

Whenever possible, criteria defining the severity of a disorder are presented in the text. "Indeterminate" is to be used when the severity is unable to be determined at the time that the diagnosis is stated.

The severity modifier is always stated after the diagnosis, e.g.,

    Axis A   Obstructive Sleep Apnea Syndrome,
              severe   780.53   *ICSD* Code [F3]

Duration

The second diagnosis modifier, coded at the third sleep-code-digit level, indicates the duration of the disorder:

1   acute
2   subacute
3   chronic

Whenever possible, criteria defining the duration of a disorder are presented in the text.

The duration-modifying term is always stated after the severity modifier, e.g.,

    Axis A   Obstructive Sleep Apnea Syndrome,
              severe, chronic   780.53-0   [F33]

Symptom

The symptom modifier indicates whether the disorder is asymptomatic or is associated with a major sleep symptom such as insomnia, excessive sleepiness, or other sleep-related and non-sleep-related symptoms. The symptoms may be presented by the patient, the caretaker, or another observer. These terms can be coded for research purposes at the fourth-digit level. One additional symptom for each diagnosis can be coded at the fifth-digit level. The symptom modifiers are as follows:

0   no symptom modifier
1   asymptomatic
2   with difficulty in initiating sleep
3   with difficulty in maintaining sleep
4   with difficulty in awakening
5   with excessive sleepiness

6   with an excessive sleep duration
7   other [sleep-related symptom]
8   other [non-sleep-related symptom]

Each of the symptom descriptors is defined as follows:

0   No symptom modifier

This modifier is used when the name of the condition describes the symptom and, therefore, no symptom modifier is necessary, e.g.,

Axis A   Sleepwalking, mild, chronic   307.46-0   [F13<u>0</u>]

1 Asymptomatic

There is no complaint, e.g.,

Obstructive Sleep Apnea Syndrome, mild, acute
[F11<u>1</u>]

2 With difficulty in initiating sleep

The predominant complaint is an inability to initiate sleep within a desired amount of time, e.g.,

Obstructive Sleep Apnea Syndrome, mild, acute
  with difficulty initiating sleep   [F11<u>2</u>]

3 With difficulty in maintaining sleep

The predominant complaint is an inability to sustain sleep due to:

A. Frequent awakenings,

and/or

B. Inability to sleep as long as desired.

4 With difficulty in awakening

The predominant complaint is difficulty in achieving the fully awake state after awakening from the major sleep episode.

5 With excessive sleepiness

A. The predominant complaint is usually difficulty in maintaining desired wakefulness,

with or without

B. An excessive major sleep episode duration or excessive total sleep per 24 hours, as compared to normal for the patient's age.

6 With an excessive sleep duration

   The predominant complaint is an excessive amount of sleep per 24 hours without excessive sleepiness.

7 Other [sleep-related symptom]

   When a specific symptom descriptor is stated in the text, it is stated and coded here. Otherwise, the sleep-related symptom is stated and coded here if it meets the following criteria:

   A. The symptom produces disruption of the sleep episode continuity,

   and/or

   B. An abnormal physiologic occurrence during sleep, e.g.,

   Axis A   Obstructive Sleep Apnea Syndrome, mild, acute
              with nocturnal choking episodes   780.53-0   [F117]

8 Other [non-sleep-related symptom]

   A major presenting symptom that does not directly describe a sleep or arousal complaint is stated and coded here, e.g.,

   Axis A   Delayed Sleep Phase Syndrome, moderate, chronic
              with poor school performance   780.55-0   [F238]

   Two symptom descriptors may be needed for a given diagnosis. The second descriptor would begin with the word "and" and the word "with" would be deleted. The digit for the second symptom is added to the code, making a five-digit code, e.g.,

   Axis A   Delayed Sleep-Phase Syndrome, moderate, chronic
              with excessive sleepiness, and difficulty
              in initiating sleep   780.55-0   [F2352]

   The Mental, Neurologic, or Other Medical Disorders should also be coded on axis A along with an appropriate sleep code if the disorders produce a major sleep disorder, e.g.,

   Axis A   Sleeping Sickness, moderately severe, chronic
              with excessive sleepiness   086.9   [F235]

   Medical disorders that are not listed in the Sleep Disorders that are Associated with Mental, Neurologic, or Other Medical Disorders section can be stated on axis A if the sleep disorder is due to the medical condition. The disorder should be coded under the appropriate ICD-9-CM number, e.g.,

   Axis A   Meningitis, severe, acute with difficulty
              in initiating sleep   322.9   [F312]

Axis B

Axis B comprises the *ICSD* classification of procedures and procedure features. This listing is the *ICSD* equivalent of the *ICD-9-CM*, Volume 3 procedure classification and is used to specify

    A. laboratory or operative procedures,

and

    B. normal or abnormal findings detected by polysomnographic or chronobiologic investigations.

The two specific laboratory procedures that mainly are used in sleep disorders medicine are the All-Night Polysomnogram and the Multiple Sleep Latency Test (MSLT). The polysomnogram is coded under the *ICD-9-CM* #89.17 and the MSLT under #89.18.

Procedures

Axis B can be used to state the procedure performed, as per the *ICD-9-CM*, Volume 3 Procedure Classification, Section 16, Miscellaneous Diagnostic and Therapeutic Procedures (87-99), e.g.,

Axis A	Obstructive Sleep Apnea Syndrome, severe, chronic with excessive sleepiness	780.53-0 [F335]
Axis B	Polysomnogram	89.17
	Continuous Positive Airway Pressure	93.99

Operations also can be listed here in accordance with the Procedure Classification of *ICD-9-CM*, e.g.,

Axis A	Obstructive Sleep Apnea Syndrome, severe, chronic with excessive sleepiness	780.53-0 [F335]
Axis B	Polysomnogram	89.17
	Multiple Sleep Latency Test	89.18
	Palatoplasty	27.60

A list of ICD-9-CM procedures that commonly are used or seen in the practice of sleep disorders medicine appears on page 311.

Procedure Features

The alphanumeric procedure-feature codes are derived from a letter of the alphabet that corresponds to a group of common features (e.g., polysomnogram features regarding sleep and sleep stages begin with the letter "P"). The particular features are listed on axis B in the order of importance in determining (1) the major diagnosis and (2) additional sleep diagnoses.

The *ICSD* procedure-features list is not designed to be an exhaustive listing of all possible measures. It has been chosen to enable coding of those measures believed to be most useful in objectively documenting the presence or absence of clinical sleep disorders, e.g.,

    Axis B   Sleep Latency   [P1]

Other nonspecified sleep-testing measures can be coded for at the second-digit level by the numeral "9," e.g.,

    Axis B   REM Cycle Length   [R9]

The absence, presence, or frequency of the feature is coded at the third-digit level by an alpha character derived from the following table:

P present
A absent
N normal
D decreased
I increased

For example,

    Axis B   Sleep Latency, decreased   [P1D]

Up to **six** axis B procedure features may be stated in addition to **four** axis B procedures, e.g.,

Axis A	Narcolepsy, moderate, chronic, with excessive sleepiness and cataplexy	347	[F2357]
	Periodic Limb Movement Disorder, mild, chronic, with difficulty in maintaining sleep	780.52-4	[F133]
Axis B	Polysomnogram	89.17	
	Number of Awakenings, increased		[P2I]
	Periodic Leg Movements, present		[U1P]
	Multiple Sleep Latency Test	89.18	
	Mean Sleep Latency (MSLT), decreased		[M0D]
	Two Sleep-Onset REM periods (MSLT), present		[M2P]

Axis C

Axis C diagnoses are those of the *ICD-9-CM Diagnostic Classification of Diseases* and include diagnoses in the section on mental disorders. Diagnoses in the *ICSD* should be listed and coded on axis A even though there may be an alternative diagnostic listing in *ICD-9-CM* (e.g., Narcolepsy should be coded on axis A, not axis C). More than one axis C diagnosis may be stated.

Axis C should list diagnoses suspected to be associated with axis A diagnoses, such as Hypertension associated with Obstructive Sleep Apnea Syndrome, e.g.,

Axis A	Obstructive Sleep Apnea Syndrome, severe, chronic with excessive sleepiness	780.53-0	[F335]
Axis C	Hypertension	401.0	

Other active diagnoses also should be specified; however, not every diagnosis needs to be stated in a given patient, e.g.,

Axis A	Narcolepsy, moderate, chronic, with excessive sleepiness and cataplexy	347	[F2357]
	Periodic Limb Movement Disorder, mild, chronic, with difficulty in maintaining sleep	780.52-4	[F133]
Axis B	Polysomnogram	89.17	
	Number of Awakenings, increased		[P2I]
	Periodic Leg Movements, present		[U1P]
	Multiple Sleep Latency Test	89.18	
	Mean Sleep Latency (MSLT), decreased		[M0D]
	Two Sleep-onset REM Periods (MSLT), present		[M2P]
Axis C	Reactive Depression	300.4	
	Hypertension	401.1	

Summary

Axis A

Final Diagnosis

Only the code letter "F" should be stated.

Provisional Diagnosis

The term *provisional diagnosis* should be placed in parentheses after the diagnosis and the code letter "P" should be stated.

Remission

The term *in remission* or *resolved* should be placed in parentheses after the diagnosis.

Acute Onset

The term *acute onset* should be placed in parentheses after the diagnosis.

Severity (second *ICSD* Code digit)

   0 indeterminate
   1 mild
   2 moderate
   3 severe

Duration (third *ICSD* Code digit)

   1 acute
   2 subacute
   3 chronic

Symptom (fourth or fifth *ICSD* Code digit)

   0 no symptom modifier
   1 asymptomatic
   2 with difficulty in initiating sleep
   3 with difficulty in maintaining sleep
   4 with difficulty in awakening
   5 with excessive sleepiness
   6 with an excessive sleep duration
   7 other [sleep-related symptom]
   8 other [non-sleep-related symptom]

Axis B

Procedure Feature (third *ICSD* Code digit)

   P present
   A absent
   N normal
   D decreased
   I increased

ICSD CODING SYSTEM

AXIS B PROCEDURE–FEATURE CODES

Axis B *ICSD* sleep codes are modifiers, such as the Polysomnogram (89.17) and Multiple Sleep Latency Test (89.18), that are stated in addition to the ICD-9-CM codes for procedures.

Axis B sleep codes consist of an alpha character indicating the subgroup of procedures and a numeral for the particular feature being coded. The two characters are followed by a third digit, indicating the presence, absence, or degree of the feature or abnormality according to the following mnemonic, PANDI:

    P   Present
    A   Absent
    N   Normal
    D   Decreased
    I   Increased

Not all of the above codes are appropriate for each axis B listing. Included beside each feature code, in brackets, are the alpha characters that may be appropriate to use with that particular feature. The alpha characters X, Y, and Z are reserved for use by researchers who wish to code for procedure features that are not listed here and that require greater specificity.

POLYSOMNOGRAM FEATURES

Feature	Code	Modifiers
Total Sleep Time	P0	[A, N, D, I]
Sleep Latency	P1	[A, N, D, I]
Number of Awakenings	P2	[A, N, D, I]
Wake after Sleep Onset	P3	[N, I]
Sleep Efficiency	P4	[N, D]
Stage 1 Sleep	P5	[A, N, D, I]
Stage 2 Sleep	P6	[A, N, D, I]
Stage 3 or Stage 4 Sleep	P7	[A, N, D, I]
Other Sleep Feature	P9	[P, A, N, D, I]

MULTIPLE SLEEP LATENCY TEST FEATURES

Feature	Code	Modifiers
Mean Sleep Latency (MSLT)	M0	[N, D, I]
One Sleep-Onset REM Period (SOREMP)	M1	[P, A]
Two SOREMPs (MSLT)	M2	[P, A]
Three SOREMPs (MSLT)	M3	[P, A]
Four SOREMPs (MSLT)	M4	[P, A]
Five SOREMPs (MSLT)	M5	[P, A]
Other MSLT Feature	M9	[P, A, N, D, I]

MAINTENANCE OF WAKEFULNESS TEST FEATURES

Mean Sleep Latency (MWT)	W0	[N, D, I]
One Sleep-Onset REM Period (SOREMP)	W1	[P, A]
Two SOREMPs (MWT)	W2	[P, A]
Three SOREMPs (MWT)	W3	[P, A]
Four SOREMPs (MWT)	W4	[P, A]
Five SOREMPs (MWT)	W5	[P, A]
Other MWT Feature	W9	[P, A, N, D, I]

MOTOR BEHAVIOR FEATURES

Headbanging	B0	[P, A, D, I]
Headrolling	B1	[P, A, D, I]
Bodyrocking	B2	[P, A, D, I]
Bodyrolling	B3	[P, A, D, I]
Legrolling	B4	[P, A, D, I]
Bruxism	B5	[P, A, D, I]
Restless Legs Muscle Activity	B6	[P, A]
Sleep Starts	B7	[P, A, D, I]
Periodic Leg Movements	B8	[P, A, N, D, I]
Other Motor Behavior Feature	B9	[P, A, N, D, I]

CARDIOLOGY FEATURES

Cardiac Rate in Sleep	C0	[N, D, I]
Extrasystolic Beats	C1	[P, A, D, I]
Atrial Fibrillation	C2	[P, A, D, I]
Ventricular Tachycardia	C3	[P, A]
Bradytachycardia	C4	[P, A]
Heart Block	C5	[P, A]
Sinus Arrest	C6	[P, A]
Cardiac Ischemia	C7	[P, A]
Other Cardiac Feature	C9	[P, A, N, D, I]

SLEEP ELECTROENCEPHALOGRAPHIC FEATURES

Alpha Activity	E0	[P, A, N, D, I]
Alpha-Delta Activity	E2	[P, A]
Beta Activity	E3	[P, A]
Sleep Spindles	E4	[P, A, N, D, I]
K Complexes	E5	[P, A, N, D, I]
Microarousals	E6	[P, A, N, D, I]
Electrical Status Epilepticus (ESES)	E7	[P, A]
Generalized Electroencephalographic Slowing	E8	[P, A]
Other Sleep Electroencephalographic Feature	E9	[P, A, N, D, I]

HISTOCOMPATIBILITY ANTIGENS

HLA Testing	H0	[P]
HLA-DQ1	H1	[P, A]
HLA-DR2	H2	[P, A]
Other Histocompatibility Feature	H9	[P, A]

COMPLEX-BEHAVIOR FEATURES

Sleepwalking	K0	[P, A, D, I]
Sleep Talking	K1	[P, A, D, I]
Screaming	K2	[P, A, D, I]
Sitting in Bed	K3	[P, A, D, I]
Thrashing Behavior	K4	[P, A, D, I]
Other Complex-Behavior Feature	K9	[P, A, N, D, I]

SLEEP-LOG FEATURES

Irregular Pattern	L0	[P, A, N, D, I]
Insufficient Sleep	L1	[P, A, N, D, I]
Advanced-Sleep Pattern	L2	[P, A, N, D, I]
Delayed-Sleep Pattern	L3	[P, A, N, D, I]
Incremental-Delay Pattern	L4	[P, A, N, D, I]
Prolonged Sleep Period	L5	[P, A, N, D, I]
Intermittent Sleep Episodes	L6	[P, A, N, D, I]
Other Sleep-Log Feature	L9	[P, A, N, D, I]

REM SLEEP FEATURES

REM Sleep	R0	[A, N, D, I]
REM Period Efficiency	R1	[N, D, I]
REM Period Duration	R2	[N, D, I]
REM Spindle Activity	R3	[P, A]
REM Period Latency	R4	[A, N, D, I]
REM Density	R5	[N, D, I]
REM Interruptions	R6	[P, A]
Other REM Feature	R9	[P, A, N, D, I]

PENILE TUMESCENCE

Penile Tumescence–Base	T0	[P, A, N, D, I]
Penile Tumescence–Tip	T1	[P, A, N, D, I]
Penile Rigidity	T2	[P, A, N, D]
Tumescence Duration	T3	[N, D, I]
Tumescence Episodes	T4	[P, A, N, D, I]
Penile Circumference	T5	[P, A, N, D, I]
Other Penile Feature	T9	[P, A, N, D, I]

MUSCLE FEATURES

Brief Leg Myoclonus	U0	[P, A]
Movement Stage Shifts	U1	[P, A, N, D, I]
Movement Awakenings	U2	[P, A, N, D, I]
Atonia in Non-REM Sleep	U3	[P, A, N, D, I]
Muscle Tone in REM Sleep	U4	[P, A, N, D, I]
Other Muscle Feature	U9	[P, A, N, D, I]

VENTILATION FEATURES

Obstructive Apnea	V0	[P, A]
Central Apnea	V1	[P, A]

Hypopnea	V2	[P, A]
Respiratory Rate	V3	[D, I]
Nonapneic Hypoventilation	V4	[P, A]
Cheyne-Stokes Breathing	V5	[P, A]
Oxygen-Saturation Value	V6	[N, D]
Carbon-Dioxide Value	V7	[N, D, I]
Other Respiratory Feature	V9	[P, A, N, D, I]

OTHER FEATURES

Circadian Temperature Rhythm	O0	[P, A]
Gastroesophageal pH Acidity	O1	[P, A, N, D, I]
Other	O9	[P, A, N, D, I]

ICSD CODING SYSTEM

DATABASE

A database containing information concerning demographics, methodology, and concomitant pathology associated with the various sleep disorders would be useful clinically, administratively, and for research. The adoption of "*ICD*-style" coding further emphasizes the utility of a system for tracking epidemiologic data. It is planned to develop a database specification and create computer software for this purpose.

The primary purpose of this database is to establish a format for epidemiologic tracking of sleep disorders at sleep-disorders centers. This standardized data processing tool will facilitate data pooling in cooperative intercenter ventures. The resulting overall multicenter database will also serve as a valuable information resource in several ways. It will provide data for updating the classification system and assessing the usefulness of the proposed classifications. It will also furnish additional detail on the statistical criteria used in classification. Specifically, factors such as duration, associated features, severity, and diagnostic criteria, will be available for careful examination and reevaluation.

To facilitate record keeping on the sleep disorders that clinicians encounter, a database system has been devised. Two formats are available. One is simple and allows for data entry of minimal identification, demographic, and diagnostic information. The other is more complex and allows for storage and retrieval of detailed information concerning the outcome of sleep studies and other examinations.

In addition to providing the specification of each data field, the database was developed with several specific design goals. The first and foremost was to provide maximal flexibility of the data. This flexibility will allow for transporting the actual data out of the database in several forms so that other computer software can use the information. Flexibility also allows upward compatibility as revisions and new versions become available. The next design goal was compatibility with widely available computing machinery. The IBM-PC or a compatible machine was selected as the target machine because of its universal availability. Finally, ease of use was a design priority. The system incorporates various approaches to data logging, including selection from menus, checklist entry, and code-book entry.

It is also expected that the general availability of a custom-tailored database system will encourage good clinical record-keeping practices. It has been suggested that a report generator be developed so that simple patient summaries can be produced. The database system will help during field trials. Finally, the system will undoubtedly have inadvertent value in training and mastery of this new database for the classification of sleep disorders.

The following is a suggested manner in which the codes could be entered into a computerized database (the example given corresponds to the clinical example given on page 322).

Sleep Codes

Pickup 1, pp. 709, 710

DIFFERENTIAL DIAGNOSIS

Differential Diagnosis of Insomnia, Excessive Sleepiness, and Other Sleep Disturbances

The ICSD axis A classifies the sleep disorders mainly for coding and statistical purposes; it is not a differential-diagnostic list. In this section, we present a differential-diagnostic listing of the sleep disorders that cause the primary sleep symptoms, insomnia and excessive sleepiness. Because many sleep disorders produce both symptoms, names in the lists are duplicated. Some sleep disorders can be asymptomatic or can produce other symptoms, and they are listed, therefore, in the Other Sleep Disturbances group. This third list is included to assist the clinician in diagnosing a complaint of an abnormal event occurring during sleep such as a movement disorder.

The organization of the differential diagnoses follows the method presented in the 1979 *Diagnostic Classification of Sleep and Arousal Disorders*. The lists include the disorders of initiating and maintaining sleep and the disorders of excessive somnolence. Additional subdivisions are included, and some entries have been reorganized. The sleep-wake schedule disorders, now called the circadian rhythm sleep disorders, are included within the differential-diagnostic listing for insomnia and excessive sleepiness where appropriate.

The symptoms are defined in the following standard manner:

A. Insomnia

> A complaint of the inability to either initiate or maintain sleep.

B. Excessive Sleepiness

> A complaint of difficulty in maintaining desired wakefulness, or a complaint of an excessive amount of sleep.

C. Other Sleep Disturbance

> An abnormal physiologic occurrence during sleep or during arousal from sleep that does not usually cause a primary complaint of insomnia or excessive sleepiness.

A. INSOMNIA

1. Associated with Behavior or Psychophysiologic Disorders
   a. Adjustment Sleep Disorder
   b. Psychophysiologic Insomnia
   c. Inadequate Sleep Hygiene
   d. Limit-Setting Sleep Disorder
   e. Sleep-Onset Association Disorder
   f. Nocturnal Eating (Drinking) Syndrome
   g. Other

2. Associated with Mental Disorders
   a. Psychoses
   b. Mood Disorders
   c. Anxiety Disorders
   d. Panic Disorder
   e. Alcoholism
   f. Other

3. Associated with Environmental Factors
   a. Environmental Sleep Disorder
   b. Food Allergy Insomnia
   c. Toxin-Induced Sleep Disorder
   d. Other

4. Associated with Drug Dependency
   a. Hypnotic-Dependent Sleep Disorder
   b. Stimulant-Dependent Sleep Disorder
   c. Alcohol-Dependent Sleep Disorder
   d. Other

5. Associated with Sleep-Induced Respiratory Impairment
   a. Obstructive Sleep Apnea Syndrome
   b. Central Sleep Apnea Syndrome
   c. Central Alveolar Hypoventilation Syndrome
   d. Chronic Obstructive Pulmonary Disease
   e. Sleep-Related Asthma
   f. Altitude Insomnia
   g. Other

6. Associated with Movement Disorders
   a. Sleep Starts
   b. Restless Legs Syndrome
   c. Periodic Limb Movement Disorder
   d. Nocturnal Leg Cramps
   e. Rhythmic Movement Disorder
   f. REM Sleep Behavior Disorder
   g. Nocturnal Paroxysmal Dystonia
   h. Other

7. Associated with Disorders of the Timing of the Sleep-Wake Pattern
   a. Short Sleeper
   b. Time Zone Change (Jet Lag) Syndrome
   c. Shift Work Sleep Disorder
   d. Delayed Sleep-Phase Syndrome
   e. Advanced Sleep-Phase Syndrome
   f. Non-24-Hour Sleep-Wake Syndrome
   g. Irregular Sleep-Wake Pattern
   h. Other

8. Associated with Parasomnias (not otherwise classified)
   a. Confusional Arousals
   b. Sleep Terrors
   c. Sleepwalking
   d. Nightmares
   e. Sleep Hyperhidrosis
   f. Other

9. Associated with Neurologic Disorders (not otherwise classified)
   a. Parkinsonism
   b. Dementia
   c. Cerebral Degenerative Disorders
   d. Sleep-Related Epilepsy
   e. Fatal Familial Insomnia
   f. Sleep-related Headaches
   g. Other

10. Associated with No Objective Sleep Disturbance
    a. Sleep-State Misperception
    b. Sleep Choking Syndrome
    c. Other

11. Idiopathic Insomnia

12. Other Causes of Insomnia
    a. Sleep-Related Gastroesophageal Reflux
    b. Fibromyalgia
    c. Menstrual-Associated Sleep Disorder
    d. Pregnancy-Associated Sleep Disorder
    e. Terrifying Hypnagogic Hallucinations
    f. Sleep-Related Abnormal Swallowing Syndrome
    g. Sleep-Related Laryngospasm
    h. Nocturnal Cardiac Ischemia
    i. Peptic Ulcer Disease
    j. Other

B. EXCESSIVE SLEEPINESS

1. Associated with Behavioral/Psychophysiologic Disorders
   a. Inadequate Sleep Hygiene
   b. Insufficient Sleep Syndrome
   c. Limit-Setting Sleep Disorder
   d. Adjustment Sleep Disorder
   e. Other

2. Associated with Mental Disorders
   a. Mood Disorders
   b. Psychoses
   c. Alcoholism
   d. Other

3. Associated with Environmental Factors
   a. Environmental Sleep Disorder
   b. Toxin-Induced Sleep Disorder
   c. Other

4. Associated with Drug Dependency
   a. Hypnotic-Dependent Sleep Disorder
   b. Stimulant-Dependent Sleep Disorder
   c. Alcohol-Dependent Sleep Disorder
   d. Other

5. Associated with Sleep-Induced Respiratory Impairment
   a. Obstructive Sleep Apnea Syndrome
   b. Central Sleep Apnea Syndrome
   c. Central Alveolar Hypoventilation Syndrome
   d. Sleep-Related Neurogenic Tachypnea
   e. Other

6. Associated with Movement Disorders
   a. Periodic Limb Movement Disorder
   b. Restless Legs Syndrome
   c. Other

7. Associated with Disorders of the Timing of the Sleep-Wake Pattern
   a. Long Sleeper
   b. Time Zone Change (Jet Lag) Syndrome
   c. Shift Work Sleep Disorder
   d. Delayed Sleep-Phase Syndrome
   e. Advanced Sleep-Phase Syndrome
   f. Non-24-Hour Sleep-Wake Syndrome
   g. Irregular Sleep-Wake Pattern
   h. Other

8. Associated with Neurologic Disorders (not otherwise classified)
   a. Narcolepsy
   b. Idiopathic Hypersomnia
   c. Post-traumatic Hypersomnia
   d. Recurrent Hypersomnia
   e. Subwakefulness Syndrome
   f. Fragmentary Myoclonus
   g. Parkinsonism
   h. Dementia
   i. Sleeping Sickness
   j. Sleep-Related Epilepsy
   k. Other

9. Other Causes of Excessive Sleepiness
   a. Menstrual-Associated Sleep Disorder
   b. Pregnancy-Associated Sleep Disorder
   c. Other

C. OTHER SLEEP DISTURBANCES

1. Associated with Behavior or Psychophysiologic Disorders
   a. Nocturnal Eating (Drinking) Syndrome
   b. Other

2. Associated with Mental Disorders
   a. Panic Disorder
   b. Other

3. Associated with Sleep-Induced Respiratory Impairment
   a. Primary Snoring
   b. Obstructive Sleep Apnea Syndrome
   c. Central Sleep Apnea Syndrome
   d. Central Alveolar Hypoventilation Syndrome
   e. Sleep-Related Asthma
   f. Chronic Obstructive Pulmonary Disease
   g. Sleep-Related Neurogenic Tachypnea
   h. Other

4. Associated with Movement Disorders
   a. Sleep Starts
   b. Sleepwalking
   c. Sleep Terrors
   d. Sleep Bruxism
   e. Periodic Limb Movement Disorder
   g. Restless Legs Syndrome
   h. Rhythmic Movement Disorder
   i. Sleep Paralysis

j. Nocturnal Leg Cramps
k. REM Sleep Behavior Disorder
l. Nocturnal Paroxysmal Dystonia
m. Other

5. Associated with Parasomnias (not otherwise classified)
   a. Nightmares
   b. Sleep Talking
   c. Sleep Enuresis
   e. Sleep-Related Painful Erections
   f. Other

6. Associated with the Neurologic Disorders (not otherwise classified)
   a. Sleep-Related Epilepsy
   b. Electrical Status Epilepticus of Sleep
   c. Fragmentary Myoclonus
   d. Other

7. Other Causes of Sleep Disturbance
   a. Sleep-Related Gastroesophageal Reflux
   b. Sleep-Related Sinus Arrest
   c. Sleep-Related Abnormal Swallowing Syndrome
   d. Sleep-Related Laryngospasm
   e. Sleep Choking Syndrome
   f. Terrifying Hypnagogic Hallucinations
   g. Other

GLOSSARY

Glossary of Terms Used in Sleep Disorders Medicine

Actigraph: A biomedical instrument used to measure body movement.

Active Sleep: A term used in the phylogenetic and ontogenetic literature for the stage of sleep that is considered to be equivalent to REM (rapid eye movement) sleep. *See* REM Sleep.

Alpha Activity: An alpha electroencephalographic wave or sequence of waves with a frequency of 8 to 13 Hz.

Alpha-Delta Sleep: Sleep in which alpha activity occurs during slow-wave sleep. Because alpha-delta sleep is rarely seen without alpha occurring in other sleep stages, the term alpha sleep is preferred.

Alpha Intrusion (-Infiltration, -Insertion, -Interruption): A brief superimposition of electroencephalographic alpha activity on sleep activities during a stage of sleep.

Alpha Rhythm: In human adults, an electroencephalographic rhythm with a frequency of 8 to 13 Hz, which is most prominent over the parieto-occipital cortex when the eyes are closed. The rhythm is blocked by eye opening or other arousing stimuli. It is indicative of the awake state in most normal individuals. It is most consistent and predominant during relaxed wakefulness, particularly with reduction of visual input. The amplitude is variable but typically below 50 µV in the adult. The alpha rhythm of an individual usually slows by 0.5 to 1.5 Hz and becomes more diffuse during drowsiness. The frequency range also varies with age; it is slower in children and older age groups relative to young and middle-aged adults.

Alpha Sleep: Sleep in which alpha activity occurs during most, if not all, sleep stages.

Apnea: Cessation of airflow at the nostrils and mouth lasting at least 10 seconds. The three types of apnea are obstructive, central, and mixed. Obstructive apnea is secondary to upper-airway obstruction; central apnea is associated with a cessation of all respiratory movements; mixed apnea has both central and obstructive components.

Apnea-Hypopnea Index: The number of apneic episodes (obstructive, central, and mixed) plus hypopneas per hour of sleep, as determined by all-night polysomnography.

Apnea Index: The number of apneic episodes (obstructive, central, and mixed) per hour of sleep, as determined by all-night polysomnography. A separate obstructive apnea index or central apnea index sometimes is stated.

Arise Time: The clock time at which an individual gets out of bed after the final awakening of the major sleep episode. This is distinguished from final wake-up.

Arousal: An abrupt change from a "deeper" stage of non-REM (NREM) sleep to a "lighter" stage, or from REM sleep toward wakefulness, with the possibility of awakening as the final outcome. Arousal may be accompanied by increased tonic electromyographic activity and heart rate, as well as by an increased number of body movements.

Arousal Disorder: A parasomnia disorder presumed to be due to an abnormal arousal mechanism. Forced arousal from sleep can induce episodes. The "classic" arousal disorders are sleepwalking, sleep terrors, and confusional arousals.

Awakening: The return to the polysomnographically defined awake state from any NREM or REM sleep stages. It is characterized by alpha and beta electroencephalographic activity, a rise in tonic electromyographic activity, voluntary rapid eye movements, and eye blinks. This definition of awakenings is valid only insofar as the polysomnogram is paralleled by a resumption of a reasonably alert state of awareness of the environment.

Axial System: A means of stating different types of information in a systematic manner by listing on several "axes," to ensure that important information is not overlooked by the statement of a single major diagnosis. *The International Classification of Sleep Disorders* uses a three-axial system: axes A, B, and C.

Axis A: The first level of the *International Classification of Sleep Disorders* axial system on which the sleep-disorder diagnoses, modifiers, and associated code numbers are stated.

Axis B: The second level of the *International Classification of Sleep Disorders* axial system on which the sleep-related procedures and procedure features, and associated code numbers, are stated.

Axis C: The third level of the *International Classification of Sleep Disorders* axial system on which *ICD-9-CM* nonsleep diagnoses and associated code numbers are stated.

Baseline: The typical or normal state of an individual or of an investigative variable before an experimental manipulation.

Bedtime: The clock time when one attempts to fall asleep, as differentiated from the clock time when one gets into bed.

Beta Activity: A beta electroencephalographic wave or sequence of waves with a frequency of greater than 13 Hz.

Beta Rhythm: An electroencephalographic rhythm in the range of 13 to 35 Hz, when the predominant frequency, beta rhythm, is usually associated with alert wakefulness or vigilance and is accompanied by a high tonic electromyogram. The amplitude of beta rhythm is variable but usually is below 30 μV. This rhythm may be drug induced.

Brain Wave: Use of this term is discouraged. The suggested term is electroencephalographic wave.

Cataplexy: A sudden decrement in muscle tone and loss of deep tendon reflexes, leading to muscle weakness, paralysis, or postural collapse. Cataplexy usually is precipitated by an outburst of emotional expression—notably laughter, anger, or startle. One of the tetrad of symptoms of narcolepsy. During cataplexy, respiration and voluntary eye movements are not compromised.

Cheyne-Stokes Respiration: A breathing pattern characterized by regular "crescendo-decrescendo" fluctuations in respiratory rate and tidal volume.

Chronobiology: The science relating to temporal, primarily rhythmic, processes in biology.

Circadian Rhythm: An innate daily fluctuation of physiologic or behavior functions, including sleep-wake states, generally tied to the 24-hour daily dark-light cycle. This rhythm sometimes occurs at a measurably different periodicity (e.g., 23 or 25 hours) when light-dark and other time cues are removed.

Circasemidian Rhythm: A biologic rhythm that has a period length of about half a day.

Conditioned Insomnia: An insomnia that is produced by the development of conditioned arousal during an earlier experience of sleeplessness. Causes of the conditioned stimulus can include the customary sleep environment or thoughts of disturbed sleep. A conditioned insomnia is one component of psychophysiologic insomnia.

Constant Routine: A chronobiologic test of the endogenous pacemaker that involves a 36-hour baseline-monitoring period, followed by a 40-hour waking episode of monitoring with the individual on a constant routine of food intake, position, activity, and light exposure.

Cycle: A characteristic of an event that exhibits rhythmic fluctuations. One cycle is defined as the activity from one maximum or minimum to the next.

Deep Sleep: A common term for combined NREM stage 3 and stage 4 sleep. In some sleep literature, the term deep sleep is applied to REM sleep because during REM sleep, individuals have a high awakening threshold to nonsignificant stimuli. *See* "Intermediary" Sleep Stage; Light Sleep.

Delayed Sleep Phase: A condition that occurs when the clock hour at which sleep normally occurs is moved back in time within a given 24-hour sleep-wake cycle. This results in a temporarily displaced, that is delayed, occurrence of sleep within the 24-hour cycle. The same term denotes a circadian rhythm sleep disturbance, called the delayed sleep-phase syndrome.

Delta Activity: Electroencephalographic activity with a frequency of less than 4 Hz (usually 0.1-3.5 Hz). In the scoring of human sleep, the minimum characteristics for scoring delta waves are conventionally 75 µV (peak-to-peak) amplitude and 0.5-second duration (2 Hz) or less.

Delta Sleep Stage: This stage is indicative of the stage of sleep in which electroencephalographic delta waves are prevalent or predominant (sleep stages 3 and 4, respectively). *See* Slow-Wave Sleep.

Diagnostic Criteria: Specific criteria established in *the International Classification of Sleep Disorders* to aid in determining the unequivocal presence of a particular sleep disorder.

Diurnal: Pertaining to the daytime.

Drowsiness: A state of quiet wakefulness that typically occurs before sleep onset. If the eyes are closed, diffuse and slowed alpha activity usually is present, which then gives way to early features of stage 1 sleep.

Duration Criteria: Criteria established in the *International Classification of Sleep Disorders* for determining the duration of a particular disorder as acute, subacute, or chronic.

Dyssomnia: A primary disorder of initiating and maintaining sleep or of excessive sleepiness. The dyssomnias are disorders of sleep or wakefulness per se; they are not a parasomnia.

Early Morning Arousal (Early a.m. Arousal): Synonymous with premature morning awakening.

Electroencephalogram (EEG): A recording of the electrical activity of the brain by means of electrodes placed on the surface of the head. With the electromyogram and electrooculogram, the electroencephalogram is one of the three basic variables used to score sleep stages and waking. Sleep recording in humans uses surface electrodes to record potential differences between brain regions and a neutral reference point, or simply between brain regions. Either the C3 or C4 (central region) placement, according to the International 10 to 20 System is referentially (referred to an earlobe) recorded as the standard electrode derivation from which sleep-state scoring is performed.

Electromyogram (EMG): A recording of electrical activity from the muscular system; in sleep recording, synonymous with resting muscle activity or potential. The chin EMG, along with the electroencephalogram and electrooculogram, is one of the three basic variables used to score sleep stages and waking. Sleep recording in humans typically uses surface electrodes to measure activity from the submental muscles. These positions reflect maximally the changes in resting activity of axial body muscles. The submental muscle EMG is tonically inhibited during REM sleep.

Electrooculogram (EOG): A recording of voltage changes resulting from shifts in position of the ocular globes; this is possible because each globe is a positive (anterior) and negative (posterior) dipole. Along with the electroencephalogram and the electromyogram, one of the three basic variables used to score sleep stages and waking. Sleep recording in humans uses surface electrodes placed near the eyes to record the movement (incidence, direction, and velocity) of the eyeballs. Rapid eye movements in sleep form one part of the characteristics of the REM-sleep state.

End-Tidal Carbon Dioxide: The carbon dioxide value that is usually determined at the nares by an infrared carbon dioxide gas analyzer. The value reflects the carbon-dioxide level in alveolar or pulmonary artery blood.

Entrainment: Synchronization of a biologic rhythm by a forcing stimulus such as an environmental time cue (zeitgeber). During entrainment, the frequencies of the two cycles are the same or are integral multiples of each other.

Epoch: A measure of duration of the sleep recording that typically is 20 or 30 seconds in duration, depending on the paper speed of the polysomnograph, and that corresponds to one page of the polysomnogram.

Excessive Sleepiness (Somnolence, Hypersomnia, Excessive Daytime Sleepiness): A subjective report of difficulty in maintaining the alert awake state, usually accompanied by a rapid entrance into sleep when the person is sedentary. Excessive sleepiness may be due to an excessively deep or prolonged major sleep episode. It can be quantitatively measured by use of subjectively defined rating scales of sleepiness or physiologically measured by electrophysiologic tests such as the multiple sleep latency test (*see* MSLT). Excessive sleepiness most commonly occurs during the daytime, but it may be present at night in a person, such as a shift worker, who has the major sleep episode during the daytime.

Extrinsic Sleep Disorders: Disorders that either originate, develop, or arise from causes outside of the body. The extrinsic sleep disorders are a subgroup of the dyssomnias.

Final Awakening: The amount of wakefulness that occurs after the final wake-up time until the arise time (lights on).

Final Wake-Up: The clock time at which an individual awakens for the last time before the arise time.

First-Night Effect: The effect of the environment and polysomnographic-recording apparatus on the quality of the subject's sleep the first night of recording. Sleep is usually of reduced quality compared to that which would be expected in the subject's usual sleeping environment, without electrodes and other recording-procedure stimuli. The subject usually will habituate to the laboratory by the time of the second night of recording.

Fragmentation (Pertaining to Sleep Architecture): The interruption of any stage of sleep due to the appearance of another stage or to wakefulness, leading to disrupted NREM-REM sleep cycles; this term is often used to refer to the interruption of REM sleep by movement arousals or stage 2 activity. Sleep fragmentation connotes repetitive interruptions of sleep by arousals and awakenings.

Free Running: A chronobiologic term that refers to the natural endogenous period of a rhythm when zeitgebers are removed. In humans, it most commonly is seen in the tendency to delay some circadian rhythms, such as the sleep-wake cycle, by approximately one hour every day; this delay occurs when a person has an impaired ability to entrain or is without time cues.

Hertz (Hz): A unit of frequency; the use of this term is preferred over the use of the synonym, cycles per second (cps).

Hypercapnia: Elevated carbon dioxide level in blood.

Hypersomnia (Excessive Sleepiness): Excessively deep or prolonged major sleep period, which may be associated with difficulty in awakening. The term is primarily used as a diagnostic term (e.g., idiopathic hypersomnia) and the term excessive sleepiness is preferred to describe the symptom.

Hypnagogic: Occurrence of an event during the transition from wakefulness to sleep.

Hypnagogic Imagery (Hallucinations): Vivid sensory images that occur at sleep onset but are particularly vivid with sleep-onset REM periods. Hypnagogic imagery is a feature of narcolepsy, in which REM periods occur at sleep onset.

Hypnagogic Startle: A "sleep start" or sudden body jerk (hypnic jerk), observed normally just at sleep onset and usually resulting, at least momentarily, in an awakening.

Hypnopompic (Hypnopomic): Occurrence of an event during the transition from sleep to wakefulness at the termination of a sleep episode.

Hypopnea: An episode of shallow breathing (airflow reduced by at least 50%) during sleep, lasting 10 seconds or longer, usually associated with a fall in blood oxygen saturation.

ICSD Sleep Code: A code number of the *International Classification of the Sleep Disorders* that refers to modifying information of a diagnosis, such as associated symptom, severity, and duration of a sleep disorder.

Insomnia: Difficulty in initiating or maintaining sleep. This term is employed ubiquitously to indicate any and all gradations and types of sleep loss.

"Intermediary" Sleep Stage: A term sometimes used for NREM stage 2 sleep. *See* Deep Sleep; Light Sleep. The term is often used, especially in the French literature, for stages combining elements of stage 2 and REM sleep.

Into-Bed Time: The clock time at which a person gets into bed. The into-bed time (IBT) will be the same as the bedtime for many people but not for those who spend time in wakeful activities in bed such as reading, before attempting to sleep.

Intrinsic Sleep Disorders: Disorders that either originate or develop from within the body or that arise from causes within the body. The intrinsic sleep disorders are a subgroup of the dyssomnias.

K-Alpha: A K-complex followed by several seconds of alpha rhythm; K-Alpha is a type of microarousal.

K-Complex: A sharp, biphasic electroencephalographic wave followed by a high-voltage slow wave. The complex duration is at least 0.5 seconds and may be accompanied by a sleep spindle. K-complexes occur spontaneously during NREM sleep and begin and define stage 2 sleep. They are thought to be evoked responses to internal stimuli. K-complexes can also be elicited during sleep by external (particularly auditory) stimuli.

Light-Dark Cycle: The periodic pattern of light (artificial or natural) alternating with darkness.

Light Sleep: A common term for NREM sleep stage 1, and sometimes stage 2.

Maintenance of Wakefulness Test (MWT): A series of measurements of the interval from "lights out" to sleep onset that are used in the assessment of an individual's ability to remain awake. Subjects are instructed to try to remain awake in a darkened room while in a semireclined position. Long latencies to sleep are indicative of the ability to remain awake. This test is most useful for assessing the effects of sleep disorders or of medication upon the ability to remain awake.

Major Sleep Episode: The longest sleep episode that occurs on a daily basis. This sleep episode typically is dictated by the circadian rhythm of sleep and wakefulness; also known as the conventional or habitual time for sleeping.

Microsleep: An episode lasting up to 30 seconds during which external stimuli are not perceived. The polysomnogram suddenly shifts from waking characteristics to sleep. Microsleeps are associated with excessive sleepiness and automatic behavior.

Minimal Criteria: Criteria of the *International Classification of Sleep Disorders* derived from the diagnostic criteria that provide the minimum features necessary for making a particular sleep-disorder diagnosis.

Montage: The particular arrangement by which a number of derivations are displayed simultaneously in a polysomnogram.

Movement Arousal: A body movement associated with an electroencephalographic pattern of arousal or a full awakening; a sleep-scoring variable.

Movement Time: The term used in sleep-record scoring to denote when electroencephalographic and electrooculographic tracings are obscured for more than half the scoring epoch because of movement. This time is only scored when the preceding and subsequent epochs are in sleep.

Multiple Sleep Latency Test (MSLT): A series of measurements of the interval from "lights out" to sleep onset that is used in the assessment of excessive sleepiness. Subjects are allowed a fixed number of opportunities (typically four or five) to fall asleep during their customary awake period. Excessive sleepiness is characterized by short latencies. Long latencies are helpful in distinguishing physical tiredness or fatigue from true sleepiness.

Muscle Tone: This term is sometimes used for resting muscle potential or resting muscle activity. *See* Electromyogram (EMG).

Myoclonus: Muscle contractions in the form of abrupt "jerks" or twitches that generally last less than 100 milliseconds. The term should not be applied to the periodic leg movements of sleep that characteristically have a duration of 0.5 to 5 seconds.

Nap: A short sleep episode that may be intentionally or unintentionally taken during the major episode of habitual wakefulness.

Nightmare: This term is used to denote an unpleasant and frightening dream that usually occurs in REM sleep. Nightmares are occasionally called dream anxiety attacks and are distinguished from sleep (night) terrors. In the past, the term nightmare has been used to indicate both sleep terrors and dream anxiety attacks.

Nocturnal Confusion: Episodes of delirium and disorientation that occur close to or during nighttime sleep; nocturnal confusion is often seen in the elderly and is indicative of organic central nervous system deterioration.

Nocturnal Dyspnea: Respiratory distress that may be minimal during the day but becomes quite pronounced during sleep.

Nocturnal penile tumescence (NPT): The natural periodic cycle of penile erections that occur during sleep, typically associated with REM sleep. The preferred term is sleep-related erections.

Nocturnal Sleep: This term is synonymous with the typical "nighttime" or major sleep episode related to the circadian rhythm of sleep and wakefulness; it is also known as the conventional or habitual time for sleeping.

Non-Rapid Eye Movement (NREM, Non-REM) Sleep: *See* Sleep Stages.

NREM-REM Sleep Cycle (Synonymous with Sleep Cycle): A period during sleep composed of a NREM sleep episode and the subsequent REM sleep episode; each NREM-REM sleep couplet is equal to one cycle. Any NREM sleep stage suffices as the NREM sleep portion of a cycle. An adult sleep period of 6.5 to 8.5 hours generally consists of four to six cycles. The cycle duration increases from infancy to young adulthood.

NREM Sleep Intrusion: An interposition of NREM sleep, or a component of NREM sleep physiology (e.g., elevated electromyographic activity, K-complex, sleep spindle, delta waves), in REM sleep; a portion of NREM sleep not appearing in its usual sleep-cycle position.

NREM Sleep Period: The NREM sleep portion of NREM-REM sleep cycle; such an episode consists primarily of sleep stages 3 and 4 early in the night and of sleep stage 2 later in the night. *See* Sleep Cycle; Sleep Stages.

Obesity-Hypoventilation Syndrome: A term applied to obese individuals who hypoventilate during wakefulness. Because the term can apply to several different disorders, its use is discouraged.

Paradoxical Sleep: This term is synonymous with REM sleep, which is the preferred term.

Parasomnia: A disorder of arousal, partial arousal, or sleep-stage transition. It represents an episodic disorder in sleep (such as sleepwalking) rather than a disorder in the quantity or timing of sleep or wakefulness per se. A parasomnia may be induced or exacerbated by sleep; a parasomnia is not a dyssomnia.

Paroxysm: Phenomenon of abrupt onset that rapidly attains a maximum level and terminates suddenly; paroxysm is distinguished from background activity. This term commonly refers to an epileptiform discharge on the electroencephalogram.

Paroxysmal Nocturnal Dyspnea (PND): Respiratory distress and shortness of breath that are due to pulmonary edema; the dyspnea appears suddenly and often awakens the sleeping individual.

Penile buckling Pressure: The amount of force applied to the glans of the penis that is sufficient to produce at least a 30° bend in the shaft.

Penile Rigidity: The firmness of the penis as measured by the penile-buckling pressure. Normally, the fully erect penis has maximum rigidity.

Period: The interval in time between the recurrence of a defined phase or moment of a rhythmic or periodic event. The time that occurs between one peak or trough and the next.

Periodic Leg Movement (PLM): A rapid partial flexion of the foot at the ankle, extension of the big toe, and partial flexion of the knee and hip that occurs during sleep. The movements occur with a periodicity of 20 to 60 seconds in a stereotyped pattern, lasting 0.5 to 5.0 seconds. PLMs are a characteristic feature of the periodic limb movement disorder.

Periodic Movements of Sleep (PMS): *See* Periodic Leg Movement.

Phase Advance: The shift of an episode of sleep or wake to an earlier position in the 24-hour sleep-wake cycle, A shift of sleep from 11 p.m.–7 a.m. to 8 p.m.–4 a.m. represents a three-hour phase advance. *See* Phase Delay.

Phase Delay: A shift of an episode of sleep or wake to a later position of the 24-hour sleep-wake cycle. A shift of sleep from 11 p.m.–7 a.m. to 2 a.m.–10 a.m. represents a three-hour phase delay. *See* Phase Advance.

Phase Transition: One of the two junctures of the major sleep and wake phases in the 24-hour sleep-wake cycle.

Phasic Event (Activity): Brain, muscle, or autonomic events of a brief and episodic nature that occur in sleep; a phasic event (such as eye movements or muscle twitches) is a characteristic of REM sleep; the usual duration is milliseconds to one to two seconds.

Photoperiod: The duration of light in a light-dark cycle.

Pickwickian: A term applied to an individual who snores, is obese and sleepy, and has alveolar hypoventilation. The term has been applied to many different disorders and, therefore, its use is discouraged.

PLM-Arousal Index: The number of sleep-related periodic leg movements per hour of sleep that are associated with an electroencephalographic arousal. *See* Periodic Leg Movement.

PLM Index: The number of periodic leg movements per hour of total sleep time as determined by all-night polysomnography; the index is sometimes expressed as the number of movements per hour of NREM sleep because the movements are usually inhibited during REM sleep. *See* Periodic Leg Movement.

PLM Percentage: The percentage of total sleep time occupied with recurrent episodes of periodic leg movements.

Polysomnogram: The continuous and simultaneous recording of multiple physiologic variables during sleep, i.e., electroencephalogram, electrooculogram, electromyogram (these are the three basic stage-scoring parameters), electrocardiogram, respiratory air flow, respiratory movements, leg movements, and other electrophysiologic variables.

Polysomnograph: A biomedical instrument used to measure physiologic variables of sleep.

Polysomnographic (as in Recording, Monitoring, Registration, or Tracings): Describes a recording on paper, computer disc, or tape of a polysomnogram.

Premature Morning Awakening (Early Morning Awakening): Early termination of the sleep episode, accompanied by an inability to return to sleep, sometimes after the last of several awakenings. It reflects interference at the end rather than at the commencement of the sleep episode. This awakening is a characteristic sleep disturbance of some people with depression.

Proposed Sleep Disorder: A disorder in which insufficient information is available in the medical literature to confirm the unequivocal existence of the disorder. This is a category of the International Classification of Sleep Disorders.

Quiet Sleep: A term used for describing NREM sleep in infants and animals when specific NREM sleep stages 1 through 4 cannot be determined.

Rapid Eye Movement Sleep (REM Sleep): *See* Sleep Stages.

Record: The end product of the polysomnograph recording process.

Recording: The process of obtaining a polysomnographic record. The term is also applied to the end product of the polysomnograph recording process.

REM Density (-Intensity): A function that expresses the frequency of eye movements per unit of time during sleep stage REM.

REM Sleep Episode: The REM sleep portion of a NREM-REM sleep cycle; early in the night it may be as short as 30 seconds, whereas in later cycles, it may be longer than an hour. *See* Sleep Stage REM.

REM Sleep Intrusion: A brief interval of REM sleep appearing out of its usual position in the NREM-REM sleep cycle; an interposition of REM sleep in NREM sleep; the intrusion can sometimes be the appearance of a single, dissociated component of REM sleep (e.g., eye movements, "drop out" of muscle tone) rather than all REM sleep parameters.

REM Sleep Latency: The interval from sleep onset to the first appearance of stage REM sleep in the sleep episode.

REM Sleep Onset: The designation for commencement of a REM sleep episode. This term can sometimes be used as a shorthand term for a sleep-onset REM-sleep episode. *See* Sleep Onset; Sleep-Onset REM Period (SOREMP).

REM Sleep Percent: The proportion of total sleep time constituted by the REM stage of sleep.

REM Sleep Rebound (Recovery): The lengthening and increase in frequency and density of REM sleep episodes, which result in an increase in REM sleep percent above baseline. REM sleep rebound follows REM sleep deprivation once the depriving influence is removed.

Respiratory-Disturbance Index (RDI) (Apnea-Hypopnea Index): The number of apneas (obstructive, central, or mixed) plus hypopneas per hour of total sleep time, as determined by all-night polysomnography.

Restlessness (Referring to a Quality of Sleep): Persistent or recurrent body movements, arousals, and brief awakenings that occur in the course of sleep.

Rhythm: An event that occurs at an approximately constant period length.

Saw-Tooth Waves: A form of theta rhythm that occurs during REM sleep and is characterized by a notched appearance in the waveform. The waves occur in bursts that last up to 10 seconds.

Severity Criteria: Criteria for establishing the severity of a particular sleep disorder, according to the following categories: mild, moderate, or severe.

Sleep Architecture: The NREM-REM sleep-stage and cycle infrastructure of sleep understood from the vantage point of the quantitative relationship of these components to each other. Often plotted in the form of a histogram.

Sleep Cycle: Synonymous with the NREM-REM Sleep Cycle.

Sleep Efficiency (or Sleep-Efficiency Index): The proportion of sleep in the episode potentially filled by sleep (i.e., the ratio of total sleep time to time in bed).

Sleep Episode: An interval of sleep that may be voluntary or involuntary. In the sleep laboratory, the sleep episode occurs from the time of "lights out" to the time of "lights on." The major sleep episode is usually the longest daily sleep episode.

Sleep Hygiene: The conditions and practices that promote continuous and effective sleep. These include regularity of bedtime and arise time; conformity of time spent in bed to the time necessary for sustained and individually adequate sleep (i.e., the total sleep time sufficient to avoid sleepiness when awake); restriction of alcohol and caffeine beverages before bedtime; and employment of exercise, nutrition, and environment factors so that they enhance, not disturb, restful sleep.

Sleepiness (Somnolence, Drowsiness): Difficulty in maintaining alert wakefulness so that the person falls asleep if not actively kept aroused. The sleepiness is not simply a feeling of physical tiredness or listlessness. When sleepiness occurs in inappropriate circumstances, it is considered to be excessive sleepiness.

Sleep Interruption: Breaks in sleep that result in arousal and wakefulness. *See* Fragmentation; Restlessness.

Sleep Latency: The duration of time from "lights out," or bedtime, to the onset of sleep.

Sleep Log (Diary): A daily, written record of a person's sleep-wake pattern that contains such information as time of retiring and arising, time in bed, estimated total sleep time, number and duration of sleep interruptions, quality of sleep, daytime naps, use of medications or caffeine-containing beverages, and the nature of waking activities.

Sleep Maintenance DIMS (Insomnia): A disturbance in maintaining sleep after sleep onset is achieved; persistently interrupted sleep without difficulty falling asleep; a disorder characterized by sleep-continuity disturbance.

Sleep Mentation: The imagery and thinking experienced during sleep. Sleep mentation usually consists of combinations of images and thoughts during REM sleep. Imagery is vividly expressed in dreams involving all the senses in approximate proportion to their waking representations. Mentation is experienced generally less distinctly in NREM sleep, but it may be quite vivid in stage 2 sleep, especially toward the end of the sleep episode. Mentation at sleep onset (hypnagogic reverie) can be as vivid as that which occurs during REM sleep.

Sleep Onset: The transition from awake to sleep, normally to NREM stage 1 sleep but in certain conditions, such as infancy and narcolepsy, into stage REM sleep. To establish sleep onset, most polysomnographers accept electroencephalographic slowing, reduction, and eventual disappearance of alpha activity, presence of electroencephalographic vertex sharp transients, and slow rolling eye movements (the components of NREM stage 1) as sufficient for sleep onset; others require appearance of stage 2 patterns. *See* Latency; Sleep Stages.

Sleep-Onset REM Period (SOREMP): The beginning of sleep by entrance directly into stage REM sleep. The onset of REM sleep occurs within 10 minutes of sleep onset.

Sleep Paralysis: Immobility of the body that occurs in the transition from sleep to wakefulness (i.e., atonia); this is a partial manifestation of REM sleep.

Sleep Pattern (24-Hour Sleep-Wake Pattern): A person's clock-hour schedule of bedtime and arise time as well as nap behavior; the sleep pattern may also include time and duration of sleep interruptions. *See* Sleep-Wake Cycle; Circadian Rhythm; Sleep Log.

Sleep-Related Erections: The natural periodic cycle of penile erections that occur during sleep, typically associated with REM sleep. Sleep-related erectile activity can be characterized by four phases: T-up (ascending tumescence), T-max (plateau maximal tumescence), T-down (detumescence), and T-zero (no tumescence). Polysomnographic assessment of sleep-related erections is useful for differentiating organic from nonorganic erectile dysfunction.

Sleep Spindle: Spindle-shaped bursts of 11.5- to 15-Hz electroencephalographic waveforms that last 0.5 to 1.5 seconds. The spindles bursts are generally diffuse, but they are of highest voltage over the central regions of the head. The amplitude is generally less than 50 µV in the adult. These waveforms are one of the identifying electroencephalographic features of NREM stage 2 sleep; they may persist into NREM stages 3 and 4 but generally are not seen in REM sleep.

Sleep-Stage Demarcation: The significant polysomnographic characteristics that distinguish the boundaries of the sleep stages. In certain conditions and with the use of certain drugs, sleep-stage demarcations may be blurred or lost, making it difficult to identify certain stages with certainty or to distinguish the temporal limits of sleep-stage lengths.

Sleep-Stage Episode: A sleep-stage interval that represents the stage in a NREM-REM sleep cycle; this concept is easiest to comprehend in relation to REM sleep, which is a homogeneous stage, i.e., the fourth REM sleep episode is in the fourth sleep cycle (unless a prior REM episode was skipped). If one interval of REM sleep is separated from another by more than 20 minutes, they constitute separate REM sleep episodes (and are in separate sleep cycles); a sleep-stage episode may be of any duration.

Sleep Stage NREM: One of the two major sleep states, distinguished from REM sleep; this stage comprises sleep stages 1 through 4, which constitute levels in the spectrum of NREM sleep "depth" or physiologic intensity.

Sleep Stage REM: The stage of sleep with the highest brain activity, characterized by enhanced brain metabolism and vivid hallucinatory imagery or dreaming. There are spontaneous rapid eye movements, resting muscle activity is suppressed, and awakening threshold to nonsignificant stimuli is high. The electroencephalogram is a low-voltage, mixed-frequency, nonalpha record. REM sleep is usually 20% to 25% of total sleep time. It is also called "paradoxical sleep."

Sleep Stages: Distinctive stages of sleep, best demonstrated by polysomnographic recordings of the electroencephalogram, electrooculogram, and electromyogram.

Sleep Stage 1 (NREM Stage 1): A stage of NREM sleep that occurs at sleep onset or that follows arousal from sleep stages 2, 3, 4, or REM. It consists of a relatively low-voltage electroencephalographic recording with mixed frequency, mainly theta activity, and alpha activity of less than 50% of the scoring epoch. It contains electroencephalographic vertex waves and slow rolling eye movements and no sleep spindles, K complexes, or REMs. Stage 1 sleep normally represents 4% to 5% of the major sleep episode.

Sleep Stage 2 (NREM Stage 2): A stage of NREM sleep characterized by the presence of sleep spindles and K complexes present in a relatively low-voltage, mixed-frequency electroencephalographic background; high-voltage delta waves may comprise up to 20% of stage 2 epochs. Stage 2 sleep usually accounts for 45% to 55% of the major sleep episode.

Sleep Stage 3 (NREM Stage 3): A stage of NREM sleep defined by at least 20% and not more than 50% of the episode consisting of electroencephalographic waves less than 2 Hz and more than 75 µV (high-amplitude delta waves). This is also known as a "delta" sleep stage. In combination with stage 4, it constitutes "deep" NREM sleep or slow-wave sleep; this stage is often combined with stage 4 into NREM sleep stage 3/4 because of the lack of documented physiologic differences between the two stages. Stage 3 sleep usually appears only in the first third of the sleep episode and usually comprises 4% to 6% of total sleep time.

Sleep Stage 4 (NREM Stage 4): All statements concerning NREM sleep stage 3 apply to sleep stage 4 except that high-voltage, electroencephalographic slow waves persist during 50% or more of the epoch in stage 4 sleep. NREM sleep stage 4 usually represents 12% to 15% of the total sleep time. Sleepwalking, sleep terrors, and confusional-arousal episodes generally begin in stage 4 or during arousals from this stage. *See* Sleep Stage 3.

Sleep Structure: This term refers to sleep architecture. In addition to encompassing sleep stages and sleep cycle relationships, however, sleep structure assesses the within-stage qualities of the electroencephalogram and other physiologic attributes.

Sleep Talking: Talking in sleep that usually occurs in the course of transitory arousals from NREM sleep. The talking can occur during stage REM sleep, at which time it represents a motor breakthrough of dream speech. Full consciousness is not achieved, and no memory of the event remains.

Sleep-Wake Cycle: Basically, the clock-hour relationships of the major sleep and wake episodes in the 24-hour cycle. *See* Phase Transition; Circadian Rhythm.

Sleep-Wake Shift (Change, Reversal): A shift that occurs when sleep as a whole, or in part, is moved to a time of customary waking activity, and the latter is moved to the time of the major sleep episode. This shift is common during periods of jet lag and shift work.

Sleep-Wake Transition Disorder: A disorder that occurs during the transition from wakefulness to sleep or from one sleep stage to another. This disorder is a form of the parasomnias and is not a dyssomnia.

Slow-Wave Sleep (SWS): Sleep characterized by electroencephalographic waves of duration slower than 8 Hz. This term is synonymous with sleep stages 3 plus 4 combined. *See* Delta Sleep Stage.

Snoring: A noise produced primarily with inspiratory respiration during sleep that is due to vibration of the soft palate and the pillars of the oropharyngeal inlet. All snorers have incomplete obstruction of the upper airway, and many habitual snorers have complete episodes of upper-airway obstruction.

Spindle REM Sleep: A condition in which sleep spindles persist atypically in REM sleep; this finding is seen in patients with chronic insomnia conditions and occasionally in the first REM period.

Synchronized: A chronobiologic term used to indicate that two or more rhythms recur with the same phase relationship. In electroencephalography, it is used to indicate an increased amplitude and usually a decreased frequency of the dominant activities.

Theta Activity: Electroencephalographic activity with a frequency of 4 to 8 Hz, generally maximal over the central and temporal cortex.

Total Recording Time (TRT): The duration of time from sleep onset to final awakening. In addition to total sleep time, it comprises the time taken up by wake periods and movement time until final awakening. *See* Sleep Efficiency.

Total Sleep Episode: This is the total time available for sleep during an attempt to sleep. It comprises NREM and REM sleep, as well as wakefulness. This term is synonymous with and preferred to the term total sleep period.

Total Sleep Time (TST): The amount of actual sleep time in a sleep episode; this time is equal to the total sleep episode less the awake time. Total sleep time is the total of all REM and NREM sleep in a sleep episode.

Trace Alternant: An electroencephalographic pattern of sleeping newborns, characterized by bursts of slow waves, at times intermixed with sharp waves, and intervening periods of relative quiescence with extreme low-amplitude activity.

Tumescence (Penile): Hardening and expansion of the penis (penile erection). When associated with REM sleep, it is referred to as a sleep-related erection.

Twitch (Body Twitch): A very small body movement such as a local foot or finger jerk; this movement usually is not associated with arousal.

Vertex Sharp Transient: Sharp negative potential, maximal at the vertex, occurring spontaneously during sleep or in response to a sensory stimulus during sleep or wakefulness. The amplitude varies but rarely exceeds 250 µV. Use of the term vertex sharp wave is discouraged.

Wake Time: The total time occurring between sleep onset and final wake-up time that is scored as wakefulness in a polysomnogram.

Waxing and Waning: A crescendo-decrescendo pattern of activity, usually electroencephalographic activity.

Zeitgeber: An environmental time cue, such as sunlight, noise, social interaction, alarm clocks, that usually helps an individual entrain to the 24-hour day.

List of Abbreviations

AHI	Apnea-Hypopnea Index	MWT	Maintenance of Wakefulness Test
AI	Apnea Index		
ASDA	American Sleep Disorders Association	NPT	Nocturnal Penile Tumescence
CNS	Central Nervous System	NOS	Not Otherwise Specified
DIMS	Disorder of Initiating and Maintaining Sleep	NREM	Non-Rapid Eye Movement (Sleep)
DOES	Disorder of Excessive Somnolence	PLM	Periodic Leg Movement
		PND	Paroxysmal Nocturnal Dystonia
DSM	Diagnostic and Statistical Manual	PSG	Polysomnogram
EEG	Electroencephalogram	RDI	Respiratory-Disturbance Index
EMG	Electromyogram		
EOG	Electrooculogram	REM	Rapid Eye Movement (Sleep)
Hz	Hertz (Cycles per Second)		
ICD	International Classification of Diseases	REMs	Rapid Eye Movements
		RLS	Restless Legs Syndrome
ICSD	International Classification of Sleep Disorders	SDB	Sleep-Disordered Breathing
		SOREMP	Sleep-Onset REM Period
MSLT	Multiple Sleep Latency Test	SWS	Slow-Wave Sleep
		TST	Total Sleep Time

GENERAL BIBLIOGRAPHY

Recommended Books, Monographs, and Reviews on Sleep and Sleep Disorders

Anch AM, Browman CP, Mitler MM, Walsh JK. Sleep: A scientific perspective. New Jersey: Prentice Hall, 1988.

Association of Sleep Disorders Centers. Diagnostic classification of sleep and arousal disorders, 1st ed. Prepared by the Sleep Disorders Classification Committee, H. P. Roffwarg, Chairman. Sleep 1979; 2: 1–137.

Barnes C, Orem J. Physiology in sleep. New York: Academic Press, 1980.

Benoit O, ed. Physiologie du sommeil: Sur exploration fonctionnelle. Paris: Masson, 1984.

Degen R, Niedermeyer E, eds. Epilepsy, sleep and sleep deprivation. Amsterdam: Elsevier, 1983.

Dinges DF, Broughton RJ. Sleep and alertness: chronobiological, behavioral and medical aspects of napping. New York: Raven Press, 1989.

Erman MK, ed. Psychiatric clinics of North America: Sleep disorders. Philadelphia: WB Saunders, 1987; 10(4): 517–724.

Fairbanks DNF, Fujita S, Ikematsu T, Simmons FB, eds. Snoring and obstructive sleep apnea. New York: Raven Press, 1987.

Ferber R. Solve your child's sleep problems. New York: Simon and Schuster, 1985.

Fletcher EC, ed. Abnormalities of respiration during sleep. Diagnosis, pathophysiology, and treatment. Orlando: Grune & Stratton, 1986.

Guilleminault C, ed. Sleeping and waking disorders. Menlo Park, California: Addison-Wesley, 1982.

Guilleminault C, ed. Sleep and its disorders in children. New York: Raven Press, 1987.

Guilleminault C, Dement WC, eds. Sleep apnea syndromes. New York: Alan R. Liss, 1978.

Guilleminault C, Dement WC, Passouant P, eds. Advances in sleep research, Volume 3: Narcolepsy. New York: Spectrum Publications, 1976.

Guilleminault C, Lugaresi E, eds. Sleep/wake disorders: Natural history, epidemiology, and long-term evolution. New York: Raven Press, 1983.

Kryger MH, ed. Clinics in chest medicine: Sleep disorders. Philadelphia: WB Saunders, 1985; 6(4): 553–730.

Kryger MH, Roth T, Dement WC, eds. Principles and practice of sleep medicine. Philadelphia: WB Saunders, 1989.

Lugaresi E, Coccagna G, Mantovani M. Advances in sleep research, hypersomnia with periodic apneas, Volume 4. New York: Spectrum Publications, 1978.

McGinty DJ, Drucker-Colín R, Morrison A, Parmeggiani PL. Brain mechanisms of sleep. New York: Raven Press, 1985.

Mendleson WB. Human sleep: research and clinical care. New York: Plenum Press, 1987.

Parkes JD. Major problems in neurology. Sleep and its disorders. London: WB Saunders, 1985; Vol. 14.

Peter JH, Podszus T, von Wichert P, eds. Sleep related disorders and internal diseases. Berlin: Springer-Verlag, 1987.

Riley TL, ed. Clinical aspects, sleep and nap disturbance. London: Butterworth, 1985.

Roth B. Narcolepsy and hypersomnia. Revised and edited by R. Broughton. Basel: Karger, 1980.

Saunders NA, Sullivan CE, eds. Lung biology in health and disease. Sleep and breathing. New York: Marcel Dekker, 1984; Vol. 21.

Sterman MB, Shouse MN, Passouant P, eds. Sleep and epilepsy. New York: Academic Press, 1982.

Thawley SE, ed. Medical clinics of North America: Sleep apnea disorders. Philadelphia: WB Saunders, 1985; 69(6): 1121–1412.

Thorpy MJ, ed. Handbook of sleep disorders. In: Koller W, series ed. Neurological disease and therapy series. New York: Marcel Dekker, 1990.

Thorpy MJ, Yager J. The encyclopedia of sleep and sleep disorders. New York: Facts on File, 1990.

Williams RL, Karacan I, Moore C, eds. Sleep disorders: Diagnosis and treatment, 2nd ed. New York: John Wiley & Sons, 1988.

APPENDIX A

ICSD Listing by *ICD-9-CM* Medical System

The listing of the *International Classification of Sleep Disorders* by medical system is to aid the clinician in categorizing the sleep disorders according to the headings of the *International Classification of Diseases (ICD)*, 9th revision. The list given here does not conform strictly to the ICD structure as presented in the *ICD-9-CM* because some disorders have been placed in the section considered to be more appropriate.

Many sleep disorders do not fit neatly into traditional medical classification systems because more than one medical system can be involved in a particular disorder and the exact cause is often unknown. In addition, differential diagnoses of the sleep disorders cross medical systems (e.g., the differential diagnosis of excessive sleepiness usually involves narcolepsy and obstructive sleep apnea syndrome). The main differential diagnosis of obstructive sleep apnea syndrome only rarely includes other pulmonary disorders, such as sarcoidosis. For classification purposes, a separate systematic category for the sleep disorders based on sleep features, as presented in axis A of the *ICSD* (sleep diagnoses), is regarded as preferable, and would be more suitable for future editions of the *ICD*. For differential diagnostic purposes, a different listing is given in Appendix A.

Subcategories are listed under the Mental Disorders because many sleep disorders can have developmental or behavioral components and may not be caused by mental disease. Developmental, behavioral, environmental, and circadian rhythm sleep disorders subcategories are presented. They are listed under the Mental Disorders because another more appropriate category does not exist in the *ICD*. However, some of these disorders, such as sleep terrors, may be exacerbated or produced by psychopathology.

1. MENTAL DISORDERS
   a. Developmental Sleep Disorders
      Rhythmic Movement Disorder................... 307.3
      Sleep Bruxism................................ 306.8
      Sleepwalking................................. 307.46-0
      Sleep Terrors................................ 307.46-1
      Confusional Arousals......................... 307.46-2
      Nightmares 307.47-0
      Sleep Starts................................. 307.47-2
      Sleep Talking................................ 307.47-3
      Sleep Enuresis............................... 788.36
      Sleep Paralysis 780.56-0

356 MEDICAL SYSTEM

    b. Behavioral Sleep Disorders
       Adjustment Sleep Disorder 307.41-0
       Inadequate Sleep Hygiene 307.41-1
       Psychophysiologic Insomnia 307.42-0
       Sleep Choking Syndrome 307.42-1
       Limit-Setting Sleep Disorder................... 307.42-4
       Sleep-Onset Association Disorder 307.42-5
       Terrifying Hypnagogic Hallucinations 307.47-4
       Sleep-State Misperception..................... 307.49-1
       Insufficient Sleep Syndrome 307.49-4
       Hypnotic-Dependent Sleep Disorder 780.52-0
       Stimulant-Dependent Sleep Disorder............ 780.52-1
       Alcohol-Dependent Sleep Disorder 780.52-3
       Idiopathic Insomnia........................... 780.52-7
       Nocturnal Eating (Drinking) Syndrome 780.52-8

    c. Circadian Rhythm Sleep Disorders
       Time Zone Change (Jet Lag) Syndrome........... 307.45-0
       Shift Work Sleep Disorder..................... 307.45-1
       Irregular Sleep-Wake Pattern 307.45-3
       Short Sleeper................................. 307.49-0
       Long Sleeper................................. 307.49-2
       Delayed Sleep-Phase Syndrome................. 780.55-0
       Advanced Sleep-Phase Syndrome 780.55-1
       Non-24-Hour Sleep-Wake Disorder.............. 780.55-2

    d. Environmental Sleep Disorders
       Food Allergy Insomnia 780.52-2
       Environmental Sleep Disorder.................. 780.52-6
       Toxin-Induced Sleep Disorder 780.54-6

    e. Psychopathologic Disorders
       Psychoses 290-299
       Mood Disorders.............................. 296, 300, 301, 311
       Anxiety Disorders 300, 308, 309
       Panic Disorder............................... 300
       Alcoholism 303, 305

2. DISEASES OF THE RESPIRATORY SYSTEM

       Altitude Insomnia 289.0
       Chronic Obstructive Pulmonary Disease 490-496
       Sleep-Related Asthma........................ 493
       Central Sleep Apnea Syndrome 780.51-0
       Central Alveolar Hypoventilation Syndrome 780.51-1
       Obstructive Sleep Apnea Syndrome.............. 780.53-0
       Primary Snoring 786.9
       Sleep-Related Neurogenic Tachypnea 780.53-2
       Sleep-Related Abnormal Swallowing Syndrome 780.56-6
       Sleep-Related Laryngospasm................... 780.57-4

3. DISEASES OF THE CIRCULATORY SYSTEM
   - Nocturnal Cardiac Ischemia 411-414
   - REM Sleep-Related Sinus Arrest 780.56-8
   - Sudden Unexplained Nocturnal Death Syndrome 780.59-3

4. DISEASES OF THE NERVOUS SYSTEM
   - Sleeping Sickness 086.9
   - Subwakefulness Syndrome 307.49-3
   - Cerebral Degenerative Disorders 330-337
   - Dementia 331
   - Parkinsonism 332-333
   - Fatal Familial Insomnia 337.9
   - Sleep-Related Epilepsy 345
   - Electrical Status Epilepticus of Sleep 345.8
   - Sleep-Related Headaches 346
   - Narcolepsy 347
   - Recurrent Hypersomnia 349.89-0
   - Nocturnal Leg Cramps 729.82
   - Periodic Limb Movement Disorder 780.52-4
   - Restless Legs Syndrome 780.52-5
   - Idiopathic Hypersomnia 780.54-7
   - Posttraumatic Hypersomnia 780.54-8
   - REM-Sleep Behavior Disorder 780.59-0
   - Nocturnal Paroxysmal Dystonia 780.59-1
   - Fragmentary Myoclonus 780.59-7
   - Sleep Hyperhidrosis 780.8

5. DISEASES OF THE DIGESTIVE SYSTEM
   - Sleep-Related Gastroesophageal Reflux 530.81
   - Peptic Ulcer Disease 531-534

6. DISEASES OF THE GENITOURINARY SYSTEM
   - Menstrual-Associated Sleep Disorder 780.54-3
   - Menopausal Sleeplessness 627.2
   - Impaired Sleep-Related Penile Erections 780.56-3
   - Sleep-Related Painful Erections 780.56-4

7. DISEASES OF PREGNANCY, CHILDBIRTH, AND THE PUERPERIUM
   - Pregnancy-Associated Sleep Disorder 780.59-6

8. DISEASES OF THE MUSCULOSKELETAL SYSTEM AND CONNECTIVE TISSUE
   - Fibromyalgia 729.1

9. CERTAIN CONDITIONS ORIGINATING IN THE PERINATAL PERIOD
   - Infant Sleep Apnea 770.80
   - Congenital Central Hypoventilation Syndrome 770.81
   - Benign Neonatal Sleep Myoclonus 780.59-5
   - Sudden Infant Death Syndrome 798.0

ICD-9-CM Listings

ICSD Alphabetical Listing

Adjustment Sleep Disorder	307.41-0
Advanced Sleep-Phase Syndrome	780.55-1
Alcohol-Dependent Sleep Disorder	780.52-3
Alcoholism	303, 305
Altitude Insomnia	289.0
Anxiety Disorders	300, 308, 309
Benign Neonatal Sleep Myoclonus	780.59-5
Central Alveolar Hypoventilation Syndrome	780.51-1
Central Sleep Apnea Syndrome	780.51-0
Cerebral Degenerative Disorders	330-337
Chronic Obstructive Pulmonary Disease	490-496
Circadian Rhythm Sleep Disorder NOS	780.55-9
Confusional Arousals	307.46-2
Congenital Central Hypoventilation Syndrome	770.81
Delayed Sleep-Phase Syndrome	780.55-0
Dementia	331
Electrical Status Epilepticus of Sleep	345.8
Environmental Sleep Disorder	780.52-6
Extrinsic Sleep Disorder NOS	780.52-9
Fatal Familial Insomnia	337.9
Fibromyalgia	729.1
Food Allergy Insomnia	780.52-2
Fragmentary Myoclonus	780.59-7
Hypnotic-Dependent Sleep Disorder	780.52-0
Idiopathic Hypersomnia	780.54-7
Idiopathic Insomnia	780.52-7
Impaired Sleep-Related Penile Erections	780.56-3
Inadequate Sleep Hygiene	307.41-1
Infant Sleep Apnea	770.80
Insufficient Sleep Syndrome	307.49-4
Intrinsic Sleep Disorder NOS	780.52-9
Irregular Sleep-Wake Pattern	307.45-3
Limit-Setting Sleep Disorder	307.42-5
Long Sleeper	307.49-2
Menstrual-Associated Sleep Disorder	780.54-3
Mood Disorders	296, 300, 301, 311
Narcolepsy	347
Nightmares	307.47-0
Nocturnal Cardiac Ischemia	411-414
Nocturnal Eating (Drinking) Syndrome	780.52-8
Nocturnal Leg Cramps	729.82
Nocturnal Paroxysmal Dystonia	780.59-1
Non-24-Hour Sleep-Wake Syndrome	780.55-2

Obstructive Sleep Apnea Syndrome	780.53-0
Other Parasomnia, NOS	780.59-9
Parkinsonism	332-333
Panic Disorder	300
Peptic Ulcer Disease	531-532
Periodic Limb Movement Disorder	780.52-4
Posttraumatic Hypersomnia	780.54-8
Pregnancy-Associated Sleep Disorder	780.59-6
Primary Snoring	780.53-1
Psychophysiologic Insomnia	307.42-0
Psychoses	292-299
Recurrent Hypersomnia	780.54-2
REM-Sleep Behavior Disorder	780.59-0
REM Sleep-related Sinus Arrest	780.56-8
Restless Legs Syndrome	780.52-5
Rhythmic Movement Disorder	307.3
Shift Work Sleep Disorder	307.45-1
Short Sleeper	307.49-0
Sleep Bruxism	306.8
Sleep Choking Syndrome	307.42-1
Sleep Enuresis	345.8
Sleep Hyperhidrosis	780.8
Sleeping Sickness	086.9
Sleep-Onset Association Disorder	307.42-4
Sleep Paralysis	780.56-2
Sleep-Related Abnormal Swallowing Syndrome	780.56-6
Sleep-Related Asthma	493
Sleep-Related Epilepsy	345
Sleep-Related Gastroesophageal Reflux	530.81
Sleep-Related Headaches	346
Sleep-Related Laryngospasm	780.59-4
Sleep-Related Painful Erections	780.56-4
Sleep-Related Neurogenic Tachypnea	780.53-2
Sleep Starts	307.47-2
Sleep-State Misperception	307.49-1
Sleep Talking	307.47-3
Sleep Terrors	307.46-1
Sleepwalking	307.46-0
Stimulant-Dependent Sleep Disorder	780.52-1
Subwakefulness Syndrome	307.49-3
Sudden Infant Death Syndrome	798.0
Sudden Unexplained Nocturnal Death Syndrome	708.59-3
Terrifying Hypnagogic Hallucinations	307.47-4
Time Zone Change (Jet Lag) Syndrome	307.45-0
Toxin-Induced Sleep Disorder	780.54-6

ICD-9-CM Numerical Listing

086.9	Sleeping Sickness
289.0	Altitude Insomnia
290-319	Mental Disorders
290-299	Psychoses
296, 300, 301, 311	Mood Disorders
300, 308, 309	Anxiety Disorders
300	Panic Disorders
303, 305	Alcoholism
306.8	Sleep Bruxism
307.3	Rhythmic Movement Disorder
307.41-0	Adjustment Sleep Disorder
307.41-1	Inadequate Sleep Hygiene
307.42-0	Psychophysiologic Insomnia
307.42-1	Sleep Choking Syndrome
307.42-4	Sleep-Onset Association Disorder
307.45-5	Limit-Setting Sleep Disorder
307.45-0	Time Zone Change (Jet Lag) Syndrome
307.45-1	Shift Work Sleep Disorder
307.45-3	Irregular Sleep-Wake Pattern
307.46-0	Sleepwalking
307.46-1	Sleep Terrors
307.46-2	Confusional Arousals
307.47-0	Nightmares
307.47-2	Sleep Starts
307.47-3	Sleep Talking
307.47-4	Terrifying Hypnagogic Hallucinations
307.49-0	Short Sleeper
307.49-1	Sleep-State Misperception
307.49-2	Long Sleeper
307.49-3	Subwakefulness Syndrome
307.49-4	Insufficient Sleep Syndrome
320-389	Nervous System Diseases
330-337	Cerebral Degenerative Disorders
331	Dementia
332-333	Parkinsonism
337.9	Fatal Familial Insomnia
345	Epilepsy
345.8	Electrical Status Epilepticus of Sleep
346	Headaches
347	Narcolepsy
411-414	Nocturnal Cardiac Ischemia
460-519	Respiratory Disorders
490-496	Chronic Obstructive Pulmonary Disease
493	Sleep-Related Asthma
530.81	Sleep-Related Gastroesophageal Reflux

NUMERICAL LISTING

531-534	Peptic Ulcer Disease
627.2	Menopausal Sleeplessness
729.1	Fibromyalgia
729.82	Nocturnal Leg Cramps
770.80	Infant Sleep Apnea
770.81	Congenital Central Hypoventilation Syndrome
780.51-0	Central Sleep Apnea Syndrome
780.51-1	Central Alveolar Hypoventilation Syndrome
780.52-0	Hypnotic-Dependent Sleep Disorder
780.52-1	Stimulant-Dependent Sleep Disorder
798.00	Sudden Infant Death Syndrome
780.52-2	Food Allergy Insomnia
780.52-3	Alcohol-Dependent Sleep Disorder
780.52-4	Periodic Limb Movement Disorder
780.52-5	Restless Legs Syndrome
780.52-6	Environmental Sleep Disorder
780.52-7	Idiopathic Insomnia
780.52-8	Nocturnal Eating (Drinking) Syndrome
780.52-9	Intrinsic-Extrinsic Sleep Disorder, NOS
780.53-0	Obstructive Sleep Apnea Syndrome
780.53-2	Sleep-Related Neurogenic Tachypnea
780.54-2	Recurrent Hypersomnia
780.54-3	Menstrual-Associated Sleep Disorder
780.54-6	Toxin-Induced Sleep Disorder
780.54-7	Idiopathic Hypersomnia
780.54-8	Posttraumatic Hypersomnia
780.55-0	Delayed Sleep-Phase Syndrome
780.55-1	Advanced Sleep-Phase Syndrome
780.55-2	Non-24-Hour Sleep-Wake Syndrome
780.55-9	Circadian Rhythm Sleep Disorder, NOS
780.56-2	Sleep Paralysis
780.56-3	Impaired Sleep-Related Penile Erections
780.56-4	Sleep-Related Painful Erections
780.56-6	Sleep-Related Abnormal Swallowing Syndrome
780.56-8	REM Sleep-Related Sinus Arrest
780.59-0	REM Sleep Behavior Disorder
780.59-1	Nocturnal Paroxysmal Dystonia
780.59-3	Sudden Unexplained Nocturnal Death Syndrome
780.59-4	Sleep-Related Larynogospasm
780.59-5	Benign Neonatal Sleep Myoclonus
780.59-6	Pregnancy-Associated Sleep Disorder
780.59-7	Fragmentary Myoclonus
780.59-9	Other Parasomnia, NOS
780.8	Sleep Hyperhidrosis
786.09	Primary Snoring
788.36	Sleep Enuresis

ICD-9-CM Sleep Listings:
307.4 Specific Disorders of Sleep of Nonorganic Origin
and
780.5 Sleep Disturbances

The listing here is based upon the headings of the major sleep sections in the *ICD-9-CM*, Volume 1, and contains the *ICSD* diagnoses presented under each heading with the appropriate code number. This listing is not part of the official *ICD-9-CM* publication but is the proposed coding system for the disorders contained in the *ICSD*. The system is fully compatible with the respective *ICD-9-CM* sections, and the five-digit code numbers and subheading statements are those of the *ICD-9-CM;* however, the *ICD-9-CM* subheadings are not used in the *ICSD*. The disorders listed here do not comprise a complete listing of all the disorders presented in the *ICSD*, because many disorders fall under code numbers that are classified elsewhere in the *ICD-9-CM* publication.

307.4 Specific Disorders of Sleep of Nonorganic Origin

Excludes: Narcolepsy (347)
Those of Unspecified Cause (780.50-780.59)

- 307.40 Nonorganic Sleep Disorder, Unspecified
- 307.41 Transient Disorder of Initiating or Maintaining Sleep
  - 307.41-0 Adjustment Sleep Disorder
  - 307.41-1 Inadequate Sleep Hygiene
- 307.42 Persistent Disorder of Initiating or Maintaining Sleep
  - 307.42-0 Psychophysiologic Insomnia
  - 307.42-1 Sleep Choking Syndrome
- 307.43 Transient Disorder of Initiating or Maintaining Wakefulness
- 307.44 Persistent Disorder of Initiating or Maintaining Wakefulness
- 307.45 Phase-Shift Disruption of 24-Hour Sleep-Wake Cycle
  - 307.45-0 Time Zone Change (Jet Lag) Syndrome
  - 307.45-1 Shift Work Sleep Disorder
  - 307.45-3 Irregular Sleep-Wake Pattern
- 307.46 Somnambulism or Night Terrors
  - 307.46-0 Sleepwalking
  - 307.46-1 Sleep Terrors
  - 307.46-2 Confusional Arousals
- 307.47 Other Dysfunctions of Sleep Stages or Arousal from Sleep
  - 307.47-0 Nightmares
  - 307.47-1 Subwakefu lness Syndrome
  - 307.47-2 Sleep Starts
  - 307.47-3 Sleep Talking
  - 307.47-4 Terrifying Hypnagogic Hallucinations

ICD-9-CM LISTING

307.48 Repetitive Intrusions of Sleep
307.49 Other
    307.49-0 Short Sleeper
    307.49-1 Sleep State Misperception
    307.49-2 Long Sleeper
    307.49-3 Subwakefulness Syndrome
    307.49-4 Insufficient Sleep Syndrome

780.5 Sleep Disturbances

Excludes: Those of Nonorganic Origin (307.40-307.49)

780.50 Sleep Disturbance, Unspecified
780.51 Insomnia with Sleep Apnea
    780.51-0 Central Sleep Apnea Syndrome
    780.51-1 Central Alveolar Hypoventilation Syndrome
780.52 Other Insomnia
    627.2 Menopausal Sleeplessness
    780.52-0 Hypnotic-Dependent Sleep Disorder
    780.52-1 Stimulant-Dependent Sleep Disorder
    780.52-2 Food Allergy Insomnia
    780.52-3 Alcohol-Dependent Sleep Disorder
    780.52-4 Periodic Limb Movement Disorder
    780.52-5 Restless Legs Syndrome
    780.52-6 Environmental Sleep Disorder
    780.52-7 Idiopathic Insomnia
    780.52-8 Nocturnal Eating (Drinking) Syndrome
    780.52-9 Intrinsic-Extrinsic Sleep Disorder, NOS
780.53 Hypersomnia with Sleep Apnea
    780.53-0 Obstructive Sleep Apnea Syndrome
    780.9 Primary Snoring
    780.53-2 Sleep-Related Neurogenic Tachypnea
780.54 Other Hypersomnia
    780.54-2 Recurrent Hypersomnia
    780.54-3 Menstrual-Associated Sleep Disorder
    780.54-6 Toxin-Induced Sleep Disorder
    780.54-7 Idiopathic Hypersomnia
    780.54-8 Posttraumatic Hypersomnia
    780.54-9 Intrinsic-Extrinsic Sleep Disorder, NOS
780.55 Disruptions of 24-Hour Sleep-Wake Cycle
    780.55-0 Delayed Sleep-Phase Syndrome
    780.55-1 Advanced Sleep-Phase Syndrome
    780.55-2 Non-24-Hour Sleep-Wake Syndrome
    780.55-9 Circadian Rhythm Sleep Disorder, NOS

780.56   Dysfunctions Associated with Sleep Stages or Arousal from Sleep
    788.36   Sleep Enuresis
    780.56-2   Sleep Paralysis
    780.56-3   Impaired Sleep-Related Penile Erections
    780.56-4   Sleep-Related Painful Erections
    780.56-6   Sleep-Related Abnormal Swallowing Syndrome
    780.53-2   Sleep-Related Neurogenic Tachypnea

780.54   Other Hypersomnia
    780.54-2   Recurrent Hypersomnia
    780.54-3   Menstrual-Associated Sleep Disorder
    780.54-6   Toxin-Induced Sleep Disorder
    780.54-7   Idiopathic Hypersomnia
    780.54-8   Post-traumatic Hypersomnia
    780.54-9   Intrinsic-Extrinsic Sleep Disorder, NOS

780.55   Disruptions of 24-Hour Sleep-Wake Cycle
    780.55-0   Delayed Sleep-Phase Syndrome
    780.55-1   Advanced Sleep-Phase Syndrome
    780.55-2   Non-24-Hour Sleep-Wake Syndrome
    780.55-9   Circadian Rhythm Sleep Disorder, NOS

780.56   Dysfunctions Associated with Sleep Stages or Arousal from Sleep
    788.36   Sleep Enuresis
    780.56-2   Sleep Paralysis
    780.56-3   Impaired Sleep-Related Penile Erections
    780.56-4   Sleep-Related Painful Erections
    780.56-6   Sleep-Related Abnormal Swallowing Syndrome
    780.56-8   REM Sleep-Related Sinus Arrest

780.59   Other
    780.59-0   REM Sleep Behavior Disorder
    780.59-1   Nocturnal Paroxysmal Dystonia
    780.59-3   Sudden Unexplained Nocturnal Death Syndrome
    780.59-4   Sleep-Related Laryngospasm
    780.59-5   Benign Neonatal Sleep Myoclonus
    780.59-6   Pregnancy-Associated Sleep Disorder
    780.59-7   Fragmentary Myoclonus
    780.59-9   Other Parasomnia, NOS

Current Procedural Terminology (CPT) Codes

The American Medical Association maintains a listing of descriptive terms and identifying codes for reporting medical services and procedures performed by physicians. The resulting publication, the *Current Procedural Terminology* (CPT), is updated each year to provide a uniform language that will accurately designate medical, surgical, and diagnostic services and thereby provide an effective means for reliable nationwide communication among physicians, patients, and third parties. The *CPT* code is not compatible with the *ICD* (or *ICD-9-CM*) procedure classification. Those tests that are pertinent to sleep disorders medicine are listed here.

Sleep Testing

Sleep studies and polysomnography refer to the continuous and simultaneous monitoring and recording of various physiological and pathophysiological parameters of sleep for six or more hours with physician review, interpretation, and report. The studies are performed to diagnose a variety of sleep disorders and to evaluate a patient's response to therapies such as nasal continuous positive airway pressure (NCPAP). Polysomnography is distinguished from sleep studies by the inclusion of sleep staging which is defined to include a 1-4 lead electroencephalogram (EEG), electro-oculogram (EOG), and a submental electromyogram (EMG). Additional parameters of sleep include: 1) ECG; 2) airflow; 3) ventilation and respiratory effort; 4) gas exchange by oximetry, transcutaneous monitoring or end tidal gas analysis; 5) extremity muscle activity, motor activity-movement; 6) extended EEG monitoring; 7) penile tumescence; 8) gastroesophageal monitoring; 10) snoring; 11) body positions; etc.

For a study to be reported as polysomnography, sleep must be recorded and staged.

(Report with a -52 modifier if less than six hours of recording or in other cases of reduce services as appropriate)
(For unattended sleep study/polysomnography use 94799)

95805 Multiple sleep latency testing (MSLT), recording, analysis and interpretation of physiological measurements of sleep during multiple nap opportunities
95807 Sleep study, three or more parameters of sleep other than sleep staging, attended by a technologist
95808 Polysomnography; sleep staging with one-three additional parameters of sleep, attended by a technologist
95810 Polysomnography; sleep staging with four or more additional parameters of sleep, attended by a technologist

From *cpt'95 Physician's Current Procedural Terminology*, 4th ed, revised. Chicago: American Medical Association, 1995.

Clinical Field Trials

Clinical field trials will form an important part of the further development of the *ICSD* nosology. They are needed, first, to evaluate the performance characteristics of the nosology and its diagnostic criteria, such as the reliability of application among raters and across sleep disorders centers. The second, broader goal of the field trials will be to evaluate the clinical and research utility of the classification. That is, does the *ICSD* enhance communication among clinicians and researchers? More specifically, does it have validity with respect to the prediction of treatment response and long-term outcome, or with respect to other measures of heterogeneity, such as genetic data or laboratory findings?

One possible informative approach to field trials will involve comparing the relative performance characteristics and the utility of the *DSM-III-R* "lumping" approach to the *ICSD* "splitting" approach. Specifically, the trial should be multisite and could address the interrater reliability and the utility of lumping vs. splitting classificatory systems (e.g., *DSM-III-R* vs. *ICSD*). The methodology for such a comparative approach to field trials has already been partially developed at the University of Pittsburgh (Reynolds, Buysse, and Kupfer, in consultation with Hauri and Kraemer), where, in a small field trial involving a review of approximately 20 cases of chronic insomnia by six raters, interrater reliability appeared to be higher for the application of *DSM-III-R* criteria than for *ASDC* (1979) criteria. This was not unexpected, because *DSM-III-R* lumps while *ASDC* splits. On the other hand, treatment recommendations based on *ASDC* diagnoses were perhaps more targeted, or focused, than treatment recommendations based on *DSM-III-R* diagnoses.

Another issue that could and should be addressed in multisite field trials is the extent to which polysomnographic data enhance diagnostic precision, particularly in patients with chronic free-standing insomnia not associated with other medical or psychiatric illness. In the Pittsburgh trial, raters were randomly assigned to blind or nonblind status regarding laboratory data. Differences among blind vs. nonblind raters with respect to final diagnosis and treatment recommendations were then compared. Such an approach allows one to assess whether the availability of polysomnographic data affects interrater reliability of diagnosis and has an impact on treatment recommendations. Because polysomnographic measures have been incorporated into the *ICSD*, field trials should attempt to assess their utility and validity vis-à-vis differential diagnostic issues.

APPENDIX B

Introduction to the First Edition of the *Diagnostic Classification of Sleep and Arousal Disorders*

Diagnostic Classification of Sleep and Arousal Disorders

1979
First Edition

Association of Sleep Disorders Centers
and the
Association for the Psychophysiological Study of Sleep

Introduction

Disturbed sleep and inadequate wakefulness are inestimable sources of human misery. Many individuals have had their chances for predictable social functioning, gratifying family life, and achievement in work wrecked by the symptoms of sleep and arousal disorders. The impetus for development of this *Diagnostic Classification of Sleep and Arousal Disorders* grew out of many years of requests from patients to medical practitioners for help with sleep problems, requests that for want of information traditionally fell upon deaf ears.

Medical causes of sleep disturbance do not customarily attract a great deal of interest or study, and the complaint of sleepiness is given only passing attention in most case presentations and records. The general physician is not alone, however, in turning aside or misunderstanding patient complaints about sleep. The workers who chose to enter the new research field of sleep physiology in the late 1950s and early 1960s by and large also believed themselves unable to interpret or help sleep symptoms, and all but a few stood apart from investigation and treatment of the clinical sleep disorders. However, this situation has recently undergone a dramatic change.

There can be little disagreement with the proposition that if a clinician is unable to diagnose or even suspect an existing sleep pathology, his treatment of the patient cannot be suitable. The practitioner, because of his customary uncertainty about the significance of sleep symptoms, has a tendency to treat sleep complaints as trifling or annoying. Characteristically, he both underestimates the etiology of sleep disorders and overtreats the symptoms with drugs.

Most doctors are astonished to discover that their accepted approach to exploring clinical problems is marked by an easily overlooked inconsistency, depending on the nature of the patient's complaint. Confronted with a traditional medical problem, the doctor—whose training emphasizes a primary objective of uncovering the source of symptoms—typically initiates a thorough workup aimed at identifying underlying pathology. By means of examination and medical tests, he attempts to document a diagnosis or isolate one or more possibilities. Only if therapy may be specifically related to reversing or neutralizing pathological mechanisms does the physician feel prepared to prescribe treatment. In contrast, when dealing with a sleep disturbance, he acts in uncharacteristic fashion in terms of his usual procedural standards: typically without verifying the patient's description of symptoms—which may be grossly inaccurate—or undertaking a diagnostic protocol to discriminate the etiology of the symptoms, he will prescribe a drug for the symptoms. In this circumstance, the practitioner is in effect treating a condition he has not investigated with an agent whose pharmacokinetics, sites of action, and effects on mental and motor performance he likely does not know and whose actual impact on the sleep of the patient he lacks the means to determine with certainty. He generally also fails to arrange for follow-up observation. Accordingly, it must be acknowledged that the time-honored exhortation to physicians to "do no harm" has been trampled in the customary medical approach to the sleep disorders.

This situation–at the same time lamentable and understandable—results chiefly from ignorance and confusion, not from a disinclination on the part of medical practitioners to respond to the needs of their patients. If anything, the physician so wishes to provide relief that he tries to alleviate symptoms before he investigates their determinants.[1] Of course, the recipient of treatment also plays a role. The patient is commonly eager, often demanding, for help from the doctor, frequently preferring that assistance be undertaken solely at the symptom level.

Much is currently written about the attitudes and qualities of physicians, but one thing is clear—physicians are sensible pragmatists. Those who have had an opportunity to observe physicians in operation are repeatedly reassured that if practitioners are alerted to information they need to know in order to understand and treat their patients' illnesses more efficiently, and if the concepts are scientifically sound, meaningfully taught, and most of all salient to increased clinical effectiveness, the practitioners will lose little time in learning the information and applying it. There is no question that the findings now being made by sleep disorders specialists are beginning to be used in this manner by the general medical community.

It is therefore with humility that we recognize that a whole realm of intimately experienced human difficulties—the disturbances and disorders of sleep–has only desultorily played upon our attention for centuries. The recent advances in knowledge about sleep resemble the pattern of advance in other medical fields–it has waited until the very last decades to emerge. Be that as it may, these breakthroughs now make possible a coherent categorization of the sleep disorders and the construction of a rational system of diagnosis. We believe that the new diag-

---

[1] This is not uncommon with many medical problems: The difference in the sleep disturbances is that little consideration is ever given to efforts at diagnosis.

nostic classification system contained in this volume will permit the sleep and arousal disorders to be finally "demystified" for the practitioner. The gain for the physician will be that rather than having to view sleep symptoms as inconsequential, obscure, or unfathomable phenomena, he can learn the elements that go into accurate diagnosis of sleep disorders. The physician will also be in a position to use findings of abnormal sleep patterns and symptoms to increase his awareness of the existence of related medical and psychiatric illnesses in his patients.

Antecedents of the Diagnostic Classification System

The mid- to late 1970s have witnessed a sharp expansion in the number and geographic spread of sleep disorder investigation-treatment facilities and a corresponding rise in the numbers of patients assessed. That the sleep disorders field has emerged as a true medical subspecialty—one in which research stands astride clinical work–is demonstrated also by the increase in practitioners working in the sleep disorders discipline, the inauguration of training programs and courses of instruction, the rapidly rising count of specific publications on clinical sleep problems, and the appearance of new scientific journals devoted to sleep studies.

The attention of sleep physiology research to clinical issues began slowly in the United States. In the 1960s a small group of investigators trained in electrophysiology began to be concerned with the nature of complaints about disturbed sleep, the physiological anatomy of sleeplessness, the patterns of excessive sleep and sleepiness, the pathophysiological disturbances linked to certain sleep stages and the process of arousal, and the effects of hypnotic agents. Since then a growing number of researchers have become clinician-investigators and have turned their efforts towards studying patients with sleep problems. Some began diagnosing and treating sleep pathologies in individual practice; others established hospital-based sleep disorders centers and clinics. Both sources have contributed heavily in recent years to the sharp increase in our data base for these conditions.

In 1972, at the tenth annual meeting of the Association for the Psychophysiological Study of Sleep (APSS), a workshop was organized on the "nosology and nomenclature of the sleep disorders." This panel marked the first, formal group attempt to share concepts concerning the "definition of the primary and secondary sleep disorders." The invitation to participate was sent to the thirteen international researchers who had a working interest in the area. The progress in our knowledge since this 1972 session has been remarkable, as indicated by the absence of sleep apnea as a condition in any of the diagnostic classification schemes submitted for discussion by the participants.

In 1975 two notable events occurred that spurred the growth of the sleep disorders discipline: one was the decisive Montpellier conference on narcolepsy, which established international conventions for the diagnosis of this condition; the other was the formation of the Association of Sleep Disorders Centers (ASDC), which has provided a continuing forum for scientific communication in the sleep disorders and has now set standards of certification for diagnostic-treatment units and clinical polysomnographers. During the February 1976 meeting, a "Nosology Committee" (later designated the Sleep Disorders Classification Committee) was appointed to begin the task of creating a diagnostic system for the sleep and arousal disorders, one that would include all conditions encountered clinically.

Classifications of the pathologies of sleep had been devised even in ancient times. The organization of these categorizations has varied widely. A number of recent, excellent classifications have been offered by individual investigators currently working in the field, to which the ASDC-APSS nosology is indebted.

Necessity for a Diagnostic Classification System

Optimization of understanding and investigative headway is only realized in a sphere of medical-scientific activity when colleagues share the same concepts about the constitution and terminology of presenting entities. They must also agree as to the lines of subdivision of clinical phenomena, how to group the conditions, and on common criteria of measurement. These agreements are not the end of knowledge in the field, rather somewhere near the beginning; they are simply a set of operating hypotheses and conventions, a working platform upon which to gain a foothold for efficient, future study.

The decision of the ASDC to develop a new classification system stems from the manifest need for an inclusive framework of sleep and arousal disorders, one that would be equal to ordering and recording the full spectrum of maladies presenting in general, as well as in specialized, clinical experience. In addition to inclusiveness, the classification and its contents, we hoped, would represent a true consensus among working specialists in the field as to the most heuristically valuable categorization of the disorders into major groupings. Another objective was that the characterizations of the diagnostic entities incorporate not only the best clinical descriptions in the scientific literature, but, when possible, also recent studies that throw light on the interrelationship of the character of the patient complaint, the clinical signs, and the invaluable physiological data furnished by polysomnographic recording.

A working assumption of the ASDC was that the nosology should be developed by a broad cross section of professionals. Varied inputs were sought from clinicians and clinician-investigators, many with strong roots in fundamental research, who served as committee members, contributors, and consultants. Moreover, all publications pertaining to the conditions were carefully reviewed and considered. Accordingly, both the overall structure of the classification system, as well as the material written on each disorder, represent amalgams of the best empirical data at hand and the shared judgments of experienced diagnosticians. Clearly, this classification system is a consequence, as well as a hopeful forerunner, of advances in our knowledge.

The value of a broad consensus is that accepted and, hopefully, the most valid, diagnostic conventions will now be standard in the evaluation of patients. Great constraints have existed on the inferences derived from needed case series investigations and other types of research owing to uncertainties and disagreements about diagnostic criteria. Only with concurrence in regard to essential diagnostic criteria can the status of clinical diagnosis, treatment, and future research in the sleep disorders be raised. Utilization of the nosology, we believe, will reduce the contamination in clinical studies introduced by data gathered from putatively identical, but in fact impure, diagnostic groupings. It is the faith of this enterprise in nosology that intra- and interfacility research will increase and be more comparable across studies. In addition, since future study populations identified in accord with this nosological system should be more homogeneous, their responses to investigative manipulations and treatments may be expected to be more uniform. This will enhance the opportunities for research to acquire insights into the pathophysiology and etiology of the sleep disorders—the ultimate goal of this classification system and the final step before the sleep disorders can be eradicated.

Limitations of a New Sleep Disorders Nosology

It is well known that standardization of diagnostic criteria is not equivalent to diagnostic validity. The purpose of an exclusive and agreed-on set of diagnostic divisions is to establish concrete entities that may then be challenged and tested on validity grounds in future research. If standardized diagnostic criteria do not agree with the pathological features appearing in nature, nature will let us know. Diagnostic "variants" of certain conditions will soon reveal themselves. The appearance of many will suggest that the original diagnostic criteria were too narrow or aberrant. In short, a diagnostic classification system guarantees only that individuals who fit (and those who do not) are at least operationally specifiable and that research commentaries about groups of patients, categorized as within (or without) particular criteria, have a chance at consistent applicability to the defined populations.

As described above, the Sleep Disorders Classification Committee used the best evidence and judgments at its command to clarify and cluster diagnostic entities. But is must be remembered that a consensus arrangement of diagnoses simply establishes a focused synchronization of viewpoints, not validity. Diagnostic boundaries must continue to be appraised as research explores the mechanisms of disorders. It is to be hoped that many of the conditions proposed—and their diagnostic criteria—will prove valid, but we hold no brief for the permanence or organizational positioning of any diagnosis. The latter merely represent today's best judgments. Concepts of classification will surely change as new findings and improved conceptual frameworks evolve.

Undoubtedly, the wisest orientation to maintain towards the sleep disorders classification system is that it is a provisional, working construct. Many conditions will require revision or elimination; others will be added. The committee anticipates that more than a few of its judgments will have to be corrected. A case in point is the decision not to create two additional diagnostic entries: "primary" disorders of initiating and maintaining sleep (DIMS) in adolescence and in old age. Some evidence is accumulating that—because of biological factors—both periods are "at risk" for the development of disturbed sleep. The committee, however, concluded that the data were insufficient at this time to warrant these unique diagnoses. It judged other DIMS in the classification sufficient to explain the insomnias presenting in adolescence and in old age, as well as in other age groups. However, this decision may someday be seen as an instance in which the committee's choice lagged behind the evidence.

In other cases, our judgments may have led the evidence. For example, though the diagnoses of childhood onset DIMS (A.7) and advanced sleep phase (C.2.c) lack the specificity of more definitive diagnoses in the classification, we believe that, like Pirandello's six characters in search of an author, two pathological conditions—approximating the two diagnoses—are "out there" in nature, shadowing diagnostic actualization. Accordingly, it was decided to include these two diagnostic entities in the classification.

To restate our view, the committee believes that not all conditions described in the nosology can lay a sure claim to eventual verification, at least in their present form; some may be merely "holding operations." However, an approximate diagnosis is superior to no diagnosis, when one is needed. The approximate diagnosis also provides a lattice upon which additional findings can be hung, allowing for a process that often leads to eventual refinement of the diagnostic picture. In this way, the nosological system assists in its own upgrading at the same time that it permits better research into the biological underpinnings of the conditions.

Structure of the Classification System

The members of the classification committee were confronted with developing a meaningful arrangement of the diverse conditions that the field encompasses. Though the partitioning of the syndromes that was arrived at seems simple enough, the reasons for the ultimate divisions and diagnostic entries had to be thought through carefully.

A leading question was whether to segregate the disturbances of sleep and the excessive somnolence conditions at all. It is well known that abnormalities of either one affect the other; that is, insomnia and hypersomnia are both sleep-wake syndromes. The argument was made that they are, in fact, inseparable and that separate categorization amounts to an artificial distinction. Nevertheless, there are problems in not separating DIMS and disorders of excessive somnolence (DOES). One is that unless other criteria of categorization—which, as discussed below, have their own deficiencies—are employed, the classification consists only of a listing of disorders and not a nosological system. There is the benefit, however, of the one-list approach that each diagnostic entity need appear only once.

As to whether the DIMS and DOES conditions are conceptually separable, the committee believes that they are at least symptomatically separable. Classification into disturbed sleep and excessive somnolence conditions allows emphasis to be placed on the apparent sleep or wake period of initiation of symptoms. We also felt that the dangers of viewing DIMS and DOES syndromes too narrowly may be avoided by drafting the clinical descriptions of the conditions in the classification to span the 24 hour symptomatology and functioning of the patient.

The committee evaluated the partitioning of sleep problems also along the lines of primary and secondary disorders, functional and organic, and by means of polysomnographic variables. Primary versus secondary is a traditional discrimination and has the advantage of appearing to take etiology into consideration. However, in virtually no sleep disorder are the true etiological antecedents of the clinical picture known. Hence, use of the term, primary, is either misapplied or confusing and is of little help in clinical evaluations. Similar arguments may be made in the case of partitioning along functional versus organic lines. It would certainly be ideal to construct a nosology of sleep disorders by etiology, as in infectious diseases. But, as mentioned, we are as yet nowhere near etiological understandings in our area of inquiry.

As to the use of the polysomnogram, the sleep research field underwent a paradigmatic change with the advent of multiple-channel electrophysiological recording and sleep-stage scoring. The committee would have been pleased to use the polysomnographic parameter, which has been so illuminating to our comprehension of the sleep disorders, as a tool in classification (similar to cardiological disease classification according to electrocardiographic findings). However, with the exception of its pattern in a few conditions, the polysomnogram is not sufficiently specific to be adequate as a diagnostic differentiator. It would also not be available in every clinical patient evaluation.

Turning to the classification schema that was developed, it is composed of four sections. (The prefatory notes to each section give additional information about features of these categories.) *Section A* classifies the disorders of initiating and maintaining wakefulness (DIMS), comprising types of disturbed and inadequate sleep; *Section B* covers the disorders of excessive somnolence (DOES), discussing types of excessive sleep and inappropriate sleepiness; *Section C* examines disorders of the sleep-wake schedule; and *Section D* describes the dysfunctions associated with sleep, sleep stages, or partial arousal, comprising abnormal behaviors and medical symptoms appearing in sleep. The classification system was designed to be reasonably comprehensive, though not encyclopedic, with respect to abnormal sleep. It emphasizes commonly observed conditions and omits very rare and unconfirmed diagnoses. The discussions of differential diagnosis are restricted to the major clinical situations requiring a discrimination of conditions.

Thus it might be assumed from the classification outline that the DIMS and DOES divisions of the nosology were assigned by *type of pathology*, the ordering of diagnoses is actually according to *type of complaint*. For example, in obstructive sleep apnea, the polysomnogram informs us that the patient may be awakened more than a hundred times in the course of sleep. However, the individual complains only of sleepiness and has no recollection of the arousals. This syndrome—which by polysomnographic criteria should be viewed as a disorder of maintaining sleep, a DIMS—is rather classified as a DOES in the new classification system.

It would seem that categorizing by sign would be sufficiently regressive (akin to discussing certain pulmonary disorders under "the cough" or infections under "the fevers"), but categorization simply by symptom—especially since the patient may be unaware of important features of the condition—would appear to be wholly indefensible. What is the justification for this system?

The fact is that this seemingly antiquated approach has many benefits. We have determined that the greatest yield of data comes from the patient's expressed reasons for seeking help. The chief complaints of insomnia and notable daytime sleepiness are found to predict reliably two nonoverlapping groupings of sleep pathologies.[2] Though this does not necessarily dictate a nosological partitioning

---

[2] Despite the fact that disturbed sleep (disorders of initiating and maintaining sleep, DIMS) leads to some daytime symptoms, these are not described by the patient in the same way as the "sleepiness" reported in disorders of excessive somnolence (DOES). If the clinician reserves the designation of the term sleepiness not for physical fatigue, lack of energy, poor concentration, etc., but for literal inability to remain awake even in stimulating circumstances, he will be in a position to differentiate the DIMS and DOES clusters.

along such lines, the committee decided that at the present stage of development of this field, a classification system that gives first priority to "listening to the patient" may be for now the most justifiable. It disposes to two superb logic-tree sets of inquiry about other attributes of the symptom picture, which offer a rational path for arriving at correct diagnosis and differential diagnosis. A symptom category classification—by providing such a means for the teaching of sleep disorders identification—has great potential at this time for upgrading diagnostic skills. Additional subcategorizations of the two symptom sets—e.g., sleep-onset DIMS versus early morning DIMS and obligatory napping versus sleepiness—are helpful in final specification of the diagnosis. (These types of symptom details are insufficient in themselves as a total basis for a classification system.)

This schema confesses rather than covers up its rudimentary nature. To summarize, it leaves the classification of DIMS and DOES as loose confederations of syndromes, whose only structural lines derive from empirical findings regarding the diagnostic utility of patient complaints. Clearly, the field is wide open for additional findings. It was our wish to let needed tests of concepts in the field and new data govern future subcategorizations, rather than have them imposed by intuition or dicta. We should, of course, be alert to any possibility. Whatever the current benefits of clustering by symptom, this system has its dangers–syphilis has taught us that several disparate symptom pictures may have a single etiology.

One other exception should be noted to the highlighting of symptoms in the classification system. Such an approach would have been counterproductive if applied to the sleep schedule disturbances, which have been isolated for separate attention in Section C of the nosology. Patients do not enter a clinic complaining of a sleep schedule or sleep-wake cycle disturbance. The currency of their presenting symptoms is, indeed, disturbed sleep, inappropriate somnolence, or both. However, with the sleep schedule disturbances, it is crucial that one not be confused by the apparent abnormalities of sleep or waking and that one learn how to collect the symptom data so as to identify, when present, the problem of misplaced (in circadian terms) sleep and waking.

Guidelines for the Coding of Diagnoses

Disorders may be coded according to two systems. First, the coding designations may be used that are inherent in the outline form of the ASDC-APSS classification system. For example, persistent psychophysiological DIMS (A.1.b) appear under A. Disorders of Initiating and Maintaining Sleep (DIMS), 1. psychophysiological, b. persistent. This method of coding has the advantage of utilizing the conceptual clusterings of the sleep disorders among and within the four major rubrics of the classification. It is likely to be used in facilities such as sleep disorders investigative units that plan to keep records on the flow of their clinical experience in terms of the whole spectrum of sleep disorders conditions. Second, a coding system has been devised that utilizes the coding numerals of the current *International Classification of Diseases, 9th revision, Clinical Modification* (*ICD-9-CM*) and which may be used concurrently or alternatively with the ASDC-APSS outline. *ICD-9-CM* is the official classification manual used by hospital record rooms in the United States. A section at the end of this classification system describes how *ICD-9-CM* codes may be used for the sleep disorders, that is, their correspondence to the ASDC-APSS rubrics. It is recommended that the *ICD-9-CM* designations be used in hospital records and in supplying diagnostic information to agencies and insurers.

The classification committee suggests that all clinically relevant and useful sleep disorder diagnoses be made, but parsimony is also to be encouraged. Those who have the responsibility for making diagnoses in general medical or psychiatric units should not feel themselves under an injunction to make all possible diagnoses relating to sleep. To illustrate, chronic schizophrenic patients commonly experience mild to moderate sleep disturbances. A formal diagnostic entry of a DIMS, separate from the diagnosis of schizophrenia, may be irrelevant (though notation of the symptom is not) unless a focus of interest exists in the facility concerning the status of sleep behavior in schizophrenia. In general, the decision to make the diagnosis of a sleep disturbance under such circumstances rests on grounds of the relationship of the symptom to the primary (non-sleep disorder) condition, the need for distinctiveness of the symptom apart from the major diagnosis, and the level of disability contributed by the symptom.

The issue of single versus multiple sleep disorders codings will be encountered with certain patients. In general, it is advisable to assign one diagnosis that can account for the entire spectrum of symptoms in the patient, but this is not always possible. *It is axiomatic that the condition, not the patient, is coded.* Though most patients seen for a sleep problem will yield only a single diagnosis for coding, some patients have multiple conditions requiring entry. For example, a few patients with narcolepsy will have sleep-related enuresis or sleepwalking as well.

There is one distinct situation in which multiple coding is required: when a parasomnia, in turn, disturbs sleep repeatedly, to the extent that the patient complains of insomnia. The parasomnia is first entered under section D, and then the DIMS induced by the parasomnia is coded under A.6.

In terms of the compatibility of diagnoses, there may exist not only simultaneous presentation of conditions of different types, but also superimposition of conditions within the same group of disorders. To illustrate, a tense patient with a long-standing and stable difficulty in maintaining sleep, diagnosed as having persistent psychophysiological DIMS (A.1.b), hears of the unexpected death of his father. The patient now develops an inability to fall asleep in less than two hours for several nights, and, in addition, his repeated awakenings continue. The criteria for the diagnosis of transient and situational DIMS (A.1.a) are clearly present along with the persistent psychophysiological DIMS, and both should be coded (if relevant).

Though multiple diagnoses may be compatible, determining whether to use them is often complicated in clinical situations. The question of entering two diagnoses arises whenever features of one condition are present along with features of another. The decision to code one or more diagnoses rests, in part, on the determination of whether, in a specific case, the different clinical features are pathognomonic, or whether some of them may have less than diagnostic implication.

Sleep-related (nocturnal) myoclonus is an example of a condition that itself is an accepted cause of DIMS and DOES, but the leg jerks that typify this disorder also appear in conjunction with other conditions such as narcolepsy, sleep apnea, and drug abuse. It is not likely that the myoclonus—when it is observed with the other conditions–represents the myoclonus disorder so much as a secondary event. However, this question is controversial and is not at all well understood. Accordingly, the condition should be individually coded as a diagnosis whenever the criteria for its diagnosis are achieved (see A.5.a and B.5.a). The less-than-criteria episodes of leg twitching should also be noted, but not as a diagnostic entry. (Data such as these, if recorded will ultimately help to unravel the role of sleep-related (nocturnal) myoclonus in symptom formation.)

A less complicated decision may be made in those cases in which an unambiguous case of sleep apnea DOES syndrome displays sleep-onset REM sleep. Though REM sleep at sleep onset is a diagnostic sign in narcolepsy, it can occur in other situations (e.g., heightened REM sleep "pressure" or unusual sleep scheduling) and is not an absolute indication of narcolepsy. The phenomenon has been described—without attribution of narcolepsy—in connection with other conditions. Accordingly, it would be inadvisable in this case to diagnose narcolepsy separately. However, the possibility of the existence of unique and independent conditions exists. If after resolution of the sleep apnea, repeat recordings continue to show sleep-onset REM periods in the presence of symptoms, the diagnosis of narcolepsy should be entertained.

Some Additional Points about the Nosology

The classification committee elected not to provide a listing of operational criteria for each diagnosis. However, the write-ups of the conditions contain the key diagnostic inclusion and exclusion points. It may be helpful to abstract, and more tightly codify, the diagnostic features of particular conditions for the purposes of some research projects.

The acronyms DIMS and DOES are generally used as nouns in the body of the classification but may also be found as adjectives (e.g., DIMS symptoms). This is admittedly infelicitous. At times it is resorted to in order to reduce use of the terms insomnia and hypersomnia–designations that have distorted meanings because they have lost all specificity and, worse, signify homogeneous symptoms in some people's minds. DIMS and DOES may eventually suffer the same fate, but at least when they are decoded, they remind us that a group of heterogeneous disorders is being referred to.

In an effort to acknowledge that people are increasingly unconfined to sleeping at night and waking by day, and because many symptoms are actually related to sleep, not night, the terms "nocturnal" and "night" (e.g., night terrors) have been replaced by "sleep-related." Exceptions and transitional terms are used in certain cases to avoid confusion (e.g., sleep-related (nocturnal) myoclonus).

Similarly, modifiers of sleep—such as "nighttime" and "night"—used to indicate the major sleep period of the 24 hour day are no longer justifiable. With some exceptions, the appellations "major sleep period" and "major wake period" have been employed.

Whenever possible, psychiatric conditions are described with the designations employed by the forthcoming *Diagnostic and Statistical Manual, 3rd edition (DSM III)*, of the American Psychiatric Association.

The outline of the classification system makes use of the phrase "not otherwise specified" (see, for example, A.8.c and C.2.f), which is to be understood in the sense of "unspecified." This entry is intended to leave place in the classification for (1) undiagnosed ("don't know") conditions and (2) additional—as yet undocumented (i.e., new)—conditions that may be described in the future.

A Note on the Bibliography of the Classification System

Literature references are grouped under the individual disorders in the classification. In addition, a number of excellent books and reviews are included under the general bibliography heading because they contribute carefully annotated summaries and syntheses of a broad range of syndromes.

The data contained in the descriptions of disorders that were written for this classification understandably derive from many sources. It should be emphasized that the data in the descriptions are not drawn solely from the citations given for each condition. These references were selected only to provide additional detail and to support certain key facts. The reader will note that a few conditions have no references listed simply because none are as yet available in print.

A related matter that warrants mention is our inability—in view of the need to limit the references for most of the conditions to two or three—to cite for many of the disorders the primary or "classical" sources. This is unfortunate, but is not our intention to slight the critical, seminal efforts of the past. However, we were frequently forced to make the alternative choice, that is, to refer to more recent and comprehensive articles in the faith that they will not only inform the reader about the disorder, but also lead him to the excellent, earlier reports in the literature.

Howard P. Roffwarg, M.D., Chairman
Sleep Disorders Classification Committee, ASDC

Reprinted from *Sleep,* Volume 2, Number 1, pages 5-15. © 1979 Raven Press, New York. Reprinted by permission of the ASDC and Raven Press.

Diagnostic Classification of Sleep and Arousal Disorders (1979 Edition)

ASDC Code		Recommended ICD-9-CM Code
	A. DIMS: Disorders of Initiating and Maintaining Sleep (Insomnias)	
	1. Psychological	
A.1.a	a. Transient and Situational	307.41-0
A.1.b	b. Persistent	307.42-0
A.2	2. Associated with Psychiatric Disorders	
A.2.a	a. Symptom and Personality Disorders	307.42-1
A.2.b	b. Affective Disorders	307.42-2
A.2.c	c. Other Functional Psychoses	307.42-3
A.3	3. Associated with Use of Drugs and Alcohol	
A.3.a	a. Tolerance or Withdrawal from CNS Depressants	780.52-0
A.3.b	b. Sustained Use of CNS Stimulants	780.52-1
A.3.c	c. Sustained Use or Withdrawal from Other Drugs	780.52-2
A.3.d	d. Chronic Alcoholism	780.52-3
A.4	4. Associated with Sleep-Induced Respiratory Impairment	
A.4.a	a. Sleep Apnea DIMS Syndrome	780.51-0
A.4.b	b. Alveolar Hypoventilation DIMS Syndrome	780.51-1
A.5	5. Associated with Sleep-Related (Nocturnal) Myoclonus and "Restless Legs"	
A.5.a	a. Sleep-Related (Nocturnal) Myoclonus DIMS Syndrome	780.52-4
A.5.b	b. "Restless Legs" DIMS Syndrome	780.52-5
A.6	6. Associated with Other Medical, Toxic, and Environmental Conditions	780.52-6
A.7	7. Childhood-Onset DIMS	780.52-7
A.8	8. Associated with Other DIMS Conditions	
A.8.a	a. Repeated REM Sleep Interruptions	307.48-0
A.8.b	b. Atypical Polysomnographic Features	307.48-1
A.8.c	c. Not Otherwise Specified	307.42-9 or 780.52-9
A.9	9. No DIMS Abnormality	
A.9.a	a. Short Sleeper	307.49-0
A.9.b	b. Subjective DIMS Complaint without Objective Findings	307.49-1
A.9.c	c. Not Otherwise Specified	307.40-1

B. DOES: Disorders of Excessive Somnolence

B.1	1. Psychophysiological	
B.1.a	a. Transient and Situational	307.43-0
B.1.b	b. Persistent	307.44-0
B.2	2. Associated with Psychiatric Disorders	
B.2.a	a. Affective Disorders	307.44-1
B.2.b	b. Other Functional Disorders	307.44-2
B.3	3. Associated with Use of Drugs and Alcohol	
B.3.a	a. Tolerance to or Withdrawal from CNS Stimulants	780.54-0
B.3.b	b. Sustained Use of CNS Depressants	780.54-1
B.4	4. Associated with Sleep-Induced Respiratory Impairment	
B.4.a	a. Sleep Apnea DOES Syndrome	780.53-0
B.4.b	b. Alveolar Hypoventilation DOES Syndrome	780.53-1
B.5	5. Associated with Sleep-Related (Nocturnal) Myoclonus and "Restless Legs"	
B.5.a	a. Sleep-Related (Nocturnal) Myoclonus DOES Syndrome	780.54-4
B.5.b	b. "Restless Legs" DOES Syndrome	780.54-5
B.6	6. Narcolepsy	347
B.7	7. Idiopathic CNS Hypersomnolence	780.54-7
B.8	8. Associated with Other Medical, Toxic, and Environmental Conditions	780.54-6
B.9	9. Associated with Other DOES Conditions	
B.9.a	a. Intermittent DOES (Periodic) Syndromes	
B.9.a.i	i. Kleine-Levin Syndrome	780.54-2
B.9.a.ii	ii. Menstrual-Associated Syndrome	780.54-3
B.9.b	b. Insufficient Sleep	307.49-4
B.9.c	c. Sleep Drunkenness	307.47-1
B.9.d	d. Not Otherwise Specified	307.44-9 or 780.54-9
B.10	10. No DOES Abnormality	
B.10.a	a. Long Sleeper	307.49-2
B.10.b	b. Subjective DOES Complaint without Objective Findings	307.49-3
B.10.c	c. Not Otherwise Specified	307.40-2

C. Disorders of the Sleep-Wake Schedule

C.1	1. Transient	
C.1.a	a. Rapid Time Zone Change ("Jet Lag") Syndrome	307.45-0
C.1.b	b. "Work Shift" Change in Conventional Sleep-Wake Schedule	307.45-1
C.2	2. Persistent	
C.2.a	a. Frequently Changing Sleep-Wake Schedule	307.45-2
C.2.b	b. Delayed Sleep Phase Syndrome	780.55-0

C.2.c	c. Advanced Sleep Phase Syndrome	780.55-1
C.2.d	d. Non-24-Hour Sleep-Wake Syndrome	780.55-2
C.2.e	e. Irregular Sleep-Wake Pattern	307.45-3
C.2.f	f. Not Otherwise Specified	307.45-9 or 780.55-9
	D. Dysfunctions Associated with Sleep, Sleep Stages, or Partial Arousals (Parasomnias)	
D.1	1. Sleepwalking (Somnambulism)	307.46-0
D.2	2. Sleep Terror (Pavor Nocturnus, Incubus)	307.46-1
D.3	3. Sleep-Related Enuresis	307.46-2 or 780.56-0
D.4	4. Other Dysfunctions	
D.4.a	a. Dream Anxiety Attacks (Nightmares)	307.47-0
D.4.b	b. Sleep-Related Epileptic Seizures	780.56-1
D.4.c	c. Sleep-Related Bruxism	306.8
D.4.d	d. Sleep-Related Headbanging (Jactatio Capitis Nocturna)	307.3
D.4.e	e. Familial Sleep Paralysis	780.56-2
D.4.f	f. Impaired Sleep-Related Penile Tumescence	780.56-3
D.4.g	g. Sleep-Related Painful Erections	780.56-4
D.4.h	h. Sleep-Related Cluster Headaches and Chronic Paroxysmal Hemicrania	780.56-5
D.4.i	i. Sleep-Related Abnormal Swallowing Syndrome	780.56-6
D.4.j	j. Sleep-Related Asthma	780.56-7
D.4.k	k. Sleep-Related Cardiovascular Symptoms	780.56-8
D.4.l	l. Sleep-Related Gastroesophageal Reflux	780.56-9
D.4.m	m. Sleep-Related Hemolysis (Paroxysmal Nocturnal Hemoglobinuria)	283.2
D.4.n	n. Asymptomatic Polysomnographic Finding	780.59
D.4.o	o. Not Otherwise Specified	307.47-9 or 780.56

Adapted from the Association of Sleep Disorders Centers Classification Committee, *Diagnostic Classification of Sleep and Arousal Disorders,* 1st ed. © 1979 Raven Press, New York. Reprinted by permission of the ASDC and Raven Press.

Alphabetical Listing of the *Diagnostic Classification of Sleep and Arousal Disorders* (1979 Edition) and Comparison with the *International Classification of Sleep Disorders*

Diagnostic Classification of Sleep and Arousal Disorders	International Classification of Sleep Disorders	ICD-9-CM Code
Advanced Sleep Phase Syndrome	Advanced Sleep Phase Syndrome	780.55-1
Alveolar Hypoventilation DIMS Syndrome	Central Alveolar Hypoventilation Syndrome	780.51-1
Alveolar Hypoventilation DOES Syndrome	Central Alveolar Hypoventilation Syndrome	780.53-1
Asymptomatic Polysomnographic Finding	(Use Axis B)	
Atypical Polysomnographic Features	(Use Axis B)	
Childhood-Onset DIMS	Idiopathic Insomnia	780.52-7
Delayed Sleep Phase Syndrome	Delayed Sleep Phase Syndrome	780.55-0
DIMS with Affective Disorders	Mood Disorders	296-301
DIMS with Chronic Alcoholism	Alcoholism	303
DIMS with Other Functional Psychoses	Psychoses	292-299
DIMS with Other Medical, Toxic, and Environmental DIMS Conditions	Environmental Sleep Disorder	780.52-6
DIMS with Sustained Use of CNS Stimulants	Stimulant-Dependent Sleep Disorder	780.52-1
DIMS with Sustained Use or Withdrawal from Other Drugs	(Use appropriate ICD listing)	
DIMS with Symptom and Personality Disorders	Anxiety Disorders Panic Disorders	300-316 300
DIMS with Tolerance to or Withdrawal from CNS Depressants	Hypnotic-Dependent Sleep Disorder	780.52-0
DOES with Affective Disorders	Mood Disorders	296-301
DOES with Menstrual-Associated Syndrome	Menstrual-Associated Sleep Disorder	780.54-3
DOES with Other Functional Disorders	(Use appropriate ICD listing)	
DOES with Other Medical, Toxic, and Environmental DOES Conditions	(Use appropriate ICD listing)	
DOES (Periodic) with Kleine-Levin Syndrome	Recurrent Hypersomnia	780.54-2

DOES with Sustained Use of CNS Depressants	Hypnotic-Dependent Sleep Disorder	780.52-0
DOES with Tolerance to or Withdrawal from CNS Stimulants	Stimulant-Dependent Sleep Disorder	780.52-1
Dream Anxiety Attacks (Nightmares)	Nightmares	307.47-0
Familial Sleep Paralysis	Sleep Paralysis	780.56-2
Frequently Changing Sleep-Wake Schedule	(Use specific Circadian Rhythm Sleep Disorder diagnosis)	
Idiopathic CNS Hypersomnolence	Idiopathic Hypersomnia	780.54-7
Impaired Sleep-Related Penile Tumescence	Impaired Sleep-Related Penile Tumescence	780.56-3
Insufficient Sleep	Insufficient Sleep Syndrome	307.49-4
Irregular Sleep-Wake Pattern	Irregular Sleep-Wake Pattern	307.45-3
Long Sleeper	Long Sleeper	307.49-2
Narcolepsy	Narcolepsy	347
Non-24-Hour Sleep-Wake Syndrome	Non-24-Hour Sleep-Wake Syndrome	780.55-2
Not Otherwise Specified DIMS Disorder	Intrinsic Sleep Disorder NOS or Extrinsic Sleep Disorder NOS	780.52-9
Not Otherwise Specified DOES Disorder	Intrinsic Sleep Disorder NOS or Extrinsic Sleep Disorder NOS	780.52-9
Not Otherwise Specified Non-DIMS Condition	Intrinsic Sleep Disorder NOS or Extrinsic Sleep Disorder NOS	780.52-9
Not Otherwise Specified Non-DOES Condition	Intrinsic Sleep Disorder NOS or Extrinsic Sleep Disorder NOS	780.52-9
Not Otherwise Specified Parasomnia	Other Parasomnia NOS	780.59-9
Not Otherwise Specified Sleep-Wake Schedule Disturbance	Circadian Rhythm Sleep Disorder NOS	780.55-9
Persistent Psychophysiological DIMS	Psychophysiological Insomnia	307.42-0
Persistent Psychophysiological DOES	Intrinsic Sleep Disorder NOS or Extrinsic Sleep Disorder NOS	780.52-9
Rapid Time Zone Change ("Jet Lag") Syndrome	Time Zone Change (Jet Lag) Syndrome	307.45-0
Repeated REM Sleep Interruptions	(Use Axis B)	
"Restless Legs" DIMS Syndrome	Restless Legs Syndrome	780.52-5
"Restless Legs" DOES Syndrome	Restless Legs Syndrome	780.52-5
Short Sleeper	Short Sleeper	307.49-0
Sleep Apnea DIMS Syndrome	Obstructive Sleep Apnea Syndrome or	780.53-0
	Central Sleep Apnea Syndrome	780.51-0
Sleep Apnea DOES Syndrome	Obstructive Sleep Apnea Syndrome or	780.53-0
	Central Sleep Apnea Syndrome	780.51-0
Sleep Drunkenness	Confusional Arousals	307.46-2
Sleep-Related Abnormal Swallowing Syndrome	Sleep-Related Abnormal Swallowing Syndrome	780.56-6
Sleep-Related Asthma	Sleep-Related Asthma	493
Sleep-Related Bruxism	Sleep Bruxism	306.8
Sleep-Related Cardiovascular Symptoms	REM Sleep-Related Sinus Arrest	780.56-8
	Nocturnal Cardiac Ischemia	411-414

Sleep-Related Cluster Headaches	Headaches	346
Sleep-Related Enuresis	Sleep Enuresis	307.46-2
Sleep-Related Epileptic Seizures	Sleep-Related Epilepsy	345
Sleep-Related Gastroesophageal Reflux	Sleep-Related Gastroesophageal Reflux	780.56-9
Sleep-Related Hemolysis (Paroxysmal Nocturnal Hemoglobinuria)	(Entry deleted)	
Sleep-Related (Nocturnal) Myoclonus DIMS Syndrome	Periodic Limb Movement Disorder	780.52-4
Sleep-Related (Nocturnal) Myoclonus DOES Syndrome	Periodic Limb Movement Disorder	780.52-4
Sleep-Related Painful Erections	Sleep-Related Painful Erections	780.56-4
Sleep-Related Headbanging (Jactatio Capitis Nocturna)	Rhythmic Movement Disorder	307.3
Sleep Terror (Pavor Nocturnus, Incubus)	Sleep Terrors	307.46-1
Sleepwalking (Somnambulism)	Sleepwalking	307.46-0
Subjective DIMS Complaint without Objective Findings	Sleep State Misperception	307.49-1
Subjective DOES Complaint without Objective Findings	Subwakefulness Syndrome	307.47-1
Transient and Situational Psychophysiological DIMS	Adjustment Sleep Disorder	307.41-0
Transient and Situational Psychophysiological DOES	Adjustment Sleep Disorder	307.43-0
"Work Shift" Change in Conventional Sleep-Wake Schedule	Shift Work Sleep Disorder	307.45-1

Adapted from the Association of Sleep Disorders Centers Classification Committee, *Diagnostic Classification of Sleep and Arousal Disorders*, 1st ed. © 1979 Raven Press, New York. Reprinted by permission of the ASDC and Raven Press.

Comparative Listing of the *Diagnostic Classification of Sleep and Arousal Disorders* (1979 Edition) and the *International Classification of Sleep Disorders*

ASDC Code	Diagnostic Classification of Sleep and Arousal Disorders	International Classification of Sleep Disorders	ICD-9-CM Code
	A. DIMS: Disorders of Initiating and Maintaining Sleep (Insomnias)		
	1. Psychological		
A.1.a	a. Transient and Situational	Adjustment Sleep Disorder	307.41-0
A.1.b	b. Persistent	Psychophysiological Insomnia	307.42-0
A.2	2. Associated with Psychiatric Disorders		
A.2.a	a. Symptom and Personality Disorders	Anxiety Disorders Panic Disorders	300-316 300
A.2.b	b. Affective Disorders	Mood Disorders	296-301
A.2.c	c. Other Functional Psychoses	Psychoses	292-299
A.3	3. Associated with Use of Drugs and Alcohol		
A.3.a	a. Tolerance or Withdrawal from CNS Depressants	Hypnotic-Dependent Sleep Disorder	780.52-0
A.3.b	b. Sustained Use of CNS Stimulants	Stimulant-Dependent Sleep Disorder	780.52-1
A.3.c	c. Sustained Use or Withdrawal from Other Drugs	(Use appropriate ICD listing)	
A.3.d	d. Chronic Alcoholism	Alcoholism	303
A.4	4. Associated with Sleep-Induced Respiratory Impairment		
A.4.a	a. Sleep Apnea DIMS Syndrome	Obstructive Sleep Apnea Syndrome or Central Sleep Apnea Syndrome	780.53-0 780.51-0
A.4.b	b. Alveolar Hypoventilation Syndrome	Central Alveolar Hypoventilation Syndrome	780.51-1
A.5	5. Associated with Sleep-Related (Nocturnal) Myoclonus and "Restless Legs"		

A.5.a	a. Sleep-Related (Nocturnal) Myoclonus DIMS Syndrome	Periodic Limb Movement Disorder	780.52-4
A.5.b	b. "Restless Legs" DIMS Syndrome	Restless Legs Syndrome	780.52-5
A.6	6. Associated with Other Medical, Toxic, and Environmental Conditions	Environmental Sleep Disorder	780.52-6
A.7	7. Childhood-Onset DIMS	Idiopathic Insomnia	780.52-7
A.8	8. Associated with Other DIMS Conditions		
A.8.a	a. Repeated REM Sleep Interruptions	(Use Axis B)	
A.8.b	b. Atypical Polysomnographic Features	(Use Axis B)	
A.8.c	c. Not Otherwise Specified	Intrinsic Sleep Disorder or Extrinsic Sleep Disorder	780.52-9
A.9	9. No DIMS Abnormality		
A.9.a	a. Short Sleeper	Short Sleeper	307.49-0
A.9.b	b. Subjective DIMS Complaint without Objective Findings	Sleep State Misperception	307.49-1
A.9.c	c. Not Otherwise Specified	Intrinsic Sleep Disorder NOS or Extrinsic Sleep Disorder NOS	780.52-9
	B. DOES: Disorders of Excessive Somnolence		
B.1	1. Psychophysiological		
B.1.a	a. Transient and Situational	Adjustment Sleep Disorder	307.41-0
B.1.b	b. Persistent	Intrinsic Sleep Disorder NOS or Extrinsic Sleep Disorder NOS	780.52-9
B.2	2. Associated with Psychiatric Disorders		
B.2.a	a. Affective Disorders	Mood Disorders	296-301
B.2.b	b. Other Functional Disorders	(Use appropriate ICD listing)	
B.3	3. Associated with Use of Drugs and Alcohol		
B.3.a	a. Tolerance to or Withdrawal from CNS Stimulants	Stimulant-Dependent Sleep Disorder	780.52-1
B.3.b	b. Sustained Use of CNS Depressants	Hypnotic-Dependent Sleep Disorder	780.52-0
B.4	4. Associated with Sleep-Induced Respiratory Impairment		
B.4.a	a. Sleep Apnea DOES Syndrome	Obstructive Sleep Apnea Syndrome or	780.53-0
		Central Sleep Apnea Syndrome	780.51-0

B.4.b	b. Alveolar Hypoventilation Syndrome	Central Alveolar Hypoventilation Syndrome	780.53-1
B.5	5. Associated with Sleep-Related (Nocturnal) Myoclonus and "Restless Legs"		
B.5.a	a. Sleep-Related (Nocturnal) Myoclonus DOES Syndrome	Periodic Limb Movement Disorder	780.52-4
B.5.b	b. "Restless Legs" DOES Syndrome	Restless Legs Syndrome	780.52-5
B.6	6. Narcolepsy	Narcolepsy	347
B.7	7. Idiopathic CNS Hypersomnolence	Idiopathic Hypersomnia	780.54-7
B.8	8. Associated with Other Medical, Toxic, and Environmental Conditions	Environmental Sleep Disorder	780.52-6
B.9	9. Associated with Other DOES Conditions		
B.9.a	a. Intermittent DOES Periodic) Syndromes		
B.9.a.i	i. Kleine-Levin Syndrome	Recurrent Hypersomnia	780.54-2
B.9.a.ii	ii. Menstrual-Associated Syndrome	Menstrual-Associated Sleep Disorder	780.54-3
B.9.b	b. Insufficient Sleep	Insufficient Sleep Syndrome	307.49-4
B.9.c	c. Sleep Drunkenness	Confusional Arousals	307.46-2
B.9.d	d. Not Otherwise Specified	Intrinsic Sleep Disorder NOS or Extrinsic Sleep Disorder NOS	780.52-9
B.10	10. No DOES Abnormality		
B.10.a	a. Long Sleeper	Long Sleeper	307.49-2
B.10.b	b. Subjective DOES Complaint without Objective Findings	Subwakefulness Syndrome	307.47-1
B.10.c	c. Not Otherwise Specified	Intrinsic Sleep Disorder NOS or Extrinsic Sleep Disorder NOS	780.52-9
	C. Disorders of the Sleep-Wake Schedule		
C.1	1. Transient		
C.1.a	a. Rapid Time Zone Change ("Jet Lag") Syndrome	Time Zone Change (Jet Lag) Syndrome	307.45-0
C.1.b	b. "Work Shift" Change in Conventional Sleep-Wake Schedule	Shift Work Sleep Disorder	307.45-1

C.2	2. Persistent		
C.2.a	a. Frequently Changing Sleep-Wake Schedule	(Use other Circadian Rhythm Sleep Disorder designation)	
C.2.b	b. Delayed Sleep Phase Syndrome	Delayed Sleep Phase Syndrome	780.55-0
C.2.c	c. Advanced Sleep Phase Syndrome	Advanced Sleep Phase Syndrome	780.55-1
C.2.d	d. Non-24-Hour Sleep-Wake Syndrome	Non-24-Hour Sleep-Wake Syndrome	780.55-2
C.2.e	e. Irregular Sleep-Wake Pattern	Irregular Sleep-Wake Pattern	307.45-3
C.2.f	f. Not Otherwise Specified	Circadian Rhythm Sleep Disorder NOS	780.55-9
	D. Dysfunctions Associated with Sleep, Sleep Stages, or Partial Arousals (Parasomnias)		
D.1	1. Sleepwalking (Somnambulism)	Sleepwalking	307.46-0
D.2	2. Sleep Terror (Pavor Nocturnus, Incubus)	Sleep Terrors	307.46-1
D.3	3. Sleep-Related Enuresis	Sleep Enuresis	307.46-2 or 780.56-0
D.4	4. Other Dysfunctions		
D.4.a	a. Dream Anxiety Attacks (Nightmares)	Nightmares	307.47-0
D.4.b	b. Sleep-Related Epileptic Seizures	Sleep-Related Epilepsy	345
D.4.c	c. Sleep-Related Bruxism	Sleep Bruxism	306.8
D.4.d	d. Sleep-Related Headbanging (Jactatio Capitis Nocturna)	Rhythmic Movement Disorder	307.3
D.4.e	e. Familial Sleep Paralysis	Sleep Paralysis	780.56-2
D.4.f	f. Impaired Sleep-Related Penile Tumescence	Impaired Sleep-Related Penile Erections	780.56-3
D.4.g	g. Sleep-Related Painful Erections	Sleep-Related Painful Erections	780.56-4
D.4.h	h. Sleep-Related Cluster Headaches	Headaches	346
D.4.i	i. Sleep-Related Abnormal Swallowing Syndrome	Sleep-Related Abnormal Swallowing Syndrome	780.56-6
D.4.j	j. Sleep-Related Asthma	Sleep-Related Asthma	493
D.4.k	k. Sleep-Related Cardiovascular Symptoms	REM Sleep-Related Sinus Arrest	780.56-8
		Nocturnal Cardiac Ischemia	413.0

D.4.l	l. Sleep-Related Gastroesophageal Reflux	Sleep-Related Gastroesophageal Reflux	530.1
D.4.m	m. Sleep-Related Hemolysis	(Entry deleted)	
D.4.n	n. Asymptomatic Polysomnographic Finding	(Use Axis B)	
D.4.o	o. Not Otherwise Specified	Other Parasomnia NOS	780.59-9

Adapted from the Association of Sleep Disorders Centers Classification Committee, *Diagnostic Classification of Sleep and Arousal Disorders,* 1st ed. © 1979 Raven Press, New York. Reprinted by permission of the ASDC and Raven Press.

INDEX

A
Abbreviations list, 351
Absence seizures, 247
Acosta's disease, 80
Actigraph, 337
Acting out of dreams, 177
Activity
  alpha, 337
  beta, 338
  delta, 339
  phasic, 345
  theta, 350
Acute brain syndrome, 237
Acute confusional state, 237
Acute coronary insufficiency, 263
Adenoidal
  hypertrophy, 52
Adjustment disorder, 224
Adjustment sleep disorder, 83
Advanced sleep-phase syndrome, 133
Agitation
  dementia and, 237
Agoraphobia, 227
AHI, 337, 351. See also Apnea-hypopnea index
AI, 337, 351. See also Apnea index
Air travel
  sleep and, 118
Alcohol
  abstinence, 230
  dependency insomnia, 111
  dependent sleep disorder, 111
  withdrawal, 230
Alcoholic psychoses, 230
Alcoholism, 230
Allergy
  insomnia and, 98
Alpha
  activity, 337
  intrusion, 337
  rhythm, 337
  sleep, 337
Alpha-delta sleep, 337
Alpha intrusion, 337
Alpha rhythm, 337

Alpha sleep, 337
Alpine sickness, 80
Altitude insomnia, 80
Alveolar hypoventilation syndrome
  central, 61
Alzheimer's disease, 237
Amnesia, 145
Amphetamine, 107
Andes disease, 80
Angina, 263
Angina, 263
  decubitus, 263
  pectoris, 263
Anxiety
  acute, 83
  disorders, 224
  dream attack, 162
Anxiety attack
  dream, 162
Anxiety disorders, 224
Apnea, 304, 337
  central, 58
  hypersomnia and, 52
  idiopathic, 198
  of infancy, 198
  infant sleep, 198
  mixed, 52
  nonobstructive sleep, 58
  obstructive, 52
  obstructive sleep, 198
  periodic, 198
  of prematurity, 198
  sleep, 52, 198
  unexplained, 198
  upper airway, 52
Apnea-hypopnea index, 337, 351
Apnea index, 337, 351
Apnea of infancy, 198
Apnea of prematurity, 198
Apparent life-threatening event, 198
Appetite loss
  altitude insomnia and, 80
Arise time, 338
Arousal, 338
  acute emotional, 83

confusional, 142
early morning, 219, 340
excessive, 35
internal, 28
movement, 343
PLM index, 345
premature, 219
psychophysiologic, 28
Arousal disorders, 16, 19, 142, 150, 338.
  See also specific disorders
Arrythmia, cardiac
  sleep-related 174
ASDC. See Association of Sleep Disorders
  Centers
Aspiration, 188
Association disorder
  sleep-onset, 94
Association of Sleep Disorders Centers
  alphabetical listing of disorders, 381-383
  disorder classification, 378-380
  ICSD comparative listing, 384-388
Asthma
  sleep-related, 269
Asynchrony
  incremental, 137
  stable, 128, 133
Asystole
  nocturnal, 175
Ataxia
  hereditary, 234
Atherosclerotic heart disease, 263
Automatism
  semipurposeful, 145
Autonomic discharge
  severe, 147
Avoidance behavior
  sleep disturbance and, 224
Awakening, 338
Axial system, 314, 338
  feature codes, 325-328
  features of, 314-323

B
Ballistic dystonia, 190
Ballistic episodes, 191
Barbiturates
  hypnotic-dependent sleep disorder
  and, 104
Bed wetting
  nocturnal, 185
Bedpartner-related sleep disorder, 77
Bedtime, 338
  inadequate enforcement, 90
  use of alcohol and, 111
Benign snoring, 195
Benzodiazepines
  hypnotic-dependent sleep disorder and, 104

Beta
  activity, 338
  rhythm, 338
Beta rhythm, 338
Binge eating, 43
Bipolar disorders, 219
Blepharospasm, 234
Blindness
  sleep and, 137
Blood oxygen saturation
  obstructive sleep apnea and, 52
Blue bloaters, 265
Body-rocking, 151
Body-rolling, 151
Brain wave, 338
Breath holding, 307
Bronchiectasis, 265
Bronchitis
  chronic, 265
Bronchopulmonary dysplasia, 265
Bruxism, 182

C
Carbon dioxide
  end-tidal, 340
Cardiac ischemia
  nocturnal, 263
Cardiac rhythm disorder
  sleep-related, 175
Cardiology features
  PANDI coding, 326
Cardiology tests
  coding, 311
Caretakers
  limit-setting sleep disorder and, 90
Cataplexy, 38, 339
Catatonica behavior, 217
Central alveolar hypoventilation
  syndrome, 61, 205
Central apnea, 58
Central hypoventilation syndrome, 205
  congenital, 205
Central sleep apnea syndrome, 58
Cerebral degenerative disorders, 234
Charley horse, 159
Chemicals, 114
Cheyne-Stokes respiration, 58, 339
Childhood insomnia, 90
Childhood-onset insomnia, 35
Childhood psychoses, 216
Choking, 188, 304, 307
Choreoathetosis
  episodes, 191
  seizures, 190
Chronic fatigue
  fibromyalgia and, 278
Chronic obstructive airway disease, 265

Chronic obstructive lung disease, 265
Chronic obstructive pulmonary
  disease, 265
Chronic paroxysmal hemicrania, 255
Chronic somatized tension, 28
Chronobiology, 339
Circadian rhythm, 339
  low-amplitude, 125
  non-existent, 125
Circadian rhythm sleep disorders, 16, 19,
  117-140. See also specific disorders
Circasemidian rhythm, 339
Classic migraine, 255
Climacteric
  insomnia, 295
Clinical field trials
  ICSD and, 366
Cluster headache, 255
Cocaine, 107
Combativeness
  dementia and, 237
Common migraine, 255
Communicating hydrocephalus, 237
Complex behavior features
  PANDI coding, 327
Complex partial seizures, 247
Conditioned insomnia, 28, 339
Conflict
  sleep and, 83
Confusion
  nocturnal, 344
Confusional arousals, 142
Congenital central hypoventilation
  syndrome, 205
Constant routine, 339
Cor pulmonale syndrome, 52
Coronary insufficiency, 263
Cot death, 209
Coughing, 188
Cow's milk allergy
  insomnia and, 98
CPT. See Current procedural terminology
  codes
Cramps
  nocturnal leg, 159
Crib death, 209
Criteria
  diagnostic, 340
  duration, 340
  minimal, 343
  severity, 347
Croup
  spasmotic, 304
Current procedural terminology (CPT)
  codes, 365
Cycle, 339
  light-dark, 342

sleep, 347
sleep-wake, 350
Cyclothymia, 219
Cystic fibrosis, 265

D
Death
  cot, 209
  crib, 209
  sudden infant, 209
  sudden unexplained nocturnal, 193
Decompensation
  psychotic, 216
Deficient swallowing, 188
Delayed sleep phase, 339
Delayed sleep-phase syndrome, 128
Delirium 237
Delirium tremens, 230
Delta
  activity, 339
  sleep stage, 339
Delusional disorder, 216
Dementia, 237
Dental therapy
  coding, 313
Dependence
  alcohol, 111
Dependent narcolepsy, 46
Depressive disorders, 219
Desynchronosis
  transmeridian flight and, 118
Diagnostic Classification of Sleep and
  Arousal Disorders
  Introduction from, 367-377
Diagnostic criteria, 340 See also specific
  disorders.
  explanation of, 21-22
Diagnostic procedures
  classification of, 311-313
Diary
  sleep, 347
Differential diagnosis
  ICSD, 331-336
DIMS, 348, 351. See also Disorder of
  initiating and maintaining sleep
Disorder of initiating and maintaining
  sleep, 348, 351
Disorganized sleeping behavior, 125
Diurnal, 340
Dorsomedial thalamic nuclei
  fatal familial insomnia and, 245
Dream
  acting out, 177
  anxiety attack, 162
  enacted, 245
  terrifying, 162, 300
Drowsiness, 340, 347

Drug abstinence
  stimulant-dependent sleep disorder and, 107
Drug-induced sleep disturbance, 107
Drug psychoses, 216
Drug-rebound insomnia, 104
Drunkenness
  sleep, 142
Duodenal ulcer, 274
Duration criteria, 340
  explanation of, 24
Dysautonomia
  fatal progressive insomnia with, 245
Dyschronism
  transmeridian, 118
Dyskinesia
  segmental, 234
Dyspepsia, 274
Dyspnea
  nocturnal, 344
  paroxysmal nocturnal, 344
Dyssomnias, 12-140, 340.
  See also specific disorders
  circadian rhythm sleep disorders, 16, 19, 117-140
  classification outline, 15-16, 18-19
  extrinsic sleep disorders, 16, 18, 72-116
  hypnotic-induced, 104
  intrinsic sleep disorders, 15-18, 27-71
  introduction to, 25-26
Dysthymia, 219
Dystonia
  ballistic, 190
  hereditary progressive, 234
  nocturnal paroxysmal, 190
  segmental, 234
  torsion, 234
Dystonic-dyskinetic episodes, 190
Dysynchronosis
  transmeridian flight, 118

E
Early morning
  arousal, 219, 340
  awakening, 346
  headaches, 255
  wakefulness, 133
Early morning awakening, 133, 219, 340, 346
EEG, 340, 351. See also Electroencephalogram
Electrical status epilepticus of sleep, 252
Electrical status of sleep, 252
Electroencephalogram, 340, 351
Electromyogram, 340, 351
Electrooculogram, 340, 351
EMG, 340, 351. See also Electromyogram
Emphysema, 265

End-tidal carbon dioxide, 340
Entrainment, 341
Enuresis
  sleep, 185
  nocturna, 185
Environment-induced sleep disorder, 77
  sleep disorder, 77
  somnolence, 77
EOG, 340, 351. See also Electrooculogram
Epigastric night pain, 274
Epilepsy, 247
Episodic reaction
  sleep and, 83
Epoch, 341
Erection
  dysfunction, 169
  failure, 169
  painful, 173
  sleep-impaired, 169
  sleep-related, 348
Esophagitis, 272
Essential enuresis, 185
Ethanol. See also Alcohol
  sleep disorders and, 111
Excessive sleepiness, 38, 121, 133, 289, 341, 342
  advanced sleep-phase syndrome and, 133
  alcoholism and, 230
  differential diagnosis, 331, 334-335
  environmental sleep disorder and, 77
  idiopathic hypersomnia and, 46
  menstrual-associated, 295
  mood disorders and, 219
  posttraumatic hypersomnia and, 49
  pregnancy-associated, 297
  psychoses and, 217
  sleeping sickness and, 260
  subwakefulness syndrome and, 285
  time-zone change syndrome and, 118
  toxin-induced sleep disorder and, 114
  transient, 121
Extrapyramidal seizures, 190
Extrinsic sleep disorders, 16, 18, 72-116, 341. See also specific disorders

F
Fatal familial insomnia, 245
Fatal progressive insomnia with dysautonomia, 245
Fatigue
  chronic, 278
Fear
  panic disorder and, 227
Fibromyalgia, 278
Fibromyositis, 278
Fibrositis, 278
Field trials
  ICSD and, 366

Final
  awakening, 341
  wake-up, 341
First-night effect, 341
Flight desynchronosis
  transmeridian, 118
Focal motor seizures, 247
Food allergy insomnia, 98
Food intolerance
  insomnia and, 98
Fragmentary myoclonus, 291
Free running, 341, 137
Free-running pattern, 137
Functionally autonomous insomnia, 28

G
Gambian sleeping sickness, 260
Gambian trypanosomiasis, 260
Gangungut, 193
Gastric ulcer disease, 274
Gastroesophageal reflux
  sleep-related, 272
Gastrojejunal ulcer, 274
Generalized anxiety disorder, 224
Glossary of terms, 337-351
Glottic spasm
  respiratory, 307
Grand mal epilepsy, 247

H
Hallucinations, 217, 342
  hypnagogic, 38
  terrifying hypnagogic, 300
Headaches
  altitude insomnia and, 80
  chronic paroxysmal hemicrania, 255
  classic migraine, 255
  cluster, 255
  common migraine, 255
  early morning, 255
  migraine, unspecified 255
  migraine with aura, 255
  migraine without aura, 255
  nocturnal migraine, 255
  sleep-related, 255
  vascular, 255
Headbanging, 151
Headrolling, 151
Heart disease
  sleep and, 263
Heartburn, 272
Heavy metals, 114
Hemicrania
  chronic paroxysmal, 255
Hereditary ataxias, 234
Hereditary progressive dystonia, 234
Hertz, 341

Histocompatibility antigens
  PANDI coding, 326
Human leukocyte antigen, 38
Huntington's disease, 234
Hyperacidity, 274
Hyperactivity
  nocturnal, 237
Hypercapnia, 341
Hyperchlorhydria, 274
Hyperhidrosis
  sleep-related, 293
Hypernycthemeral syndrome, 137
Hypersexuality, 43
Hypersomnia, 341, 342
  functional, 46
  harmonious, 46
  healthy, 285
  idiopathic, 46
  mixed, 46
  periodic, 43
  posttraumatic, 49
  recurrent, 43, 295
  secondary, 49
Hypersomnia sleep apnea syndrome, 52
Hypertrophy
  adenoidal, 52
Hypnagogic, 342
Hypnagogic hallucinations, 38, 300
  imagery, 342
  jerks, 155
Hypnagogic paralysis, 166
  startle, 342
Hypnic jerks, 155
Hypnogenic paroxysmal dystonia, 190
Hypnopomic, 342
Hypnopompic, 342
Hypnopompic paralysis, 166
Hypnotic-dependent
  insomnia, 104
  sleep disorder, 104
Hypnotic-drug-rebound insomnia, 104
Hypnotic-induced dyssomnia, 104
Hypobaropathy, 80
Hypochondriasis
  sleep, 32
Hypokinesia
  parkinsonism and, 240
Hypomania, 219
Hypopnea, 342
Hyposomnia
  healthy, 282
Hypoventilation
  central alveolar, 61
  idiopathic alveolar, 61
  nonapneic alveolar, 61
  primary alveolar, 61

syndrome,
  congenital central, 205
  obesity, 52
Hypoventilation syndrome
  congenital central, 205
  obesity, 52
Hz, 341, 351. See also Hertz

I

ICD-9-CM. See International Classification of Diseases, 9th revision
ICSD. See International Classification of Sleep Disorders
ICSD sleep code, 342
Idiopathic
Idiopathic alveolar hypoventilation, 61
  apnea, 198
Idiopathic CNS hypersomnia, 46
  enuresis, 185
Idiopathic hypersomnia, 46
Idiopathic insomnia, 35
  narcolepsy, 46
  torsion dystonia, 234
Imaging tests
  coding, 312
Impotence, 169
Inadequate
Inadequate sleep, 87
Inadequate sleep hygiene, 73
Incoherence, 217
Incremental asynchrony, 137
Incubus, 147
Index
  apnea, 337, 351
  apnea-hypopnea, 337, 351
  PLM, 345
  respiratory-disturbance, 347, 351
  sleep-efficiency, 347
Infant sleep apnea, 198
Infiltration
  alpha, 337
Insomnia, 342, 348
  alcohol-dependency, 111
  alcoholism and, 230
  altitude, 80
  anxiety disorders and, 224
  childhood, 35, 90
  chronic obstructive pulmonary disease and, 265
  climacteric, 295
  conditioned, 28, 339
  differential diagnosis, 331-333
  environmental, 77
  explanation of, 23-24
  fatal familial, 245
  food allergy, 98
  functionally autonomous, 28
  hypnotic-dependency, 104
  hypnotic drug rebound, 104
  idiopathic, 35
  learned, 28
  lifelong, 35
  maintenance, 224
  menopausal, 295
  menstruation-associated, 295
  mood disorders and, 219
  parkinsonism and, 240
  periodic, 137
  pregnancy-associated, 297
  premenstrual, 295
  psychophysiologic, 28
  psychoses and, 217
  short-term, 83
  sleep-onset, 128, 224
  sleep-wake system problems and, 35
  thalamic, 245
  toxin-induced sleep disorders and, 114
  transient, 121
  transient psychophysiologic, 83
  without objective findings, 32
Insufficient nocturnal sleep, 87
Insufficient sleep syndrome, 87
International Classification of Diseases, 9th revision
  ASDC classification and, 378-380
  ICSD alphabetical listing, 358-359
  ICSD listed medically, 355-357
  ICSD numerical listing, 360-361
  nonorganic ICSD listing, 362-363
  sleep disturbances listing, 363-364
International Classification of Sleep Disorders
  alphabetical listing, 358-359
  ASDC classification and, 378-380
  ASDC comparative listing, 381-383, 384-388
  axial system of, 13-14, 314-323, 325-328
  classification outline, 15-20
  clinical field trials and, 366
  coding system database, 329-330
  criteria definitions, 21-24
  differential diagnosis, 331-336
  ICD-9-CM listing, 355-357
  nonorganic origin listing, 362-363
  numerical listing, 360-361
  sleep disturbances listing, 363-364
Into-bed time, 342
Intrinsic asthma, 269
Intrinsic sleep disorders, 15, 18, 27-71, 342. See also specific disorders
Intrusion
  alpha, 337
Involuntary movements
  cerebral degenerative disorders and, 235

Irregular sleepwake pattern, 125
Ischemia
  nocturnal cardiac, 263
  silent, 263
Isolated sleep paralysis, 166

J
Jactatio capitis nocturna, 151
Jerks
  hypnagogic, 155
  hypnic, 155
  leg, 65
Jet lag, 118
Jet lag syndrome, 118

K
K-alpha, 342
K-complex, 342
Kleine-Levin syndrome, 43
Korsakoff's psychosis, 230

L
Larkishness
  extreme, 133
Laryngospasm
  emotional, 307
  sleep-related, 304
Leg jerks, 65
Leg cramps, 159
Leg movements, periodic, 345, 351
  jerks, 65
  muscle tightness, 159
  nocturnal cramps, 159
  nocturnal pain, 159
  periodic movement, 345, 351
  restless, 68
Levodopa-induced sleep disturbances, 240
Light-dark cycle, 342
Limb jerking
  neonatal, 212
Limb movement disorder
  periodic, 65
Limit-setting sleep disorder, 90
L'ivresse du sommeil, 142
Long sleeper, 285
Lung disease
  chronic obstructive, 265
Lymphadenopathy
  sleeping sickness and, 260

M
Maintenance insomnia
  anxiety and, 224
Maintenance of wakefulness test, 343, 351
  PANDI coding, 326
Major depression, 219
Major sleep episode, 343
Mania, 219

Manic-depressive illness, 219
Masked depression, 219
Medically related sleep disorders, 259-280.
  See also specific disorders
  classification outline, 17, 19-20, 259
  introduction to, 215, 259-260
Memory loss
  dementia and, 237
Menstrual-associated sleep disorder, 295
Menstruation-associated insomnia, 295
Mentally related sleep disorders, 216-233.
  See also specific disorders
  classification outline, 17, 19-20, 216
  introduction to, 215-216
Microsleep, 343
Micturition
  during sleep, 185
Migraine
  classic, 255
  common, 255
  nocturnal, 255
  unspecified 255
  with aura, 255
  without aura, 255, 255
Milk allergy insomnia, 98
  insomnia, 98
Minimal criteria, 343
  explanation of, 22
Miscellaneous sleep disturbances
  differential diagnosis, 331, 335-336
Miscellaneous sleep procedures
  coding, 313
Mixed apnea, 52
  apnea, 52
Mixed hypersomnia, 46
Moans, 157
Montage, 343
Mood disorders, 219
Morning sleepiness, 128
Motor
Motor behavior features
  PANDI coding, 326
Motor parasomnia, REM, 177
  REM, 177
Motor system degeneration, 235
Mountain sickness
  acute, 80
Movement arousal, 343
Movement disorder, rhythmic, 151
Movement time, 343
Movements
  during sleep, 65
MSLT, 343, 351. See also Multiple sleep latency test
Multiple sleep latency test, 343, 351
  PANDI coding, 325
Multi-system atrophy, 240

Munchhausen's stridor, 304
Muscle features
  PANDI coding, 327
Musculorum deformans, 234
Musculoskeletal pain, 278
MWT, 343, 351. See also Maintenance of wakefulness test
Myoclonus, 343
  benign neonatal sleep, 212
  fragmentary, 291
  nocturnal, 65
  partial, 212, 291
  predormital, 155
  sleep, 212, 291

N
Nap, 343
Napping
  excessive, 73
Narcolepsy, 38
  dependent, 46
  idiopathic, 46
  NREM, 46
Neonatal sleep myoclonus
  benign, 212
Neurogenic tachypnea
  sleep-related, 302
Neurologic tests
  coding, 312
Neurologically related sleep disorders, 234-258. See also specific disorders
  classification outline, 17, 19-20, 124, 234
  introduction to, 215, 234
Night eating syndrome, 100
Night shift
  sleep and, 121
Night sweats, 293
Night terrors, 147
Nightmares, 162, 343
  sleep-onset, 300
Nocturnal
  angina, 263
  asthma, 269
  asystole, 175
  bedwetting, 185
  bruxism, 182
  cardiac ischemia, 263
  confusion, 237, 344
  death syndrome, sudden unexplained, 193
  delirium, 237
  drinking syndrome, 100
Nocturnal paroxysmal dyspnea, 344
  dyspnea, paroxysmal, 344
Nocturnal
  eating/drinking syndrome, 100
  hyperactivity, 237

  leg cramps, 159
  leg pain, 159
  migraine, 255
  Nocturnal myoclonus, 65
  Nocturnal paroxysmal dystonia, 190
  Nocturnal penile tumescence, 344, 351
    impaired, 169
  pH monitoring, 274
  sleep, 344
  sleep, insufficient 87
  sleep disruption, 38
  tooth grinding, 182
Nocturnal wandering, 237
Noise-induced sleep disturbance, 77
Non-24-hour sleep-wake syndrome, 137
Nonlaita, 193
Non-rapid eye movement, see NREM, 344. See also NonREM; NREM
  narcolepsy, 46
  REM sleep cycle, 344
  sleep, 344
  sleep period, 344
Non-REM See Non-rapid eye movement, NREM sleep, 344
NonREM sleep-related dystonic-dyskinetic episodes, 190
Nonapneic alveolar hypoventilation, 61
Nonobstructive sleep apnea, 58
Nonorganic sleep disorders
  classification of, 362-363
Nonsurgical procedures
  classification of, 311-313
NPT, 344, 351. See also Nocturnal penile tumescence
NREM
  narcolepsy, 46
  REM sleep cycle, 344
  sleep, 344
  sleep period, 344
  See Non-rapid eye movement
NREM narcolepsy, 46
NREM-REM sleep cycle, 344
NREM sleep, 344
NREM sleep period, 344

O
Obesity hypoventilation syndrome, 52, 344
Obsessive-compulsive disorder, 224
Obstructive apnea, 52
Obstructive hydrocephalus, 237
Obstructive sleep apnea syndrome, 52, 198
Olivopontocerebellar degeneration, 234
Ondine's curse, 205
Oneiric stupor, 245
Oneirism, 177
Operations
  coding, 313

Otolaryngologic tests
  coding, 312
Overdosage
  alcohol, 111
Oxygen desaturation
  central alveolar hypoventilation syndrome and, 61
  central sleep apnea syndrome and, 58

P
Pain
  musculoskeletal, 278
  nocturnal leg, 159
Palsy
  progressive supranuclear, 240
  shaking, 240
PANDI mnemonic, 323, 325
Panic disorder, 227
Paradoxical sleep, 344
Paradoxical vocal cord motion, 304
Paralysis
  sleep, 38, 166
Paralysis agitans, 240
Paranoid disorder, 216
Parasomnia, 344
  REM motor, 177
Parasomnias, 141-214, 344.
  See also specific disorders
  arousal disorders, 16, 19, 142-150
  associated with REM sleep, 16, 19, 162-180
  classification outline, 16-17, 19
  introduction to, 141
  miscellaneous, 16-17, 19, 181-214
  REM motor, 177
  sleep-wake transition disorders, 16, 19, 151-161
Paresis
  functional abduction, 307
Parkinsonism, 240
Parkinson's-ALS-dementia complex, 240
Parkinson's disease, 240
Paroxysm, 344
Paroxysmal choreoathetosis, 190
Paroxysmal dystonia
  nocturnal, 190
Paroxysmal dystonic episodes, 190
Paroxysmal hemicrania
  chronic, 255
Paroxysmal kinesigenic dystonia, 190
Paroxysmal nocturnal dyspnea, 344, 351
Partial motor seizures, 247
Partial myoclonus, 212, 291
Pavor nocturnus, 147
Penile buckling pressure, 344
Penile erections
  sleep-impaired, 169

Penile pain
  sleep-related, 173
Penile rigidity, 345
Penile tumescence, 351
  impaired, 169
  nocturnal, 344, 351
  PANDI coding, 327
Peptic ulcer disease, 274
Period, 345
Periodic apnea, 198
Periodic excessive sleepiness, 137
Periodic hypersomnia, 43
Periodic insomnia, 137
Periodic leg movement, 345, 351
Periodic limb movement disorder, 65
Periodic movements of sleep, 65, 345
Petit mal epilepsy, 247
Phase
  advance, 133, 345
  delay, 128, 345
  lag, 128
  transition, 345
Phase delay, 128, 345
Phase lag, 128
Phase transition, 345
Phasic event, 345
Phenylethylamine, 107
Phobia
  simple, 224
  social, 224
Photoperiod, 345
Pick's disease, 237
Pickwickian syndrome, 52, 345
  definition, 345
Pink puffers, 265
PLM, 345, 351. See also Periodic leg movement
PLM arousal index, 345
  index, 345
  percentage, 345
PLM index, 345
PLM percentage, 345
PND, 344, 351. See also Paroxysmal nocturnal dyspnea
Poisoning, 114
Pokkuri, 193
Polypnea during sleep, 302
Polysomnogram, 345
  PANDI coding, 325
Polysomnograph, 346
Positive human leukocyte antigen DR2, 38
Posttraumatic hypersomnia, 49
Posttraumatic stress disorder, 224
Postdormital paralysis, 166
Postencephalitic parkinsonism, 240
Predormital myoclonus, 155
Predormital paralysis, 166

Pregnancy-associated
  excessive sleepiness and, 297
  insomnia and, 297
Pregnancy-associated sleep disorder, 297
Premature arousal, 219
Premature morning awakening, 346
Premenstrual insomnia, 295
Primary alveolar hypoventilation, 61, 205
Primary enuresis, 185
Primary snoring, 195
Prinzmetal's angina, 263
Progressive supranuclear palsy, 240
Prolonged-episode dystonic-dyskinetic
  episodes, 190
Proposed sleep disorders, 281-309, 346.
  See also specific disorders
  classification outline, 17, 20, 281
  introduction to, 281-282
Pseudoinsomnia, 32
PSG, 346, 351. See also Polysomnogram
Psychiatric therapy
  coding, 313
Psychogenic stridor, 307
Psychologic tests
  coding, 312
Psychophysiologic arousal, 28
Psychophysiologic insomnia, 28, 83
  transient, 83
Psychoses, 216
  alcoholic, 230
  childhood, 216
  drug, 216
  Korsakoff's, 230
  other, 216
  unspecified functional, 216
Pulmonary disease
  chronic obstructive, 265

Q
Quiet sleep, 346

R
Rapid eye movement sleep, 346.
  See also REM
RDI, 347, 351. See also Respiratory-
  disturbance index
Recording, 346
Recurrent hypersomnia, 43, 295
Reflux
  gastroesophageal, 272
Reflux esophagitis, 272
Regurgitation
  sleep-related, 272
REM
  density, 346
  parasomnia, 177
  nightmare, 162

REM sleep
  abnormal, 38
  associated parasomnias, 16, 19, 162-180.
    See also specific disorders
  behavior disorder, 177
  episode, 346
  features, PANDI coding, 327
  intrusion, 346
  latency, 346
  onset, 346
  percent, 346
  rebound, 111, 230, 346
  related sinus arrest, 175
Respiration
  Cheyne-Stokes, 58, 339
Respiratory disturbance index, 347
Respiratory glottic spasm, 307
Respiratory test
  coding, 311
Respiratory therapy
  coding, 313
Restless legs syndrome, 68
Restlessness, 347
Rett syndrome, 234
Rheumatic pain modulation disorder, 278
Rhodesian sleeping sickness, 260
Rhodesian trypanosomiasis, 260
Rhythm, 347
  alpha, 337
  beta, 338
  circadian, 339
  circasemidian, 339
Rhythmic movement disorder, 151
RLS, 351. See also Restless legs syndrome
Ryhthmie du sommeil, 151

S
Sawtooth waves, 347
Schizophrenia, 216
Schizophreniform disorder, 216
Schlaftrunkenheit, 142
Seasonal affective disorder, 219
Seasonal reaction
  sleep and, 83
Segmental dyskinesias, 234
Segmental dystonias, 234
Senile degeneration of brain, 237
Severe autonomic discharge, 147
Severity criteria, 347
  explanation of, 22
Sexual dysfunction, 169
Shaking palsy, 240
Shift work sleep disorder, 121
Shock
  emotional, 83
Short sleeper, 282
Short-term insomnia, 83

Shy-Drager syndrome, 240
Silent ischemia, 263
Sinus arrest
  REM sleep-related, 175
Situational reaction
  sleep and, 83
Sleep
  active, 337
  alpha, 337
  alpha-delta, 337
Sleep apnea, 52, 198
  infant, 198
Sleep apnea syndrome
  central, 58
  obstructive, 52
Sleep architecture, 347
Sleep bruxism, 182
Sleep choking syndrome, 307
Sleep code
  ICSD, 342, 351
Sleep curtailment, 87
Sleep cycle, 347
Sleep death, 193
Sleep diary, 347
Sleep disorder
  adjustment, 83
  alcohol-dependent, 111
  associated with forced vigilance, 77
  bedpartner-related, 77
  environment-induced, 77
  environmental, 77
  hospital-induced, 77
  hypnotic-dependent, 104
  intrinsic, 342
  limit-setting, 90
  proposed, 346
  stimulant-dependent, 107
  toxin-induced, 114
Sleep disruption
  nocturnal, 38
Sleep disturbance
  classification of, 363-364
  differential diagnosis, 331-336
  noise-induced, 77
  temperature-induced, 77
Sleep drunkenness, 142
Sleep-duration continuum, 282, 285
  extreme high end, 282
  extreme low end, 285
Sleep efficiency, 347
Sleep electroencephalographic features
  PANDI coding, 326
Sleep enuresis, 185
Sleep environment
  unfamiliar, 83
Sleep epilepsy, 247

Sleep episode, 347, 349
  major, 343
  total, 350
Sleep habits, 73
  bad, 73
  irregular, 73
Sleep hygiene, 73, 347
  inadequate, 73
Sleep hygiene abuse, 73
Sleep hyperhidrosis, 293
Sleep hypochondriasis, 32
Sleep-incompatible behaviors, 73
Sleep inertia
  excessive, 142
Sleep interruption, 347
Sleep intrusion
  NREM, 344
  REM, 346
Sleep latency, 347
  REM, 346
Sleep log, 347
  PANDI coding, 327
Sleep log features
  PANDI coding, 327
Sleep maintenance complaint
  alcohol-induced, 111
Sleep maintenance DIMS, 348
Sleep mentation, 348
Sleep myoclonus, 291
  benign neonatal, 212
Sleep onset, 348
  REM, 346
Sleep-onset association disorder, 94
Sleep-onset insomnia, 128
  anxiety and, 224
  nightmares, 300
Sleep-onset
  REM period, 219, 348
Sleep paralysis, 38, 166, 348
Sleep pattern, 348
Sleep-phase syndrome
  advanced, 133
  delayed, 128
Sleep rebound
  REM, 111
Sleep reduction, 87
Sleep-related
  abnormal swallowing syndrome, 188
  asthma, 269
  epilepsy, 247
  epileptic seizures, 247
  erections, 348
  gastroesophageal reflux, 272
  headaches, 255
  laryngospasm, 304
  neurogenic tachypnea, 302

painful erections, 173
penile erections, impaired, 169
Sleep restriction, 87
Sleep spindle, 348
Sleep-stage demarcation, 348
Sleep-stage episode, 349
Sleep stage NREM, 349
Sleep stage REM, 349
Sleep stages, 349
  delta, 339
  intermediary, 342
Sleep starts, 155
Sleep state misperception, 32
Sleep structure, 350
Sleep syndrome
  insufficient, 87
Sleep system
  inadequately developed, 35
Sleep talking, 157, 350
Sleep terrors, 147
Sleep testing
  CPT codes, 365
Sleep tests
  coding, 311
Sleep-wake cycle, 350
Sleep-wake pattern
  irregular, 125
Sleep-wake rhythm
  grossly disturbed, 125
Sleep-wake schedule
  frequently changing, 121
Sleep-wake shift, 350
Sleep-wake system problems
  insomnia and, 35
Sleep-wake transition disorders, 16, 19, 151-161, 350. See also specific disorders
Sleepiness, 347
  evening, 134
  excessive, 38, 46, 49, 77, 114, 118, 133, 217, 219, 230, 260, 289, 295, 297, 341, 342
  explanation of, 23
  morning, 128
  periodic excessive, 137
  transient excessive, 121
Sleeping-pill withdrawal, 104
Sleeping sickness, 260
Sleepwalking, 145
Slow-wave sleep, 350
Snoring, 350
  continuous, 195
  primary, 195
  without sleep apnea, 195
Social phobia, 224
Somnambulism, 145
Somniloquy, 157
Somnolence, 341, 347

environment-induced, 77
evening, 133
Spasm
  glottic, 307
Spastic torticollis, 234
Spindle sleep, 348
Spinocerebellar degeneration, 234
Stable asynchrony, 128, 133
Stage 4 nightmares, 162
Status epilepticus of sleep, 252
Stimulants, 107
Stress
  acute, 83
Striatonigral degeneration, 240
Stridor
  Munchhausen's, 304
  psychogenic, 307
Stupor
  oneiric, 245
Subjective complaint of disorder of sleep without objective findings, 32
Subjective sleep complaint, 32
Substance abuse, 107
Subvigilance syndrome, 288
Subwakefulness syndrome, 288
Sudden death, 193
Sudden infant death syndrome, 209
Sudden unexplained nocturnal death syndrome, 193
Sundown syndrome, 237
Supranuclear palsy
  progressive, 240
Surgical therapy
  coding, 313
Swallowing
  abnormal, 188
Sweats
  night, 293
Symptomatic enuresis, 185
Symptomatic torsion dystonia, 234
Synchronized, 350
Syndrome
  acute brain, 237
  advanced sleep-phase, 133
  central alveolar hypoventilation, 61, 205
  central hypoventilation, 205
  central sleep apnea, 58
  congenital central hypoventilation, 205
  cor pulmonale, 52
  delayed sleep-phase, 128
  fibromyositis, 278
  hypernycthemeral, 137
  hypersomnia sleep apnea, 52
  insufficient sleep, 87
  jet lag, 118
  Kleine-Levin, 43
  night eating, 100

nocturnal drinking, 100
nocturnal eating, 100
non-24-hour sleep-wake, 137
obesity hypoventilation, 52, 344
obstructive sleep apnea, 52, 198
Pickwickian, 52, 345
primary alveolar hypoventilation, 205
restless legs, 68
Rett, 234
Shy-Drager, 240
sleep choking, 307
sleep-related abnormal swallowing, 188
subvigilance, 288
subwakefulness, 288
sudden infant death, 209
sudden unexplained nocturnal death, 193
sundown, 237
time zone change, 118
withdrawal, 107

T
Tachypnea
  sleep-related neurogenic, 302
Talking
  during sleep, 350
Temperature-induced sleep disturbance, 77
Temporal lobe epilepsy, 247
Terrifying hypnagogic hallucinations, 300
Terror
  sleep, 147
Test
  maintenance of wakefulness, 343, 351
  multiple sleep latency, 343, 351
Thalamic insomnia, 245
Thalamus, insomnia and, 245
Theta activity, 350
Time
  arise, 338
  total sleep, 350
  wake, 351
Time zone change syndrome, 118
Tolerance
  alcohol, 111
Tonic-clonic epilepsy, 247
Tooth clenching, 182
Tooth grinding
  nocturnal, 182
Torsion dystonia, 234
Torticollis
  spastic, 234
Total recording time, 350
Total sleep episode, 350
Total sleep time, 350
Toxin-induced sleep disorder, 114
Toxins, 114

Trace alternant, 351
Transient excessive sleepiness, 121
Transient insomnia, 121
Transient psychophysiologic insomnia, 83
Transmeridian dyschronism, 118
Transmeridian flight
  desynchronosis and, 118
Tremor
  parkinsonism and, 240
Trypanosomiasis, 260
Tumescence, 351
  nocturnal penile, 344, 351
Twitching, 291, 351
  neonatal, 212

U
Ulcer, 274
Unexplained nocturnal death syndrome, 193
Unstable angina, 263
Upper airway apnea, 52
Utterances, 157

V
Variable sleeping behavior, 125
Vascular headaches, 255
Ventilation features
  PANDI coding, 327-328
Verbalization, 157
Vertex sharp transient, 351
Vocal cord motion
  paradoxical, 304
Vocal cord spasm, 304
Vocalization
  dementia and, 237

W
Wake time, 351
Wakefulness
  early morning, 133
Waking
  sleep, 145
Wandering
  dementia and, 237
Waves
  brain, 338
  sawtooth, 347
Withdrawal
  alcohol, 111
  syndromes, 107
Work-shift sleep changes, 121

Z
Zeitgeber, 351
  disregard of, 125